Psychiatric and Physical Comorbidity in Schizophrenia

Guest Editors

MICHAEL Y. HWANG, MD
HENRY A. NASRALLAH, MD

PSYCHIATRIC CLINICS OF NORTH AMERICA

www.psych.theclinics.com

December 2009 • Volume 32 • Number 4

SAUNDERS an imprint of ELSEVIER, Inc.

W.B. SAUNDERS COMPANY
A Division of Elsevier Inc.

1600 John F. Kennedy Boulevard • Suite 1800 • Philadelphia, PA 19103-2899

http://www.theclinics.com

PSYCHIATRIC CLINICS OF NORTH AMERICA Volume 32, Number 4
December 2009 ISSN 0193-953X, ISBN-13: 978-1-4160-6346-9, ISBN-10: 1-4160-6346-3

Editor: Sarah E. Barth
Developmental Editor: Donald Mumford

Psychiatric Clinics of North America (ISSN 0193-953X) is published quarterly by Elsevier Inc., 360 Park Avenue South, New York, NY 10010-1710. Months of issue are March, June, September, and December. Business and Editorial Offices: 1600 John F. Kennedy Blvd., Suite 1800, Philadelphia, PA 19103-2899. Periodicals postage paid at New York, NY and additional mailing offices. Subscription prices are $248.00 per year (US individuals), $430.00 per year (US institutions), $125.00 per year (US students/residents), $297.00 per year (Canadian individuals), $535.00 per year (Canadian Institutions), $369.00 per year (foreign individuals), $535.00 per year (foreign institutions), and $185.00 per year (international & Canadian students/residents). Foreign air speed delivery is included in all *Clinics*' subscription prices. All prices are subject to change without notice. **POSTMASTER:** Send address changes to *Psychiatric Clinics of North America*, Elsevier Health Sciences Division, Subscription Customer Service, 3251 Riverport Lane, Maryland Heights, MO 63043. Customer Service: 1-800-654-2452 (US). From outside the United States, call 1-314-447-8871. Fax: 1-314-447-8029. E-mail: journalscustomerservice-usa@elsevier.com (for print support) and journalsonlinesupport-usa@elsevier.com (for online support).

Reprints. For copies of 100 or more, of articles in this publication, please contact the Commercial Reprints Department, Elsevier Inc., 360 Park Avenue South, New York, New York 10010-1710. Tel.: (212) 633-3813, Fax: (212) 462-1935, E-mail: reprints@elsevier.com.

Psychiatric Clinics of North America is covered in *MEDLINE/PubMed (Index Medicus)*, *Current Contents/Social and Behavioral Sciences, Social Science Citation Index, Embase/Excerpta Medica,* and PsycINFO.

Printed and bound by CPI Group (UK) Ltd, Croydon, CR0 4YY

Transferred to Digital Print 2012

Contributors

GUEST EDITORS

MICHAEL Y. HWANG, MD
Associate Professor of Psychiatry, Robert Wood Johnson Medical School, University of Medicine and Dentistry of New Jersey, Piscataway, New Jersey; Clinical Professor of Psychiatry, The Commonwealth Medical College of Pennsylvania, Scranton, Pennsylvania

HENRY A. NASRALLAH, MD
Professor of Psychiatry & Neuroscience, University of Cincinnati College of Medicine, Cincinnati, Ohio

AUTHORS

GIOVANNI CARACCI, MD
Chairman, Department of Psychiatry, New Jersey Medical School, University of Medicine and Dentistry of New Jersey, Newark, New Jersey

STANLEY CAROFF, MD
Department of Psychiatry, Philadelphia VA Medical Center; Professor of Psychiatry, Department of Psychiatry, University of Pennsylvania School of Medicine, Philadelphia, Pennsylvania

ROBERT R. CONLEY, MD
Distinguished Lilly Scholar, Eli Lilly and Company, US Medical Division, Lilly Corporate Center, Indianapolis, Indiana

ARMAN DANIELYAN, MD
Department of Psychiatry, University of Cincinnati College of Medicine, Cincinnati, Ohio

JOANNE M. HAWLEY, PharmD
Clinical Associate Professor, Department of Psychiatry, Virginia Tech Carilion School of Medicine, Blacksburg, Virginia

MICHAEL Y. HWANG, MD
Associate Professor of Psychiatry, Robert Wood Johnson Medical School, University of Medicine and Dentistry of New Jersey, Piscataway, New Jersey; Clinical Professor of Psychiatry, The Commonwealth Medical College of Pennsylvania, Scranton, Pennsylvania; Mental Health Service, Franklin Delano Roosevelt Hospital, Veterans Affairs Hudson Valley Healthcare System, Montrose, New York

ISABELLA KANELLOPOULOU, MD
Clinical Assistant Professor, Mt Sinai School of Medicine, New York, New York

SUNG-WAN KIM, MD, PhD
Assistant Professor, Department of Psychiatry, Chonnam National University Medical School, Gwangju, Korea

TAK KIM, MD, PhD
Professor, Department of Obstetrics and Gynecology, Korea University Anam Hospital, Seoul, Korea

SUN KYOUNG YUM, MD
Department of Obstetrics and Gynecology, Korea University Anam Hospital, Seoul, Korea

J.P. LINDENMAYER, MD
Clinical Professor, Department of Psychiatry, New York University School of Medicine, New York University; Director, Psychopharmacology Research Unit, Nathan Kline Institute for Psychiatric Research, New York; Manhattan Psychiatric Center, New York, New York

JANICE LYBRAND, MD
Department of Psychiatry, Philadelphia VA Medical Center, Philadelphia, Pennsylvania

MARIO MAJ, MD, PhD
Professor of Psychiatry, Department of Psychiatry, University of Naples SUN, Naples, Largo Madonna delle Grazie, Napoli, Italy

VASSILIS MARTIADIS, MD
Post-doctoral Fellow, Department of Psychiatry, University of Naples SUN, Naples, Largo Madonna delle Grazie, Napoli, Italy

MAUREEN F. McCARTHY, MD
Chief of Staff, Department of Veterans Affairs Medical Center, Salem, Virginia; Clinical Associate Professor, Department of Psychiatric Medicine, University of Virginia School of Medicine, Charlottesville, Virginia

PALMIERO MONTELEONE, MD
Professor of Psychiatry, Department of Psychiatry, University of Naples SUN, Naples, Largo Madonna delle Grazie, Napoli, Italy

HENRY A. NASRALLAH, MD
Professor of Psychiatry and Neuroscience, Department of Psychiatry, University of Cincinnati College of Medicine, Cincinnati, Ohio

LEWIS A. OPLER, MD, PhD
Clinical Professor of Psychiatry, Department of Psychiatry, Columbia University College of Physicians & Surgeons, New York, New York

MAURIZIO POMPILI, MD, PhD
Professor of Suicidology, Department of Psychiatry, Sant' Andrea Hospital, Sapienza University of Rome, Rome, Italy; McLean Hospital, Harvard Medical School, Boston, Massachusetts

ALEC ROY, MD
Department of Veterans Affairs, New Jersey Healthcare System, East Orange, New Jersey

DELMAR D. SHORT, MD
Chief, Mental Health Service Line, Department of Veterans Affairs Medical Center, Salem, Virginia; Clinical Associate Professor, Department of Psychiatric Medicine, Virginia Tech Carilion School of Medicine, Roanoke, Virginia

SUN YOUNG YUM, MD
Clinical Assistant Professor of Psychiatry, The Commonwealth Medical College of Pennsylvania, Scranton, Pennsylvania; Research Physician, Lilly Pharmaceuticals, Seoul, Korea

Contents

Preface xiii

Michael Y. Hwang and Henry A. Nasrallah

Neurological Disorders in Schizophrenia 719

Arman Danielyan and Henry A. Nasrallah

Schizophrenia (SZ) is a complex, heterogeneous, and disabling psychiatric disorder that impairs multiple aspects of human cognitive, perceptual, emotional, and behavioral functioning. SZ is relatively frequent (prevalence around 1%), with onset usually during adolescence or early adulthood, and has a deteriorating course. The rapidly growing area of neuroimaging research has has found clear evidence of many cortical and subcortical abnormalities in individuals with SZ. In this article the most recent findings from multiple studies on neurological disorders in SZ are reviewed, and the authors make a strong argument for a neurological basis of the schizophrenic process.

Management of Schizophrenia with Medical Disorders: Cardiovascular, Pulmonary, and Gastrointestinal 759

Delmar D. Short, Joanne M. Hawley, and Maureen F. McCarthy

Medical illnesses are particularly common in patients who have schizophrenia and one of the major tasks for consultation-liaison psychiatrists, and others, is to determine which medications are safest in which comorbid condition. The authors review the relative risks for various antipsychotics, especially focusing on cardiovascular, pulmonary, and gastrointestinal co-morbid illnesses. The authors further review the atypical antipsychotics' cardiovascular risks, especially for prolonging QT intervals, in trying to avoid the risk for torsades de pointes. The relative risk for anticholinergic actions for these medicines is also reviewed, as this is especially important in the medically ill or elderly. The authors also review the relative safety of antipsychotics in patients who have liver disease and pulmonary disease. Finally, the authors review specific drug interactions that may be problematic when treating the medically ill with atypical antipsychotics.

Management of Schizophrenia with Obesity, Metabolic, and Endocrinological Disorders 775

Palmiero Monteleone, Vassilis Martiadis, and Mario Maj

People with schizophrenia have an increased prevalence of overweight/obesity, type 2 diabetes mellitus, dyslipidemia, and metabolic syndrome, which increases the risk for cardiovascular diseases and mortality. Part of this increased risk is attributable to the use of antipsychotic medications, especially second-generation antipsychotics. Antipsychotic drugs

differ in their potential to induce weight gain, with clozapine and olanzapine exhibiting the highest weight gain liability; evidence for differing effects of antipsychotics on glucose and lipid metabolism is less convincing. Individuals with schizophrenia may develop hyperprolactinemia, with or without clinical symptoms, after starting antipsychotic medications. This effect is particularly frequent with first-generation antipsychotics and with the second-generation antipsychotic risperidone and paliperidone. Psychiatrists should be aware of metabolic and endocrine side effects of antipsychotics and should make every effort to prevent or minimize them to improve the patients' compliance and quality of life.

Clinical Perspectives on Autoimmune Processes in Schizophrenia **795**

Sun Young Yum, Sun Kyoung Yum, Tak Kim, and Michael Y. Hwang

This article reviews the epidemiology of autoimmune conditions in schizophrenia, symptom manifestations of autoimmune conditions resembling schizophrenia, and the immunological changes observed in schizophrenia; and reflects on their associations with neurodevelopment, neurodegeneration, clinical course, and management of schizophrenia.

Schizophrenia and Eating Disorders **809**

Sun Young Yum, Giovanni Caracci, and Michael Y. Hwang

Schizophrenia requires diverse and individualized treatment approaches. Accurate identification and management of comorbid psychiatric syndromes determine outcome. Disturbances in eating and the distorted perception of body image are difficult to separate from other psychotic phenomena. Eating is a complicated integration of psychoneuroendocrinology. Despite the difficulties in defining the distinction between behaviors and cognitive perceptions that are and are not of diagnosable severity, there are patients with clearer coexistence of eating disorders and schizophrenia that carry on independent courses. This article presents clinical cases that portray a spectrum of eating pathology in patients with schizophrenia.

Management of Schizophrenia with Substance Use Disorders **821**

Janice Lybrand and Stanley Caroff

Around 50% of patients with schizophrenia develop a co-occurring substance use disorder involving alcohol or illicit substances at some time during their lives. The comorbid substance abuse will markedly affect the course of illness of schizophrenia. In this article, the authors review the epidemiology, theories of causation, effect on the course of illness, and treatment of co-occurring schizophrenia and substance use disorder.

Management of Schizophrenia with Obsessive-Compulsive Features **835**

Michael Y. Hwang, Sung-Wan Kim, Sun Young Yum, and Lewis A. Opler

Although obsessive-compulsive symptoms (OCS) in schizophrenia have been conceptually controversial and clinically challenging, recent

evidence suggests that schizophrenia with OCS may constitute a distinct schizophrenic subgroup. Recent epidemiological and clinical findings have shown that the subgroup obsessive-compulsive (OC) schizophrenia is associated with poor outcome and is more frequent than previously realized. Emerging biological evidence suggests that OCS in schizophrenia has more than one pathogenesis, with distinct mechanisms that may require different treatment interventions. Therefore, the management of OCS in patients with schizophrenia requires an individualized treatment approach based on the pathogenesis and clinical status of the patient. For example, the atypical antipsychotics that are potent serotonin antagonists sometimes induce de novo or exacerbate preexisting OCS, which resolves if the patient is switched to an antipsychotic with a different profile or if adjunctive treatment with serotonin reuptake inhibitors (SSRIs) is undergone. Regarding OC schizophrenia, SSRIs are often a necessary part of treatment, with knowledge of potential pharmacokinetic interactions with antipsychotic drugs essential. In this article, recent progress and current knowledge of OC schizophrenia is reviewed and treatment guidelines are offered for this complex and challenging subgroup of schizophrenic patients.

The Burden of Depressive Symptoms in People with Schizophrenia **853**

Robert R. Conley

People with schizophrenia and concurrent depressive symptoms have poorer long-term functional outcomes compared with the nondepressed. Their poorer quality of life, greater use of mental health services, and higher risk of involvement with law enforcement agencies underscore a need for special treatment interventions. Treatment of the nonpsychotic dimensions of schizophrenia is a critical part of recovery. In a 3-year study, the depressed cohort was significantly more likely than the nondepressed to use relapse-related mental health services (emergency psychiatric services, sessions with psychiatrists); to be a safety concern (violent, arrested, victimized, or suicidal); to have greater substance-related problems; and to report poorer life satisfaction, quality of life, mental functioning, family relationships, and medication adherence. Furthermore, changes in depressed status were associated with changes in functional outcomes.

Management of Schizophrenia with Suicide Risk **863**

Alec Roy and Maurizio Pompili

Suicidal behavior remains a major source of morbidity and mortality among schizophrenics. The National Institute of Mental Health Longitudinal Study of Chronic Schizophrenia found that over a mean of 6 years, 38% of the patients had at least one suicide attempt and 57% admitted to substantial suicidal ideation. Suicide is also a major issue among inpatients, with serious implications for clinical practice and patient-doctor relationships. The management of schizophrenic patients with suicide risk remains a difficult area for clinicians despite attempts to better understand it by gathering experts in the field. This article discusses the frequency of suicidal behavior in schizophrenia, offers a model for understanding it,

and discusses various aspects of the management of the at-risk schizophrenic patient.

Schizophrenia with Impulsive and Aggressive Behaviors **885**

J.P. Lindenmayer and Isabella Kanellopoulou

Impulsive and aggressive behaviors are important clinical challenges in the treatment of patients with schizophrenia. They occur both in the acute phase as well as in the chronic phase of the disorder and call for differentiated treatment interventions. It is important to always first consider behavioral and nonpharmacological interventions. High levels of structure and organization together with a nonconfrontational approach may be very successful interventions. In terms of acute pharmacological interventions, clinicians now have a broad spectrum of intramuscular antipsychotic compounds available with rapid onset of action and relatively little sedation. There is a need for new compounds with a more acceptable tolerability profile for the long-term treatment of these important syndromes.

Index **903**

FORTHCOMING ISSUES

March 2010

Genetics

James B. Potash, MD, MPH,
Guest Editor

June 2010

Women's Mental Health

Susan G. Kornstein, MD and
Anita Clayton, MD,
Guest Editors

September 2010

Cognitive-Behavioral Therapy

Bunmi O. Olatunji, PhD, *Guest Editor*

RECENT ISSUES

September 2009

Anxiety Disorders

Hans-Ulrich Wittchen, PhD and
Andrew T. Gloster, PhD, *Guest Editors*

June 2009

Ethics in Psychiatry: A Review

Laura Weiss Roberts, MD, MA and
Jinger G. Hoop, MD, MFA,
Guest Editors

March 2009

Child and Adolescent Psychiatry for the General Psychiatrist

Malia McCarthy, MD and
Robert L. Hendren, DO,
Guest Editors

RELATED INTEREST

Psychiatric Clinics of North America, September 2007 (Vol. 30. No. 3)
Schizophrenia: A Complex Disease Necessitating Complex Care
P.F. Buckley and E.L. Messias, *Guest Editors*

Critical Care Clinics, October 2008 (Vol. 24. No. 4)
Psychiatric Aspects of Critical Care Medicine
J.R. Maldonado, MD, *Guest Editor*

Preface

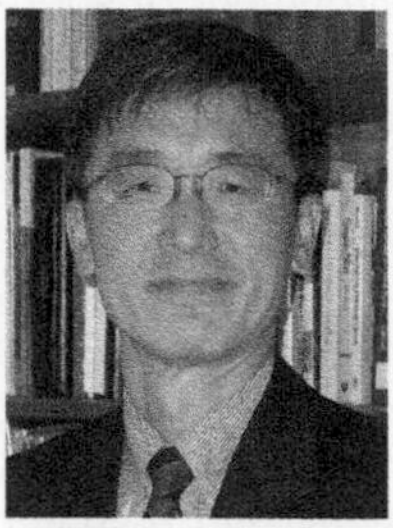

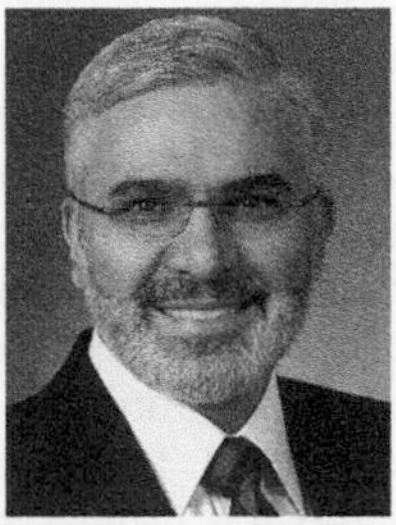

Michael Y. Hwang, MD Henry A. Nasrallah, MD
Guest Editors

Schizophrenia is associated with many psychiatric and nonpsychiatric comorbidities, such as neurologic conditions, substance abuse, and medical disorders. Some comorbid disorders may precede the onset of schizophrenia, whereas others emerge or become clinically prominent after the onset. Researchers and clinicians often have debated whether coexisting psychiatric conditions, such as mood or anxiety, are distinct disorders in their own right or should be considered components of a broader "schizophrenia spectrum disorder." A psychiatric disorder, such as obsessive-compulsive disorder or dysphoria, appears following the initiation of antipsychotic pharmacotherapy and could be regarded as an iatrogenic comorbidity. On the other hand, some neurologic comorbidities may play a role in the pathophysiology of schizophrenia, and some medical comorbidities, such as obesity, diabetes, and hypertension, may be secondary to the pharmacotherapy and unhealthy lifestyle associated with schizophrenia. Substance-use comorbidities (eg, cannabis, stimulants) may play a role in triggering the onset of schizophrenia or contribute to medical comorbidities (eg, liver disease, HIV).

This issue of *Psychiatric Clinics of North America* addresses the complexities of schizophrenia and its various comorbidities from an epidemiologic, diagnostic, biological, and treatment perspective. The presence of comorbidities certainly influences the clinical management of schizophrenia and may require polypharmacy or behavioral therapy intervention; in addition, however, the overlap between schizophrenia and various psychiatric, neurologic, and medical conditions may offer unique opportunities for research into shared neurobiology and genetics.

To start off this issue, Drs Danielyan and Nasrallah review and synthesize the extensive and complex literature about the neurologic aspects of schizophrenia, which include neurologic conditions that may co-occur with schizophrenia, neurologic disorders that may produce schizophrenia-like psychoses, iatrogenic neurologic movement disorders, and the progressive gray and white matter neurobiological deterioration associated with the psychotic-relapse schizophrenia. The evolving literature depicts schizophrenia as a neuropsychiatric brain disorder often complicated by secondary neurologic features.

Next, Dr Short and colleagues review management of major comorbid medical disorders in patients with schizophrenia, including the cardiovascular, pulmonary, and

Psychiatr Clin N Am 32 (2009) xiii–xv
doi:10.1016/j.psc.2009.10.002

gastrointestinal disorders. Although the clinical challenge has been long recognized, the intricacy of assessing and treating both medical and psychiatric conditions often challenges practicing clinicians. In the context of the current environment of short-term hospitalization and rapid advancements in psychopharmacology, the authors present a comprehensive review of the current knowledge in management of schizophrenia with comorbid medical conditions. The authors give a unique clinician perspective in symptom assessment and discuss the specific pharmacological challenges of concurrent treatment of medical conditions in schizophrenia.

Dr Monteleone and his coauthors examine and discuss various metabolic and endocrinological disorders in patients with schizophrenia. While these challenging comorbid conditions have been long recognized, the recent introduction of a new generation of antipsychotics has heightened the clinical implications and research interest in patients who have schizophrenia. Dr Monteleone and his colleagues review metabolic and endocrinological effects of current pharmacotherapy and suggest specific treatment interventions.

The long-standing and emerging clinical and research issue of schizophrenia with comorbid autoimmune disorders has drawn increasing attention in the past decade. This interest is in part derived from the increasing insight into the immunological roles of etiopathogenesis and the clinical course of schizophrenic illness. Often, schizophrenic patients with autoimmune disorders are resistant to conventional antipsychotic treatment and run volatile clinical courses frequently the result of prolonged immune suppressant treatment. Unfortunately, research and clinical data about this schizophrenic subgroup with autoimmune disorders are scarce. Dr Yum and coauthors review the published research and succinctly present the pathophysiological and clinical interface between autoimmune disorder and schizophrenia and suggest future direction for research in this complex and poorly understood clinical issue.

Mainly as a result of a heightened focus recently on obesity and metabolic disorders in schizophrenia, eating disorders in schizophrenia represent an emerging and complex clinical/research area. Using clinical vignettes, Drs Yum, Caracci and Hwang present a conceptual pathogenesis framework of comorbid eating disorders in schizophrenia incorporating psychological and biological attributes to facilitate clinical management.

The next article reviews the prevalence, pathogenesis, and impact of substance abuse in the clinical course and treatment outcome in schizophrenia. Although current evidence indicates high prevalence rates and adverse effects in clinical course and outcome, the bio-psycho-social pathogenesis for substance abuse in schizophrenia remains poorly understood and no reliably effective treatment has been found. Drs Lybrand and Caroff examine and summarize the current evidence and present a useful model in management of schizophrenic patients with substance abuse with psychosocial and drug-specific pharmacological intervention recommendations.

Obsessive-compulsive phenomena in schizophrenia have intrigued and challenged both psychoanalysts and psychopharmacologists over the years, and their management has undergone significant advances in the past decade. Driven by earlier modifications in *Diagnostic and Statistical Manual* diagnostic criteria and advances in psychopharmacology, as well as growing knowledge about the biological basis of the specific psychopathology, our understanding of obsessive-compulsive schizophrenia has greatly expanded. Earlier, the obsessive-compulsive phenomena in schizophrenia were believed to be part and parcel of the psychotic process. Now, emerging evidence suggests possible multiple causes in their pathogenesis. Dr Hwang and his coauthors have compiled the current bio-psycho-social basis of the interface in psychosis and the obsessive-compulsive phenomena and present a schema for pathogenesis and treatment options in obsessive-compulsive schizophrenia.

Depression in patients with schizophrenia is well recognized; however, research continues into its pathogenesis, treatment intervention, and outcome. The advent of novel effective antidepressant agents in the past decade has provided new treatment options for practicing clinicians. The current clinical and research evidence indicates that depression in patients with schizophrenia adversely affects the patient's course of illness and long-term outcome with worse quality of life and higher risks for suicide. Dr Conley summarizes his clinical and research experience and discusses optimal management of diverse depressive phenomena in patients with schizophrenia.

Bleuler noted early in the last century that suicide drives in schizophrenia are "the most serious schizophrenic symptoms." Such symptoms still represent the major cause of morbidity and a clinical challenge. In this next article, Drs Roy and Pompili review psychosocial factors for suicidal behavior in schizophrenia, and present an in-depth but succinct review of the biological studies of suicide in patients with schizophrenia. The authors summarize their extensive clinical experience and research findings in this important clinical and research issue and present the optimal approaches for treatment and long-term management. Finally, the authors propose biological pathogenesis of suicidal behavior in schizophrenia and future directions of research.

Finally, persistent impulsive-aggressive behavior in schizophrenia poses a serious social and management challenge, and risk to the staff and others. Dr Lindenmayer and his coauthor review the underlying causes of aggression in patients with schizophrenia and suggest general guidelines for the intervention and clinical assessment in aggressive and violent patients. The article extensively reviews all the current psychopharmacological agents commonly used in acute aggression and persistently violent schizophrenic patients. The authors review major pharmacological study findings, including the Clinical Antipsychotic Trials of Intervention Effectiveness (CATIE) study, and present data on the treatment effectiveness of all currently used antipsychotics and mood stabilizers. This article includes a treatment flow chart for the persistently aggressive and assaultive schizophrenic patient.

We hope this issue enables readers to appreciate the various medical disorders, both psychiatric and physical, that are frequently encountered in persons suffering from schizophrenia, and helps readers recognize and manage such disorders where needed.

Michael Y. Hwang, MD
F.D.R. VAMC
Mental Health Service (116)
P.O. Box 100
Montrose, NY 10548

Henry A. Nasrallah, MD
University of Cincinnati College of Medicine
260 Stetson Street, Suite 3224
Cincinnati, OH 45219, USA

E-mail addresses:
michael.hwang@va.gov (M.Y. Hwang)
henry.nasrallah@uc.edu (H.A. Nasrallah)

Neurological Disorders in Schizophrenia

Arman Danielyan, MD, Henry A. Nasrallah, MD*

KEYWORDS

• Schizophrenia • Neurological • Gray matter
• White matter • Antipsychotics • Cognitive

Schizophrenia (SZ) is a complex, heterogeneous, and disabling psychiatric disorder that impairs multiple aspects of human cognitive, perceptual, emotional, and behavioral functioning.[1,2] Schizophrenia is relatively frequent (prevalence around 1%), with onset usually during adolescence or early adulthood, and has a deteriorating course. Neurobiological pathologies driven by both genetic and environmental factors are believed to play a major etio-pathophysiological role in SZ. History of scientific interest in brain abnormalities of patients with SZ goes back as far as the history of recognition of SZ itself. Kraepelin believed that dementia praecox was due to severe and widespread disease of the frontal, motor, and temporal cortices.[3] Even before him, John Haslam[4] in Britain, and later Hecker[5] in Germany and Southard[6] in the United States, reported brain abnormalities in schizophrenic patients, including enlarged lateral ventricles and hydrocephalus. A significant body of scientific literature has accumulated since then, supporting the hypothesis that there are structural brain abnormalities in the patients with SZ, compared with matched healthy controls,[7,8] and that such abnormalities are often associated with abnormal findings on neurological examination[9,10] The rapidly growing area of neuroimaging research also found clear evidence of many cortical and subcortical abnormalities in individuals with SZ.[7,11] There are some speculations in the literature that various subtypes of SZ, for example, hallucinatory-paranoid versus nonparanoid; disorganized, with prevalence of negative symptoms, including blunted affect and social withdrawal, are associated with neurological signs specific to each of those subtypes.[12–20] However, the specificity of these findings is unclear and requires further investigation. There were also some arguments in the literature that some of the neurological brain abnormalities in patients with SZ could be a result of treatment with antipsychotic medications.[21] However, multiple studies have consistently demonstrated that a wide variety of neurological abnormalities, including dyskinesias, parkinsonian or extrapyramidal signs, neurological soft signs, and decreased pain perception are present in drug-naïve individuals with

Department of Psychiatry, University of Cincinnati College of Medicine, 260 Stetson Street, Suite 3224, Cincinnati, OH 45244, USA
* Corresponding author.
E-mail address: henry.nasrallah@uc.edu (H. Nasrallah).

Psychiatr Clin N Am 32 (2009) 719–757
doi:10.1016/j.psc.2009.08.004 psych.theclinics.com

first-episode psychosis prior to receiving any antipsychotic medications.[22] This variety was further confirmed by the data from neuroimaging studies, showing that structural brain changes are present in patients before initiation of treatment with antipsychotic medications.[23–25] Further, it has been well established that these structural brain changes are progressive, as evidenced by follow-up neuroimaging studies that demonstrate continuous ventricular dilatation and reduced gray matter volume.[26]

In this article, the authors review the most recent findings from multiple studies, making a strong argument for a neurological basis of schizophrenic process.

STRUCTURAL BRAIN ABNORMALITIES IN SCIZOPHRENIA

Structural brain changes are believed to be one of the core findings in SZ, and to be at least partly responsible for complex phenomenological presentation of patients with SZ. Structural brain abnormalities are also found more frequently in unaffected family members of patients with SZ compared with the general population, and to be associated with neurocognitive and behavioral dysfunctions found in the first-degree relatives. As such, morphometric brain changes were proposed by some investigators to be endophenotypic markers of SZ.[27,28]

Although structural brain abnormalities were historically viewed as a result of noxious effect of schizophrenic process itself, it is now believed that some morphological and volumetric abnormalities in the brain can already be present at the first outbreak of the illness, and that some other structural changes may develop as the schizophrenic process proceeds. In contrast to first-episode cases, patients with long history of SZ showed extended alterations within the frontal and temporal regions, the hippocampus, amygdala, and basal ganglia. For example, in a study of 93 first-episode and 72 recurrently ill patients with SZ, compared with 175 matched healthy controls using cross-sectional and conjunctional voxel-based morphometry of whole-brain magnetic resonance imaging (MRI) data, Meisenzahl and colleagues[29] found significant bilateral reduction in gray matter density in the temporal and prefrontal areas, including the anterior cingulate gyrus, as well as in both thalami in the first episode patients compared with healthy controls. Vita and colleagues,[30] in a meta-analysis of 21 studies with 577 SZ patients at their first psychotic episode and 692 healthy controls, confirmed the presence of specific brain abnormalities during the first episode of SZ. The abnormalities included increased size of lateral and third ventricles, as well as volume reduction of whole brain and hippocampus. However, in another functional MRI (fMRI)study of 473 individuals, including 89 patients with chronic SZ, 162 with first-episode psychosis, 135 at ultra-high risk for psychosis (of whom 39 subsequently developed a psychotic illness), and 87 controls, no significant changes in the medial temporal brain structures, including hippocampus and amygdala, were found until after the onset of a psychotic illness.[31] First-episode patients had only left hippocampal volume reductions, in contrast to bilateral hippocampal volume reduction observed in patients with chronic SZ.

Increased total ventricular volume up to 30%[8,32–36] and *decreased whole brain volumes*[7,8,32,37] were consistently reported in patients with SZ, and are believed to be associated with deficits in attention, executive functioning, and premorbid cognitive functioning in patients.[37] The most significant changes are reported in lateral ventricles, with up to 16% increase in the volume compared with controls,[33,38] followed by changes in the size of the third ventricle.[34,38–40] Increase in lateral and third ventricular volumes, as well as reduced whole brain and hippocampal volumes in patients compared with healthy controls, for example, were reported in a meta-analysis of 52 cross-sectional studies with 1424 patients with SZ.[8] Cross-sectional and

MRI studies at follow-up have also demonstrated evidence of enlarged ventricles and augmented cerebrospinal fluid (CSF) in patients with SZ.[41,42] These findings led the scientific community to believe that such anatomical and structural changes are most consistent with the neurodegenerative hypothesis of SZ. However, there have been consistent reports now showing that such changes can be found in patients with SZ at an earlier age, during the first psychotic outbreak. For example, in a study of Schulz and colleagues,[25] 7 out of 8 never-treated adolescents with SZ had enlarged ventricles, compared with the control group of 18 patients with no diagnosis of SZ. In another MRI study comparing 62 never-treated patients with 42 normal controls, Lieberman and colleagues[24] reported enlarged ventricles in 18% of the former and 2% of the latter. Similar rates were reported by Gur and colleagues,[23] who reported a 16% increase in ventricular volume in 33 never-treated patients compared with 65 normal controls, using MRI. A 20% increase in total ventricular volume of medication-naïve patients with SZ was reported by McCreadie and colleagues[43] in another MRI study, comparing 42 never-treated patients with 31 normal controls.

Gray Matter

Multiple studies consistently showed significant reduction in gray matter volume and density in numerous brain regions of patients with SZ compared with healthy controls, including first-episode cases.[8,44] The rate of gray matter changes sometimes was significant, with studies showing up to 3% reductions in the gray matter volume of the whole brain and up to 3.65% reduction in the gray matter volume of the frontal lobe as early as 2- to 3-year follow-up.[45] Brain regions affected most significantly included the frontal eye fields, supplementary motor, sensorimotor, parietal and temporal areas bilaterally, cerebellum and the cingulates, insula, both thalami, and caudates; the parahippocampal region; and the hippocampus.[44,46–48] In a study of 130 patients with SZ, including 51 medication-naïve and 79 previously treated patients, and 130 healthy controls, the investigators found gray matter volume reduction to be associated with cognitive performance, but not symptom severity.[23] Gray matter volume reduction was described in temporolimbic structures.[23] In another study done by the same group, the gray matter volume reduction was shown in the dorsolateral area in men (9%) and women (11%), in dorsomedial area only in men (9%), and in orbital regions only in women (23% and 10% for lateral and medial, respectively).[49] Higher volumes of gray matter were reported in the left temporal and right parietal regions, left cerebellum, left putamen, and left insula in patients with first-episode SZ compared with healthy subjects.[50,51] According to some reports, decrease in the gray matter volume in the temporal lobes is the most pathognomonic to SZ.[52]

The question of whether gray matter changes are the result of natural aging of the brain, are secondary to the illness process itself, are the results of treatment with psychotropic medications or are present early on, even before manifestation of psychotic illness, and hence could be causative of SZ, remains controversial. Gray matter changes due to natural aging of the brain were shown to be more prevalent in left amygdala and left hippocampus,[53] whereas frontal lobe volume reductions were shown to be more prominent in patients with SZ.[33,34] Molina and colleagues[54] reported prefrontal gray matter volume reduction only in patients with "short-term chronic and long-term chronic SZ" but not in patients with first-episode SZ or healthy controls, concluding that volume loss occurs as a result of the illness. Similar findings, demonstrating progressive loss of cortical gray matter volume in patients with SZ, were reported by others[55] at 2 years,[56] 5 years,[57] and 10 years[58] of follow-up. On the other hand, several studies also demonstrated that gray matter volume reduction can be detected in patients with SZ at first presentation. In an MRI study of 26 never-medicated adolescents, including 23 patients with *Diagnostic and Statistical Manual of Mental Disorders* (Fourth Edition) (DSM-IV) diagnosis of SZ, and 38 healthy controls, the investigators reported significantly less gray matter volume in left and right caudate nuclei, cingulate gyri, parahippocampal gyri, superior temporal gyri, cerebellum and right thalamus, and prefrontal cortex at the time of first episode of psychosis.[59] In another study, widespread abnormalities characterized by a lower fractional anisotropy neuroanatomically associated with localized reduced gray matter were reported in 25 patients with adolescent onset SZ compared with 25 healthy controls.[60] Reduction in gray matter volumes in some part of the brain, that is, right orbitofrontal, ventromedial prefrontal, and posterior cingulate cortices, as well as the left ventromedial prefrontal and anterior cingulate cortices, is believed to be associated with impaired foresight in SZ.[61]

Hippocampus and amygdala volume reductions up to 6% were found in patients with SZ.[33,62] Hippocampus and amygdala dysfunctions were found to be more significant on the left side[29] and to be significantly more altered in patients with recurrent attacks of SZ compared with first-episode cases.[29] However, even in first-episode cases, smaller volume of hippocampus in both hemispheres was already observed at the onset of childhood-onset SZ and remained so throughout the study in 29 11- to 26-year-old patients with childhood-onset SZ compared with controls.[63] In a similar study, smaller anterior hippocampal volume was reported in 24 patients with SZ compared with healthy controls, and was suggested to be at least partly causative of overall impairment of neuropsychological functioning, especially in domains of IQ, attention, and executive function reported in the patients.[64]

Decreased volume of the *thalamus* has been reported during the very first episode of SZ.[22] In particular, a volume reduction in mediodorsal nuclei of the thalamus and underdevelopment in adhesio interthalamica in female patients with SZ was reported.[65] In a study of Gur and colleagues,[66] the investigators found 10% reduction in the volume of thalamus in 42 patients compared with 94 normal controls. Gilbert and colleagues[67] similarly reported 18% reduction in the volume of the thalamus in 16 patients with SZ compared with 25 normal controls. Treatment with antipsychotic medications does not seem to impact the thalamic volume changes. Ettinger and colleagues,[68] for example, failed to find any difference in the degree of thalamus volume reduction in patients with SZ who were treatment naïve versus those treated with antipsychotics. In both cases 5% reduction was reported. Reduction of thalamic volume seems to be present in the family members of patients with SZ as well.[69] Significant reduction in the gray matter density of the thalamus was reported in familial cases of SZ compared with sporadic patients.[70]

Among the structured of *basal ganglia*, the size of the *caudate* was reported to be significantly smaller in medication naïve patients with SZ,[71–73] but some other studies failed to replicate these findings.[29,43,74] A significant increase in the size of the *globus pallidus* and the *putamen* was reported by Gur and colleagues.[66] However, Keshavan and colleagues[75] reported a trend in the opposite direction, and Karlsson and colleagues[74] found no difference. Lower gray matter concentration in the left putamen was reported in first-episode SZ patients with movement sequencing abnormalities, whereas the group of first-episode patients without such abnormalities had a higher concentration of gray matter than healthy controls in the putamen and pallidum in both hemispheres.[76]

Decreased volume of the left *fusiform gyrus,* and reversed asymmetries of the gray matter of the *parahippocampal* and fusiform gyri were reported in patients with SZ as well.[77,78] Vogeley and colleagues[79] saw this as another indicator of support for the neurodevelopmental theory of SZ.

The *entorhinal cortex* is another brain area found to be significantly reduced in antipsychotic-naïve patients with SZ compared with healthy controls.[80] Structural abnormality of the *brain membranes* were found in 14 of 62 (23%) never-treated individuals with SZ compared with 1 of 46 (2%) controls.[81] However, Keshavan and colleagues,[82] comparing 40 never-treated patients with 59 normal controls, found no difference in the incidence of this structural abnormality between the groups.

White Matter

There recently has been increasing attention paid to the question of cerebral white matter abnormalities in patients with SZ. Although it was previously believed that gray matter dysfunction was the core feature of SZ, recent knowledge suggests that morphological changes in the cerebral white matter could be major role-players in understanding of the mechanisms of development of SZ. Furthermore, an extensive body of recent literature shows that cognitive impairment, currently believed to be the core feature of SZ, could in fact be a result of disturbed white matter connectivity, or "damaged brain microcircuitry" in the presence of normal or near normal gray matter architecture.[44,83–95] In fact, only neuropsychologically impaired patients (scoring 1 standard deviation below normal on a broad spectrum of cognitive tests) had significantly smaller white matter and larger lateral ventricle volumes than healthy comparison subjects in a brain morphometric study of 54 "neuropsychologically impaired" patients with SZ compared with 21 neuropsychologically near normal subgroup patients on 4 tests of attention and verbal and nonverbal working memory.[40] Both neuropsychologically near normal and neuropsychologically impaired patients had markedly smaller gray matter and larger third ventricle volumes than healthy comparison subjects. "Disconnectivity" was explained as "impaired control of synaptic plasticity that manifests as abnormal functional integration of neural systems,"[86] as "disruption of WM integrity,"[46,47,96] and as "connectivity related to neurons connecting with erroneous targets."[35] The idea of disrupted connections in the brain in psychotic patients was noted back at the beginning of the twentieth century. Kraepelin and Wernicke[3,97] suggested that disruption of association fiber tracts was the cause of psychoses. Bleuler[98] postulated in 1911 that splitting of mental domains results in psychopathology. Although some believed that disruption in white matter connectivity appears later in the course of the illness, and by itself is a result either of the noxious effect of the schizophrenic process on the brain or of treatment with psychotropic medications, a significant body of more recent literature suggests that white matter abnormalities are in fact already present during the original manifestation of the schizophrenic illness, before treatment with antipsychotics.[42,44,99–103] For example, in a study of 29 10- to 18-year-old patients with early-onset first-episode SZ, schizotypal disorder, delusional disorder, or other nonorganic psychoses, and 29 matched controls using high-resolution 3-dimensional T1-weighted MRI of the brain, white matter changes and enlarged lateral ventricles, but not gray matter volume changes, were found in the patients.[42]

Diffusion tensor imaging (DTI) investigations in SZ have provided evidence of impairment in white matter, as indicated by reduced fractional anisotropy (FA). Mori and colleagues,[104] for example, demonstrated decreased FA in the white matter in the frontal and temporal regions, as well as in the genu and splenium of the corpus callosum in patients with SZ using DTI. A significant negative correlation between FA and duration of illness was also found in the white matter, suggesting that white matter changes are progressive in nature. In another study, Federspiel and colleagues,[105] in a study of 12 patients with first-episode SZ and 12 age- and gender-matched control groups, reported increased intervoxel coherence values in 3 brain regions, including anterior thalamic peduncle, optic radiation, and posterior part of the internal capsule; and significantly decreased intervoxel coherence in 11 other brain regions, suggestive of disturbed cerebral connectivity due to white matter changes.

There is increasing interest recently in the role of myelination process and its disruption in etiopathogenesis of SZ. This interest is not surprising because myelin is in fact an "electrical insulation" for the neuronal fibers, composing the white matter itself.[106] Normal brain development extends until approximately age 50 years, when maximal white matter volumes and myelination are reached in frontal lobes[107] and association areas. The extensive process of myelination increases the brain's capacity to process information distributed over multiple interconnected regions. Multiple lines of evidence now suggest that abnormalities in the process of myelination, and myelin maintenance and repair contribute greatly to the schizophrenic process, as evidenced by imaging and neurocytochemical studies, similarities with demyelinating diseases, age-related changes in white matter, myelin-related gene abnormalities, and morphological abnormalities in the oligodendroglia in schizophrenic brains.[108] Not surprisingly, disturbances in *corpus callosum,* a structure responsible for connection of both hemispheres, have been proposed to be in part responsible for disordered corticocortical connections and lateralization.[109,110] General as well as local changes in the corpus callosum have been reported in medication-naïve patients with SZ.[22,111,112] The mean area of corpus callosum was reported to be smaller in 25 antipsychotic-naïve patients compared with 21 normal controls.[113] These abnormalities were postulated to be at least partly responsible for cognitive deficits in this population, as a result of disturbed connection between 2 hemispheres.[111] Gasparotti and colleagues,[114] in their study of 21 medication-naïve patients with SZ compared with 21 healthy controls, reported lowered mean FA values in the splenium of the patients with respect to healthy controls, supporting the hypothesis that corpus callosum does participate in a pathology of interhemispheric connectivity that affects some first-episode SZ patients.

Effect of Psychotropic Medications on Brain Morphology

There is increasing evidence that antipsychotic medications have an independent effect on brain structure and function, contributing to their therapeutic as well as adverse event profile. Specific morphological changes in the brain are hypothesized by some investigators to correlate with the type and dose of the psychotropic medication used.[44,115] Information on the mechanisms of impact of psychotropic medications on brain morphology is limited, and theories about the difference in action between conventional versus atypical antipsychotics (AA) on brain morphology are at least controversial. Velakoulis and colleagues,[31] for example, found no significant structural volumetric changes between patients taking atypical versus conventional antipsychotics. Patients with first-episode SZ treated with risperidone, on the other hand, were reported to have both gray and white matter changes in several brain regions after 3 to 6 weeks of treatment,[116] whereas treatment with conventional antipsychotics was associated with enlargement of pituitary volume compared with atypicals.[117,118] Lieberman and colleagues[119] found significant reductions in gray matter volume in patients treated with haloperidol, but not olanzapine. It should be noted here that there is also some evidence that magnitude of response to treatment with a particular psychotropic agent may be modulated by the severity of structural abnormalities in the brain at the onset of SZ.[44]

Antipsychotic medications, specifically atypical, are also believed to enhance neuroplastic changes in the brain. Girgis and colleagues,[116] for example, found brain parenchymal changes in 15 medication-naïve patients with first psychotic episode, compared with healthy controls at 6 weeks' follow-up after treatment with risperidone. The changes were reported in gray and white matter in several brain regions, including superior temporal gyrus. There are also some data indicating that the choice of antipsychotic medications may differentially impact brain myelination in adults with SZ. In a study of 18- to 35-year-old men with SZ, Bartzokis and colleagues,[107] for example, found significantly larger white matter volume in patients treated with risperidone compared with those treated with fluphenazine decanoate.

MOVEMENT DISORDERS IN SCHIZOPHRENIA

It was believed in the past that movement disorders in SZ were primarily a result of treatment with antipsychotic medications, mostly of the first generation. However, more recent studies showed that medication-naïve patients suffering from SZ do exhibit movement disorders, including gait abnormalities, dyskinesias, and parkinsonian signs.[7] In a review of the literature, Koning and colleagues[120] compared characteristics of dyskinesia and parkinsonian signs in 213 antipsychotic-naïve patients with SZ and 242 controls, as well as in unaffected first-degree relatives (n = 395) and controls (n = 379). The investigators found a strong association between antipsychotic-naïve SZ with dyskinesia (odds ratio [OR]: 3.59, 95% confidence interval [CI]: 1.53–8.41) and parkinsonism (OR: 5.32, 95% CI: 1.75–16.23) in patients compared with controls. Significant movement abnormalities were also found in adolescents at high risk for developing SZ. In a naturalistic, prospective, longitudinal study of 121 adolescents (mean baseline age, 14.26 years), including 32 with schizotypal personality disorder, 49 nonclinical controls, and 40 with other personality disorders, the schizotypal group exhibited significantly elevated movement abnormalities in comparison with controls at baseline and 2 annual follow-ups.[121] Furthermore, dyskinesias and parkinsonian signs were found to be significantly more prevalent in healthy first-degree relatives of patients with SZ compared with healthy controls (OR: 1.38, 95% CI: 1.06–1.81, and OR: 1.37, 95% CI: 1.05–1.79, respectively), supporting the idea that movement disorders could potentially be another endophenotypic markers of SZ.[120] Patients with SZ also have significantly greater degree of motor overflow (involuntary movement occurring during voluntary movement) compared with controls.[122]

Dyskinesias

Tardive dyskinesia (TD) is a side effect of chronic antipsychotic medication exposure with mostly conventional antipsychotics, which are potent antagonists of dopamine D(2) receptors (DRD2). Abnormalities in dopaminergic activity in the nigrostriatal brain system have been most often suggested to be involved in development of TD. The rate of TD in individuals with SZ, treated with antipsychotic medications, has been estimated to range from 12% to 30%.[123–126] However, there is valid evidence that a significant percentage of dyskinesias can in fact be elicited in patients with SZ before initiation of treatment with antipsychotic medications. TD-like movement disorders were observed in one-third of 600 patients with SZ in an English asylum between 1850 and 1890, as reported in the review of the records compiled by Turner.[127] Many other pre-antipsychotic era psychiatrists provided comprehensive descriptions of dyskinetic symptoms in patients with SZ.[3] Some of the descriptions included "marked and well-observed motor disturbances," "peculiar twitching of the facial muscles," and "myoclonic jerking of forearms and hands"[128]; "choreiform manifestations" and "spasmodic movements of expression," including "making faces" or "grimacing."[129] Based on this evidence, Casey and Hansen questioned what percentage of drug-induced dyskinesias are truly drug-induced rather than simply being exacerbations of preexisting symptoms.[123] Since 1959 numerous studies have assessed the prevalence of dyskinesias in individuals with SZ who had not been treated with antipsychotics. The prevalence rates of dyskinesia in psychotropic-naïve patients vary significantly in the literature, ranging from 4.2% to 5%[123,130] up to as high as 38%.[22,126,131–134] Such discrepancy could at least partly be explained by the use of different scales and thresholds in the measurements.[7] Another factor is that in some of the older studies the patient, although medication naïve, could in fact have been treated with electroconvulsive thrapy or insulin shock therapy.[135]

Patients with SZ with symptoms of TD have been shown to have morphological brain abnormalities as well. In the MRI and DTI analysis of 20 SZ patients with TD, 20 age-, gender-, and handedness-matched schizophrenic patients without TD, and 20 matched healthy subjects, more widespread white matter abnormalities in the SZ with TD group than in the SZ without TD group were shown.[136] Differences were specifically emphasized over the inferior frontal gyrus, temporal sublobar extranuclear white matter (around the basal ganglion), parietal precuneus gyrus white matter (around somatosensory cortex), and medial frontal gyrus white matter (around the dorsolateral prefrontal cortex [DLPFC]). Several genetic studies have focused on the association of dopamine system gene polymorphisms and TD. An association between TD and the Ser9Gly polymorphism of the DRD3 gene and the TaqIA site 3′ of the DRD2 gene was one of the most consistent findings. The variable number tandem-repeat polymorphism in exon 3 of DRD4 has been associated with TD as well. More recently, Zai and colleagues[137] reported on haplotypes consisting of 4 tag polymorphisms that were associated with TD in 171 European Caucasian males.

Parkinsonian Signs

Parkinsonian or extrapyramidal motor signs (EPS) in treatment-naïve patients with SZ were described in the literature in the past. Kraepelin[3] described patients with rigidity and bradykinesia as well as those with a tremor. In 1926, Reiter[128] similarly described patients with SZ with a "well-defined parkinsonian syndrome, which overshadows all other symptoms." EPS were frequently found to be present in premorbid states before manifestation of either positive or negative symptoms.[7] The most common symptoms in this category include rigidity, tremor, gait abnormalities, including bradykinesias, and awkward, uncoordinated movements.[133] The prevalence of EPS was reported to be as high as 38% in drug-naïve patients with SZ. Presence of EPS in patients with SZ was speculated to be predictive of development of TD later in the course of schizophrenic illness. About half of the patients who developed TD were shown to have preexisting EPS in the SOHO (Schizophrenia Outpatient Health Outcomes) study.[138]

Treatment of Movement Disorders with Antipsychotic Medications

Some recent data indicate that certain psychotropic medications, including AAs, can be effective in treating movement disorders associated with Parkinson disease and other neurological conditions, as well as in improving movement disorders developed as a result of previous treatment with conventional antipsychotics. Quetiapine, for example, was demonstrated to be superior to haloperidol in treatment of patients with established TD, with sustained response over a year.[139] In another study of 39 subjects with a first episode of psychosis, quetiapine, in addition to not causing EPS, in fact improved preexisting motor dysfunction in these patients.[140] Clozapine, the very first truly AA agent, was found to be effective for the treatment of dyskinesias associated with Parkinson disease.[141] However, agranulocytosis, which is associated with clozapine treatment, limits its use.[142] Olanzapine was demonstrated to be effective in treatment of dyskinesias in patients with Parkinson disease compared with placebo.[143] However, olanzapine may worsen the symptoms of Parkinson disease itself. Risperidone, another AA, unlike most of the other medications in its class, is associated with either development or worsening of parkinsonian symptoms in patients, treated with dose of 5 mg/day or higher.[144] However, when compared with conventional antipsychotics, long-term use of risperidone was shown to prevent relapse in more patients and for a longer time, and also induces less abnormal movements than haloperidol.[145]

NEUROLOGICAL SOFT SIGNS

Up to 60% of patients diagnosed with SZ have been found to have neurological abnormalities on routine neurological examination, referred to as "equivocal" or "soft signs."[146] Neurological soft signs (NSS) are defined as "subtle neurological abnormalities comprising deficits in sensory integration, motor coordination, and sequencing of complex motor acts."[10] NSS are linked to the neuropathology that is believed to underlie SZ symptoms.[147] The name referred originally to the fact that NSS were mostly transient and often nonlocalizing in nature. In contrast to so-called hard signs, such as the patellar tendon reflex, which often are specific to dysfunction in a particular brain area, NSS represent more complex brain functions. The scientific literature regarding possible pathophysiological mechanisms of NSS is still evolving.

Recent scientific evidence suggests that NSS are most probably the result of disrupted neurodevelopment of the brain as a result of pre- or perinatal cerebral insult. Studies repeatedly showed significantly increased prevalence of NSS in SZ patients compared with controls over time.[10,148–151] NSS were consistently found in medication-naïve patients with SZ, supporting the hypothesis that NSS are intrinsic feature of SZ rather than a side effect of medication,[148,152,153] and that antipsychotic medications are not the main cause of the neurological abnormalities but rather a contributing cause.[19,154] NSS, in fact, can be found early in life (during the first 2 years) in high-risk subjects.[155] Furthermore, there is a very high prevalence of NSS (close to 100%) in cases of SZ with early and adolescent onset, compared with adult onset (55%).[156] Cross-sectional studies have consistently reported an association of NSS with baseline symptoms severity, increased symptom levels, poor premorbid adjustment, and unfavorable outcome,[10,147–149,157] as well as with neurobiological measures such as neuropsychological deficits and structural and functional cerebral abnormalities.[19,158–160] In a prospective study of 39 patients with first-episode SZ-spectrum disorders and controls, Bachmann and colleagues[161] reported NSS scores in patients to be significantly elevated relative to comparison subjects at baseline and 14 months later, despite the fact that NSS significantly decreased in patients, but remained stable in a comparison group. These investigators also reported that such an effect was more pronounced in patients with a favorable rather than a chronic course of the illness. In another prospective study, the overall severity of the NSS was found to be statistically significantly higher in nonremitters than in remitters (as measured by the Positive and Negative Syndrome Scale [PANSS]) at the 1-year follow-up in a study of 92 first-episode male schizophrenic patients.[157]

There are some data in the literature suggesting that NSS might be heritable.[28] NSS were reported in relatives of SZ patients and unaffected cotwins of monozygotic twin pairs discordant for SZ.[162–164] Relatives at increased genetic risk for SZ were found to have more frequent NSS compared with controls in a recent study of 74 offspring of persons with SZ compared with 86 healthy controls.[165] NSS have been suggested by some to qualify as potential endophenotypic markers, expressing genetic vulnerability to SZ.[166]

Neuroimaging studies have shown associations of NSS with activation changes in the sensorimotor cortex and the supplementary motor area, cerebellar abnormalities, and subcortical findings involving the basal ganglia and thalamus.[153,159,161,167] NSS were reported to be significantly associated with reduced gray or white matter densities in the pre- and postcentral gyrus, premotor area, middle and inferior frontal gyri, cerebellum, caudate nucleus, and thalamus.[151] NSS are believed to result from circuitry dysfunctions rather than overall brain dysfunction, with the pattern of cerebral changes clearly supporting the model of "cognitive dysmetria," involving disrupted corticocerebellar-thalamic-cortical circuit in patients with SZ.[151,168,169] Reduced white matter densities are consistent with hypothesis in SZ research, implying "disconnect" phenomena of the brain regions as being the major pathophysiological mechanism of SZ. Thomann and colleagues[151] conducted an MRI investigation of 42 patients with first-episode SZ or schizoaffective disorder, being treated with AAs, and compared them to 22 healthy controls. NSS scores were significantly higher in patients than in healthy controls. These investigators found a significant association between NSS and reduced gray or white matter densities in the pre- and postcentral gyrus, premotor area, middle and inferior frontal gyri, cerebellum, caudate nucleus, and thalamus in the patients. No such associations were found in controls, except for NSS and reduced frontal gyri densities.

There were also some speculations in the literature that NSS are specific to subtypes of SZ such as familial versus sporadic SZ,[170,171] chronic versus acute SZ,[172] and disorganized versus nondisorganized SZ,[173] but not paranoid versus nonparanoid SZ.[174,175] Others hypothesized that[148,176] NSS are representative of specific psychopathology, for example, negative symptoms and formal thought disorders,[12,158,177] but that severity of those reduce along with remission of the psychopathological symptoms.[177–179] However, Bachmann and colleagues,[161] in a prospective study of patients with first episode of SZ, showed that despite significant reduction in the severity of NSS, they still remained elevated in patients relative to healthy subjects.

Among NSS, *motor disturbances* in particular have been reported in more than 90% of patients with SZ, and include clumsiness, postural disturbance, stereotypic movements, mannerisms, and motor blocking; increased or decreased eye blinking,[180] rapid paroxysms and disturbed eye tracking with abnormal smooth pursuit eye movements, and abnormal saccadic eye movements have also been widely reported.[160,181,182] Disturbances of *eye movement* are also common in patients with SZ. In a study of 20 patients with SZ, Kallimani and colleagues[183] assessed oculomotor activities of these patients in the acute phase of the illness before being treated with antipsychotic medications, and then again in the remission phase, after treatment with antipsychotics. These investigators found that saccade and smooth eye pursuit dysfunction measures remained reasonably stable over time and were independent of the clinical state of SZ, that is, during the acute phase versus in remission. Another dysfunction of the eye movements, exploratory eye movement (EEM), was speculated to be specific to SZ.[184] In this study, the discriminant analysis between 251 patients with SZ compared with 389 nonschizophrenics was performed on several variables, including number of eye fixations, total eye scanning length, mean eye scanning length, and responsive search score. The total eye scanning length and responsive search score were found to be 73.3% sensitive and 79.2% specific in discriminating between schizophrenic and nonschizophrenic patients. Several forms of eye movement dysfunctions were found in first-degree relatives of patients with SZ, allowing some to speculate that eye movement disturbances could be an endophenotypic marker for the study of genetic liability in SZ. Takahashi and colleagues,[185] for example, based on the results of the study of 23 probands with SZ, 23 of their healthy siblings, and 43 unrelated normal controls, observed EEM abnormalities more frequently in SZ groups compared with unaffected siblings and normal controls. EEM abnormalities were also shown to be more frequent in the healthy siblings than in normal controls, thus putting healthy siblings in the intermediate position between the probands with SZ and normal controls.[185,186] In a meta-analytical review of the literature, Calkins and colleagues[187] reported memory-guided saccade accuracy and error rate, global smooth pursuit dysfunction, intrusive saccades during fixation, antisaccade error rate, and smooth pursuit closed-loop gain to be the best for differentiating relatives of patients with SZ.

There are numerous NSS that indicate frontal lobe dysfunction, including disturbances in the grasp and palmomental reflexes, abnormalities of face-hand tests and graphaesthesia, minor motor and sensory disturbances, recognizable choreoathetotic, dystonic, and ticlike presentations, gait disturbances, difficulties with coordination and smooth performance of motor activities, reflex changes, and variable Babinski responses.

CEREBRAL METABOLISM IN SCHIZOPHRENIA

Metabolic activity of the brain is measured by using positron emission tomography (PET), single photon emission computed tomography (SPECT), or fMRI. One of the brain areas consistently shown to be disturbed in patients with SZ is the DLPFC. The theory of "hypofrontality," referring to decreased activation of DLPFC in patients with SZ, has been consistently supported by many studies and meta-analyses. DLPFC deficits were reported to already be present at the onset of the first acute exacerbation of SZ and not to be due to current or previous medication effects.[188] In a study of 14 antipsychotic-naïve patients with SZ, Barch and colleagues[188] found that those with SZ failed to show activation of the DLPFC in response to neuropsychological tasks when compared with 12 normal controls. In a case-control study of 43 schizophrenic patients and 43 healthy volunteers, FA reduction was found in 6 frontotemporal clusters in the schizophrenic group in comparison with healthy volunteers, and 3 clusters showed fractional anisotropy increase.[88] Two of the clusters showing reduced fractional anisotropy were associated with reduced gray matter density in neuroanatomically related regions in schizophrenic subjects. Working memory deficit in patients with SZ was postulated to be a result of decreased activation of the right dorsolateral prefrontal cortex (RDLPC).[188–193] Patients with predominantly negative symptoms of SZ were shown to have lower glucose metabolism in the RDLPC.[194]

Protein abnormalities in the DLPFC were recently found in patients with SZ.[195] Using mass spectrometry, the investigators identified 15 SZ-associated proteins and 51 bipolar disorder-associated proteins, with synaptic proteins being the most affected in SZ. In another study of 31 SZ patients (12 antipsychotic-naïve first-episode and 19 antipsychotic-free multi-episode patients) and 31 healthy age- and sex-matched controls, Smesny and colleagues,[196] using phosphorus-31 magnetic resonance spectroscopy (^{31}P-MRS), reported metabolites of phospholipids (phosphomonoester and phosphodiester) and energy (phosphocreatine and inorganic phosphate) metabolism to be significantly reduced in bilateral prefrontal and medial temporal (including hippocampal) brain regions, caudate nucleus, thalamus, and anterior cerebellum in patients with SZ compared with controls, supporting the hypothesis of disturbed phospholipid metabolism in SZ.

It should also be mentioned that other brain regions also exhibit either hypo- or hyperfunctionality in patients with SZ compared with controls. Increased activation in anterior cingulate and left frontal pole regions in patients with SZ, for example, was found to be consistent in a quantitative meta-analysis of 12 functional neuroimaging studies of working memory in SZ.[197] In an fMRI study of 10 patients with SZ and 20 healthy controls, the investigators found overactivation in some brain areas, including anterior cingulate cortex, DLPFC, hippocampus, parahippocampal gyrus, and superior temporal gyrus during the auditory activation task, as well as a lack of communication between those regions.[198]

EPILEPSY

The view of SZ as a neuropsychiatric condition contributed to a scientific notion that structural brain abnormalities in these patients could directly contribute to increased risk of seizures in this population as well.[199–201] Patients with SZ were reported to have an 11-fold increase in the prevalence of comorbid epilepsy.[202] On the other hand, patients with epilepsy were found to be at increased risk of SZ (relative risk [RR] 2.48, 95% CI 2.20–2.80) and SZ-like psychosis (RR 2.93, 95% CI 2.69–3.20).[203,204] Prevalence of psychiatric comorbidities, particularly with psychotic symptoms, in patients with epilepsy, is also significantly increased compared with the general population (2.5%–8% vs 1%, respectively).[205] The onset of psychotic symptoms was reported to be slightly late in patients with epileptic psychosis (mean age 30.1 years) compared with those with SZ (mean age 26.6 years).[206] Psychotic presentation in patients with epilepsy were reported to be the most prominent in cases of frontal and temporal lobe epilepsy,[199,201,205] with cases of medial temporal areas being the most commonly associated with psychotic presentation. Psychotic symptoms in epilepsy may develop in postictal, interictal, and bimodal phases.[207]

The most recent evidence suggests that there is significant overlap in epidemiological, clinical, neuropathological, and neuroimaging features of these 2 diseases, with shared biological liability. Those include ventricular enlargement in both conditions, the leucine-rich glioma inactivated (LGI) family gene loci overlap in both conditions, and other similarities.[203]

ELECTROENCEPHALOGRAPHY

The question whether there are any electroencephalographic (EEG) abnormalities pathognomonic to SZ remains controversial. Heath[208] reported spike abnormalities in the septal region, and secondarily in the hippocampus and amydgala in 26 patients with SZ; such spikes were not found in nonpsychotic patients or Parkinson disease. Petersen and colleagues[209] similarly reported abnormal electrical activity in the "deep frontal" and "subthalamic" regions in 4 individuals with SZ. In a study of 31 adults with diagnosis of paranoid SZ, Bob and colleagues[210] found a direct relationship between wavelet phase synchronization and coherence in pairs of EEG signals recorded from frontal, temporal, central, and parietal brain areas, and positive and negative symptoms of SZ. Some other EEG abnormalities found in patients with SZ include disturbed sleep continuity, slow-wave sleep deficits, and shortened rapid eye movement sleep latency.[211,212] For example, in a sleep EEG study of 15 medication-naïve patients with DSM-IV (Revised) diagnoses of undifferentiated SZ, compared with 15 age- and sex-matched normal controls, patients with SZ appeared to have profound difficulties in sleep initiation and maintenance, poor sleep efficiency, a slow-wave sleep (SWS) deficit, and an increased rapid eye movement density.[213]

Abnormalities of EEG coherence in SZ are at least partly believed to indicate functional disconnection between the frontal and the temporal lobe in the left hemisphere,[214] and were reported in medication-naïve patients. Begré and colleagues[215] reported that first-episode SZ patients with less FA in the hippocampus had more anterior alpha activity. In the EEG of medication-naïve SZ patients, certain types of time periods of synchronous activity (the so-called microstates) have been shown to be shorter in time compared with controls,[216,217] suggesting that functionally interconnected networks are maintained for less time in SZ. It was also shown that patients with SZ have an altered sequence of microstates and thus a different sequential connectivity.[216] In a meta-analysis conducted by Boutros and colleagues,[218] the most consistent results were related to the increased preponderance of slow rhythms in SZ patients, including medication-naïve patients.

Some investigators suggested that EEG changes in patients with SZ are linked to working memory dysfunction.[219] Changes in P50 auditory evoked potentials in EEG findings of patients with SZ, for example, were proposed to be related to deficits in attention.[220] Recent data analysis showed that approximately 40% of healthy controls had P50 ratios within 1 SD below the mean compared with patients with SZ.[221]

Auditory evoked P300 was also reported to be associated with cognitive processes, such as attention and orientation. Abnormal P300 waveforms of the event-related potentials during the auditory oddball task are believed to be one of the most consistent findings in patients with SZ.[222] Reduction in P300 amplitudes was reported to begin early in the prodromal phase of SZ and to have a progressive course from prodromal to chronic state.[223] P300 was found to be reduced in both treatment-naïve and treated patients with SZ, and at least partly was believed to be caused by reduced volume of cortical gray matter.[224–227] The amplitude of event-related P300 was recently demonstrated to be significantly lower in nonmedicated prodromal ($P = .03$), first-episode ($P = .01$), and chronic patients ($P = .001$) with SZ compared with the healthy controls.[223] P300 amplitude but not latency was found to be affected in young patients with recent-onset SZ, whereas both were unaffected in healthy unaffected young siblings.[228]

Reduced N400 amplitude and worse performance in the frontal lobe function test was demonstrated in patients with SZ compared with healthy participants.[229] Statistically significant positive correlations between N400 amplitude and neuropsychological performances on the Stroop Task and Wisconsin Card Sorting Test in patients with SZ were found, suggestive of disturbed integrity of the frontotemporal network in patients with SZ.

DECREASED PAIN PERCEPTION

Pain is believed to be a result of activity of both excitatory and inhibitory endogenous modulation systems.[230] Several clinical observations indicate that pain processing might be disturbed in psychotic disorders such as SZ. Pain insensitivity was also reported in relatives of patients with SZ, suggesting that decreased pain perception may serve as one of the endophenotypes of SZ, and might serve as a prodromal predictor of susceptibility for SZ.[231] There were some speculations in the literature that decreased pain perception is a consequence of treatment with antipsychotic medications.[232,233] However, descriptions of pain insensitivity in psychotic patients were widely recognized and accepted in the scientific community many years before discovery of antipsychotic medications.[234] Descriptions of pain perception deficits in "insane" go back to the eighteenth century. In the 1798 edition of his textbook, Haslam[235] described "great degree of insensibility, so that patients have appeared hardly to feel ... the application of blisters or the operation of cupping." Later he added a description of an insane patient who amputated his own penis.[4] Other cases of severe self-mutilations, unaccompanied by expected affect, were described by Esquirol in 1838[236] and by Kraepelin.[3] Studies conducted later supported these findings. In 2 such studies in the 1950s, 87%[237] and 83%[238] of patients with SZ who suffered myocardial infarctions did not complain of pain. Smaller numbers were reported in a study at a Veterans Administration Hospital. Among those diagnosed with SZ, pain appeared to be absent in 21% of patients with an acute perforated ulcer, 37% of patients with acute appendicitis, and 41% of patients with a fractured femur.[239] A questionnaire to members of the National SZ Fellowship in England reported that 16% said they had "insensitivity to pain."[240] Patients with SZ were reported to have decreased pain sensitivity during cardiac ischemia, perforated ulcers, burns, appendicitis, and bone fractures.[22] It is still unclear, however, whether altered pain perception in patients with SZ is a result of increased pain threshold as a result of neurological brain abnormalities, or the inability of the patients to react to pain.[241] In a review of 50 articles by Bonnot and colleagues,[242] for example, it was concluded that there is significant clinical and experimental data supporting the notion of decreased behavioral reactivity to pain, but not of analgesia per se. Diminished pain sensitivity in SZ is also believed to be related to abnormal excitatory mechanisms.[230]

The effect of antipsychotic medications on pain perception in patients with SZ is underinvestigated. In a recent study assessing thresholds of warmth perception, thermal pain onset, and thermal pain tolerance, and the influence of antipsychotic medication on those processes in acute schizophrenic patients, patients with SZ were found to have significantly increased thresholds of warmth and heat pain perceptions relative to healthy controls.[243] No changes in pain perception were demonstrated after use of antipsychotics.

NEUROCOGNITIVE DEFICITS IN SCHIZOPHRENIA

Neuropsychological and cognitive deficits in patients with SZ were under intensive scientific focus for the past decade, and are now believed to be a central feature of SZ and one of the major contributors to decreased quality of life in this population.[244–246] Some even believe that cognitive performance rather than improvement in psychotic symptoms should be viewed as the primary outcome measure in SZ.[247] Even though neurocognitive deficits, including impairments in memory, executive functions, attention, and processing speed can also be observed in other psychiatric conditions, including schizoaffective disorder and bipolar disorder, only SZ patients are more impaired than the other groups in all cognitive domains.[245] According to some investigators, cognitive deficits in SZ remain relatively stable over the course of the illness,[248] whereas others report worsening of the cognitive functioning over time.[249] In one study, the investigators compared cognitive function between 20 patients with early-onset SZ and 20 healthy controls at 2 time points, when aged 15.58 and after a mean interval of 4 (±1.08) years when aged 19.46 years. No differences were found between patients and controls in the degree of change over this time period in general intellectual function and planning ability. However, there was deterioration in the verbal memory and attentional control index scores from the Wechsler Memory Scale—Revised but relative improvement in Part A of the Trail Making Test. The investigators concluded that most aspects of cognitive function remain relatively stable in cases with early-onset SZ during adolescence except for immediate verbal memory and attention.[248] The question of whether psychopharmacological interventions may improve cognitive functioning in these patients is also controversial, with some investigators contributing the improvement to practical effect.[250]

In the past it was believed that cognitive disturbances were the end result of the schizophrenic process itself or a consequence of treatment with antipsychotic medications.[251,252] More recent data suggest that impaired cognition in patients with SZ is a result of impaired activation of the DLPFC with disruption of coordinated activity between this DLPFC and a brain network that supports cognitive control.[253] A growing volume of scientific evidence also demonstrates that cognitive deficits in patients with SZ are often observed in childhood,[254] before manifestation of the first psychotic episode,[251,255,256] and could potentially be explained by morphological abnormalities of the brain, including disturbed process of myelination, leading to white matter abnormalities. First-episode cases were found to have substantial neurocognitive impairments of 1 to 2 SDs below average in working memory, episodic memory, attention, processing speed, and executive and motor functions.[257–259] Not surprisingly, children and adolescents with poor cognitive abilities in childhood were repeatedly shown to be at increased risk for developing SZ later in life. Review of birth cohort and conscript studies consistently reported strong associations between poor performance on cognitive batteries and increased risk of SZ in youth, whereas studies on school performance, although less consistent, still found strong associations across all school subjects.[254] Significant neurocognitive deficit (0.8–1.8 SDs) on every domain except for social functioning were reported in 31 adolescents with early-onset SZ compared with 67 normal controls, using the MATRICS battery.[260] The most affected cognitive functions were verbal learning, working memory, and visual learning. Patients with SZ were also found to have a reliable, medium-sized impairment in premorbid IQ many years before manifestation of psychotic symptoms, according to a meta-analysis of 18 studies performed by Woodberry and colleagues.[261] There are some speculations in the literature that measurement of an IQ could be an indicator of general cognitive ability early in the course of the illness, and may serve as more sensitive and reliable predictor of functional outcome than specific measures of memory and of executive functioning.[262]

Neurocognitive deficits are at least partly believed to be genetic in origin, as evidenced by the fact that impairments in memory, attention, and executive function are found not only in schizophrenic patients but also in their unaffected relatives.[252,263] Genetic studies involving functional polymorphisms of the catechol-*O*-methyltranferase (COMT) gene demonstrated an association between COMT Val158/108 Met polymorphism and cognitive function, particularly working memory.[190,264,265]

Major areas of neurocognitive deficits in patients with SZ are verbal memory, learning, abstraction, selective attention, spatial memory, and language abilities.[256,258,266–268] The most severely affected areas of cognitive functioning (such as executive functions and memory) are those associated with frontal and medial-temporal regions of the brain.[7]

Memory impairments were reported by Haslam[4] in his 1809 "Observations on Madness and Melancholy," where he noted that recent memory was often impaired in individuals with insanity. Various aspects of memory function are impaired in patients with SZ.

There is solid scientific evidence that patients with SZ demonstrate significant deficits of *working memory*, which has been replicated in many studies.[269–275] Working memory refers to a system for temporarily storing and managing the information required to carry out complex cognitive tasks such as learning, reasoning, and comprehension, and depends on the integrity of the prefrontal cortex. Neuroimaging studies have demonstrated correlations between functional impairment in the DLPFC and working memory performance in patients with SZ, as reported in the FBIRN (Function Biomedial Informatics Research Center) study.[276] Of interest, the DLPFC insufficiency may manifest as either hypo- or hyperfunction, depending on the task demands, and not as hypo- or hyperfrontality as previously believed.[276] Patients with SZ appear to have reduced prefrontal activity during maintenance and response phases of working memory but not during the encoding phase, as reported in another fMRI study of 14 patients with SZ (4 medication-free) and 12 healthy controls.[277] Although large deficits in working memory are demonstrated in patients with SZ across all major working memory domains, no clear differences across subdomains or between particular working memory tasks were reported.[278] Working memory deficits, including slowing of the reaction time and impaired accuracy, were found in first-episode (n = 33) as well as chronic schizophrenic patients (n = 29) compared with controls (n = 64) in a cross-sectional study of Zanello and colleagues.[279] However, no significant differences were found between the groups, suggesting stability of the deficits over time. Working memory deficits were demonstrated to be present early in the course of SZ, and have been shown to be consistently associated with reduced levels of elementary social skills and learning capacity.[280] In a study assessing task performance during a Sternberg working memory task in 23 nonaffected first-degree relatives compared with 43 matched healthy controls using fMRI, the investigators found deficits in working memory performance in the former group.[281] Reduced activation in the relatives of SZ was most remarkable in bilateral DLPFC/VLPFC and posterior parietal cortex when encoding stimuli, and in bilateral DLPFC and parietal areas during response selection. Working memory consolidation, implying the ability to form stable representations of the visual environments, also seems to be abnormally prolonged in patients with SZ.[282]

Impairment in *spatial working memory* is believed to be present at the earliest stages of the illness, and to respond only minimally to treatment with AA.[268] Face recognition deficits in patients with SZ and their families are also believed to be a result of frontotemporal impairment.[283]

Verbal and visual memory deficits are also believed to be prominent trait markers for SZ. Verbal memory impairment in patients with SZ, and their first-degree relatives, has been described extensively in the literature, and was attributed to prefrontal and hippocampal dysfunction.[263,275,284,285] The extent of gray matter changes in patients with SZ were found to be positively correlated with longitudinal changes in *verbal learning and memory*.[45] However, only disturbances in immediate encoding and stabilization of memory representations are believed to be potential SZ-associated intermediate phenotype, whereas visual recall and savings impairments are believed to be the results of the deficits caused by the illness process.[286] Impairment of both verbal fluency and memory are present in the early stages of schizophrenic disease process. In a study of 21 adolescents with SZ spectrum disorders (mean age, 15.4 years) compared with 28 healthy adolescents (mean age, 15.1 years), Landro and Ueland[287] reported that the patient group performed significantly worse than healthy controls on measures of learning and delayed recall, and on a frequency estimation task. The patient group also had impairment of phonological and semantic fluency. In the adult literature, some of the domains of verbal memory that were impaired in SZ compared with controls are difficulties recalling the first items in a list, and impaired object recognition and identification.[288,289]

Impairment in *declarative memory*, but not in nondeclarative memory, was also reported in patients with SZ.[290,291] In a recent study of episodic memory using Logical Memory and Visual Reproduction tasks of the Wechsler Memory Scale (Revised), 162 patients with SZ, their nonpsychotic siblings (n = 146), and controls (n = 205), the investigators found shared impairment in verbal learning, but not memory, for both patients and siblings. Only patients, however, had significant verbal and visual savings deficits over short delays ($P<.0001$) as well as verbal deficits over long delays ($P<.005$). No abnormalities in either measure were found in siblings.[286]

Prospective memory , the ability to remember to execute a delayed intention in the future without explicit prompts, has been found to be affected in patients with chronic SZ, possibly related to prefrontal lobe dysfunction.[292] Prospective memory was postulated to be a primary deficit rather than a secondary consequence of neurocognitive impairments in SZ.[293] *Event-episodic memory* is another area with noticeable deficit in patients with SZ.[294]

Semantic memory-based processes are believed to be mostly controlled by inferior frontal and temporal cortices, whereas particularly demanding integrative processes also require involvement of the DLPFC and sometimes parietal cortices. In a fMRI study of 16 patients with SZ and 16 healthy volunteers, Kuperberg and colleagues[295] demonstrated that although basic activation and retrieval of verbal and imagistic representations were normally modulated in patients with SZ, the patients failed to recruit the DLPFC, medial frontal, and parietal cortices to incongruous (relative to congruous) sentences, and failed to recruit the DLPFC to concrete (relative to abstract) sentences, compared with controls. Cross-sectional functional imaging studies have shown a reduced leftward language lateralization in schizophrenic patients, which do not vary over time and are not influenced by the severity of psychotic symptoms, providing further evidence for a particular organization of language typical for SZ.[296]

Speech and *language* dysfunctions have been consistently found in patients with SZ. These dysfunctions are believed to be a result of abnormal development in language-related regions of the brain, as reported from the studies of childhood-onset SZ.[1,296,297] Delays in speech,[298] and impaired language and arithmetical ability during childhood[299] were in fact reported in children who later developed SZ. Impaired language production in patients with SZ was found on both microlinguistic (lexical and morpho-syntactic skills) and macrolinguistic (pragmatic and discourse level processing) levels, with more significant impairments found in macrolinguistic variables.[300] Semantic and letter fluency are specifically affected in these patients, according to some investigators.[297,301] Others, however, reported that unlike patients with Alzheimer dementia, patients with SZ do not suffer from "degradation of semantic knowledge," but instead are unable to "use semantic knowledge appropriately, particularly when selection of salient semantic relations is required."[302] In a study of visual lexical decision task during fMRI in 15 young adults at high genetic risk for developing SZ, compared with 15 of their siblings with SZ or schizoaffective disorder and 15 age- and sex-matched individuals at low risk for SZ, Li and colleagues[303] reported more bilateral brain activation in SZ patients and their high-risk siblings than in controls. In control subjects, discrimination of words from psuedowords significantly activated Brodmann area 44 more strongly than when nonlinguistic symbols were discriminated. However, high-risk subjects and their siblings with SZ activated this region similarly for both language and nonlanguage tasks.

Deficits in *attention and concentration* are believed to be one of the core features of SZ.[304] Impairment in sustained attention, for example, as measured by the continuous performance test, was found to be a strong indicator of SZ,[305] and in fact was found also in relatives of patients with SZ.[306] Sustained attention was found to be more significantly impaired in the siblings of patients with SZ with high familial loading compared with those from simplex families.[307] Sustained attention deficits have hence been proposed as an endophenotypic marker of SZ. Recent evidence also suggests that patients with SZ have significant impairment in the control of selection part of the attention process, but little or no impairment in the implementation of selection.[308,309] On the other hand, Gur and colleagues[310] found that patients with SZ have inability both to focus on targets and to ignore distraction. Some believe that there is an association between deficits in executive control, particularly inhibitory control, and more severe negative and disorganized symptoms of SZ. O'Grada and colleagues[311] examined the contribution of sustained attention to symptom severity using the Sustained Attention to Response Task (SART) in 69 patients with SZ. These investigators found that the ability to sustain attention significantly predicted variance the severity of negative symptom.

Lack of awareness of having SZ was attributed to deficits in *executive function* and coping styles.[7] Executive functioning refers to a set of processes involved in complex, goal-directed thought and behavior involving multiple brain regions (eg, prefrontal cortex, parietal cortex, basal ganglia) and multiple neurotransmitters (eg, dopamine, glutamate, γ-aminobutyric acid [GABA]).[312] The consensus of the first Cognitive Neuroscience for Treatment Research to Improve Cognition in SZ (CNTRICS) meeting was that 2 specific cognitive mechanism seem to be impaired in SZ: (1) rule generation and selection; and (2) dynamic adjustments in control (ie, after conflict and errors).[312] Volumetric alterations in prefrontal-thalamic-cerebellar gray matter networks, including reduced dorsolateral prefrontal and anterior cingulate gray matter volumes,[313] as well as hippocampal abnormalities were postulated to be associated with executive function deficits in SZ.[314]

CHANGES IN COGNITION AFTER TREATMENT WITH ATYPICAL ANTIPSYCHOTICS

There is relatively little effect of conventional antipsychotics on cognition in patients with SZ.[315,316] There is much controversy about the role of AAs in improving cognitive functioning in patients with SZ, however. According to some investigators, treatment with AAs, in contrast to conventional antipsychotics, is associated with improvement in multiple variables of cognitive functioning, including overall intellectual functioning, auditory and visual memory, working memory, and executive functioning.[259,317–325]

Clozapine, the first atypical antipsychotic drug, was reported to be superior to conventional antipsychotics in improving insight in patients with SZ.[318] Large industry-sponsored controlled trials that examined risperidone or olanzapine in patients with first-episode SZ found significant improvement from baseline with the AAs; effect sizes ranged from 0.35 to 0.54 on composite measures of cognition.[257] In a study by Bilder and colleagues,[259] more than 50% of patients treated with risperidone and olanzapine had significant improvement in cognitive functions compared with haloperidol. In a study by Davidson and colleagues[326] comparing cognitive performance of 498 patients with schizophreniform disorder or first-episode SZ after treatment with haloperidol versus several AA, including amisulpride, olanzapine, quetiapine, or ziprasidone, improvement in composite cognitive test scores in all 5 treatment groups was observed at the 6-month follow-up evaluation, with no significant differences among the treatment groups. A weak correlation was found between the degree of cognitive improvement and changes in Positive and Negative Syndrome Scale scores. In another 12-week trial, of the 40 patients randomized to treatment with sertindole and haloperidol, patients treated with sertindole showed significant improvement on the Reaction Time Decomposition task at week 4 and continued to improve at week 12, whereas those treated with haloperidol showed marked impairment at week 4 with partial recovery by week 12.[327] In a review of literature on cognitive effects of risperidone, Houthoofd and colleagues[328] found that treatment with oral risperidone was associated with improved functioning in the cognitive domains of processing speed, attention/vigilance, verbal and visual learning and memory, and reasoning and problem solving in patients with SZ or schizoaffective disorder. Long-acting injectable risperidone was reported by the same investigators to be associated with improved functioning in the domains of attention/vigilance, verbal learning and memory, and reasoning and problem solving, as well as psychomotor functioning, in patients with SZ or schizoaffective disorder. Treatment with both quetiapine and olanzapine were associated with improvement in memory and general cognitive functions compared with treatment with first-generation antipsychotics.[1,319,320,322,323] Quetiapine alone was found to significantly improve verbal fluency, attention, and executive functioning after 6 months and 1 year of treatment.[329] Ziprasidone treatment was found to improve cognitive functioning in patients with a history of either treatment resistance or intolerance in a randomized double blind controlled study of clozapine or ziprasidone in SZ patients (n = 130) with a history of failure to respond to or intolerance of previous adequate antipsychotic treatments.[330]

However, there is a growing volume of literature suggesting that "practice effect" is responsible for most of the improvements in cognitive functioning observed in patients with SZ after treatment with AAs.[250] Goldberg and colleagues,[257] for example, argued that none of the studies that reported cognitive improvement in patients with SZ after treatment with AAs included healthy controls undergoing repeated testing to assess the possibility that improvements might reflect simple practice effects. To evaluate that hypothesis, the same group conducted a randomized controlled trial of cognitive effects of risperidone and olanzapine in 104 patients with first-episode SZ and 84 healthy controls. The patients underwent cognitive assessment, including measures of working memory and attention, speed, motor function, episodic memory, and executive function at baseline, 6 weeks later, and 16 weeks later. The study results did not support the notion that treatment with antipsychotic medications are in fact contributing to improved cognitive functioning in patients with SZ. The cognitive improvements were found to be equal to practice effects observed in healthy controls, including exposure, familiarity, or procedural learning.[257] In an earlier study, Mohamed and colleagues[331] used extensive batteries to assess neuropsychological functioning of 77 antipsychotic-naïve patients compared with 21 others who had received medications and 305 normal controls. Both patient groups displayed "substantial impairments in most aspects of cognition," especially on tests of memory, speeded cognitive tasks, attention, social cognition, and executive skills (eg, sequencing, organization, and flexibility). Neither mono- nor polypharmacotherapy seems to significantly enhance cognitive function in patients with SZ, according to Galletly.[332] In a study assessing the differential effects of risperidone and haloperidol on verbal memory, attention, and psychiatric symptoms in 28 patients with SZ compared with healthy controls, the patients with SZ did not differ on the California Verbal Learning Test and the d2 Cancellation Tests.[333] No improvement in neurocognitive performance in haloperidol or risperidone groups were reported at a 12-month follow-up either. In another prospective, randomized, double-blind, placebo-controlled, 6-week study of 30 patients with DSM-IV SZ, the investigators similarly did not find significant improvement of cognitive function in patients treated with risperidone for 6 weeks after receiving chronic treatment with clozapine.[334]

However, in a naturalistic study of 56 patients with SZ or schizoaffective disorder, assessing the cognitive effects of antipsychotics using the Brief Assessment of Cognition in SZ (BACS), Elie and colleagues[335] found that changes in cognitive functioning were related to a dose of antipsychotics used, and whether the patients were receiving mono- versus polypharmacotherapy. It seemed that increasing the antipsychotic daily dose was associated with poorer cognitive functioning.

In a recent MATRICS workshop, the classes of drugs were identified that are "most likely to be cognitive enhancers in SZ."[336] The potentially promising agents include cholinergic agents, including α-7 nicotinic receptor agonists and M1 muscarinic receptor agonists; dopaminergic agents, including D1 receptor agonists; glutamatergic agents acting on both ionotropic and metabotropic receptors; α-2 adrenergic receptor agonists; and agents acting on the GABA system and on various serotonin receptors. In a recent study, Barr and colleagues[337] investigated the effect of transdermal nicotine on attention in a randomized, double-blind, placebo-controlled crossover study of 28 patients with SZ compared with 32 normal controls. Patients receiving nicotine showed significant improvement in performance on the Continuous Performance Test Identical Pairs (CPT-IP) Version as measured by hit reaction time, hit reaction time standard deviation, and random errors in both groups. In addition, nicotine reduced commission errors on the CPT-IP and improved the performance on a Card Stroop task to a greater extent in those with SZ versus controls.

SUMMARY

Despite the fact that SZ, at least by its manifestation, is a psychiatric condition, both historical and more recent scientific evidence point to a conclusion that schizophrenic illness is a psychopathological as well as neuropathological condition. Most of the neurological disturbances in SZ could be better explained by disturbance in neurodevelopmental rather than neurodegenerative processes, as evidenced by the presence of multiple neurological symptoms, syndromes, or even nosologies in patients with SZ before manifestation of diagnosable psychopathological symptoms. NSS almost always can be elicited on close neurological examination of patients with SZ. Major brain areas have been persistently shown to be affected in patients with SZ, including periventricular area, caudate, thalamus, and so forth. Significant changes in gray and white matter, as well as disturbed process of myelinization, resulting in "disconnect" between various brain regions, have been observed in several neuroimaging studies. Morphological brain changes were shown to be present many years before the manifestation of the psychotic illness and before treatment with psychotropic agents, opposing the point of view that such changes are the result of the noxious effect of the schizophrenic process on the brain, or are the results of treatment with psychotropic medications. Genetic etiology of brain matter changes is supported by the fact that many of those pathological features are observed in the first-degree relatives of patients with SZ. Cognitive dysfunction in patients with SZ is now believed to be one of the core features of SZ. However, there is no theory that yet explains the complex pattern of psychosis, negative symptoms, cognitive impairment, and associated psychopathology seen in SZ.[332] Unfortunately, there is also no single abnormality in brain structure or function that is pathognomonic for SZ. As a result, there is no specific diagnostic test or set of tests able to be used for SZ. Most of the neurological and cognitive deficits found in patients with SZ can also be found in many other neurological and nonneurological disease processes.

Molecular psychiatry is growing fast, and will hopefully identify a complex set of genes implicated in the development of SZ. Psychopharmacogenetics is also an area of great promise, which should help in choosing "patient-specific" psychotropic agents with improved efficacy and reduced adverse event profile for SZ patients.

Detailed neurological and neuropsychological history and examination should be a key factor in psychiatric evaluation of any patient with SZ, and especially the younger patient, before initiation of medication treatments. Triggers for such thorough investigation should be the presence of known risk factors for the development of SZ in the future, including positive family history. This history taking potentially can improve early intervention, and hopefully achieve a better outcome in the treatment of this chronic psychiatric condition.

One of the initiatives currently focused on further development of more specific neuropsychological tests for assessment of SZ is MATRICS. The MATRICS initiative includes developing a consensus neuropsychological battery of 10 tests designed to evaluate performance across 7 domains previously shown to be impaired in SZ, including speed of processing; attention/vigilance; working memory; verbal learning; visual learning; reasoning and problem solving; and social cognition.[338–341] A network of 7 research sites called the Treatment Units for Research on Neurocognition in SZ (TURNS; http://www.turns.ucla.edu) has been established to undertake clinical trials of drugs with the potential to improve cognition in SZ.

REFERENCES

1. Kasai K, Iwanami A, Yamasue H, et al. Neuroanatomy and neurophysiology in schizophrenia. Neurosci Res 2002;43(2):93–110.
2. Nasrallah HA, Smeltzer DJ. Contemporary diagnosis and management of the patient with schizophrenia. Philadelphia(PA): Handbooks in Health Care; 2003.
3. Kraepelin E. Dementia praecox and paraphrenia. Edinburgh: Livingstone; 1919.
4. Haslam J. Observations on madness and melancholy. New York: The Classics of psychiatry and behavioral science library; 1809.
5. Hecker E. Die Hebephrenie. Arch Pathol Anat Physiol Klin Med 1871;52: 394–409.
6. Southard EE. On the topographical distribution of cortex lesions and anomalies in dementia praecox, with some account of their functional significance. Am J Insanity 1915;71:603–71.
7. Nasrallah HA. Neurologic comorbidities in schizophrenia. J Clin Psychiatry 2005; 66(Suppl 6):34–46.
8. Steen RG, Mull C, McClure R, et al. Brain volume in first-episode schizophrenia: systematic review and meta-analysis of magnetic resonance imaging studies. Br J Psychiatry 2006;188:510–8.
9. Cadet JL, Rickler KC, Weinberger DR. The neurologic examination in schizophrenia. In: Nasrallah HA, Weinberger DR, editors. Handbook of schizophrenia, vol.1: The neurology of schizophrenia. Amsterdam: Elsevier; 1986. p. 1–48.
10. Heinrichs DW, Buchanan RW. Significance and meaning of neurological signs in schizophrenia. Am J Psychiatry 1988;145(1):11–8.
11. Shenton ME, Dickey CC, Frumin M, et al. A review of MRI findings in schizophrenia. Schizophr Res 2001;49(1–2):1–52.
12. Arango C, Kirkpatrick B, Buchanan RW. Neurological signs and the heterogeneity of schizophrenia. Am J Psychiatry 2000;157(4):560–5.
13. Buchanan RW, Heinrichs DW. The Neurological Evaluation Scale (NES): a structured instrument for the assessment of neurological signs in schizophrenia. Psychiatry Res 1989;27(3):335–50.
14. Merriam AE, Kay SR, Opler LA, et al. Neurological signs and the positive-negative dimension in schizophrenia. Biol Psychiatry 1990;28(3):181–92.
15. Flashman LA, Flaum M, Gupta S, et al. Soft signs and neuropsychological performance in schizophrenia. Am J Psychiatry 1996;153(4):526–32.

16. Wong AH, Voruganti LN, Heslegrave RJ, et al. Neurocognitive deficits and neurological signs in schizophrenia. Schizophr Res 1997;23(2):139–46.
17. King DJ, Wilson A, Cooper SJ, et al. The clinical correlates of neurological soft signs in chronic schizophrenia. Br J Psychiatry 1991;158:770–5.
18. Mohr F, Hubmann W, Cohen R, et al. Neurological soft signs in schizophrenia: assessment and correlates. Eur Arch Psychiatry Clin Neurosci 1996;246(5): 240–8.
19. Manschreck TC, Maher BA, Rucklos ME, et al. Disturbed voluntary motor activity in schizophrenic disorder. Psychol Med 1982;12(1):73–84.
20. Rochford JM, Detre T, Tucker GJ, et al. Neuropsychological impairments in functional psychiatric diseases. Arch Gen Psychiatry 1970;22(2):114–9.
21. Breggin PR. Does clozapine treatment cause brain disease? Arch Gen Psychiatry 1998;55(9):845.
22. Torrey EF. Studies of individuals with schizophrenia never treated with antipsychotic medications: a review. Schizophr Res 2002;58(2–3):101–15.
23. Gur RE, Turetsky BI, Bilker WB, et al. Reduced gray matter volume in schizophrenia. Arch Gen Psychiatry 1999;56(10):905–11.
24. Lieberman J, Bogerts B, Degreef G, et al. Qualitative assessment of brain morphology in acute and chronic schizophrenia. Am J Psychiatry 1992;149(6): 784–94.
25. Schulz SC, Koller MM, Kishore PR, et al. Ventricular enlargement in teenage patients with schizophrenia spectrum disorder. Am J Psychiatry 1983;140(12): 1592–5.
26. Keshavan MS, Tandon R, Boutros NN, et al. Schizophrenia, "just the facts": what we know in 2008 part 3: neurobiology. Schizophr Res 2008;106(2–3): 89–107.
27. Keshavan MS, Prasad KM, Pearlson G. Are brain structural abnormalities useful as endophenotypes in schizophrenia? Int Rev Psychiatry 2007;19(4): 397–406.
28. Prasad KM, Sanders R, Sweeney J, et al. Neurological abnormalities among offspring of persons with schizophrenia: relation to premorbid psychopathology. Schizophr Res 2009;108(1–3):163–9.
29. Meisenzahl EM, Koutsouleris N, Bottlender R, et al. Structural brain alterations at different stages of schizophrenia: a voxel-based morphometric study. Schizophr Res 2008;104(1–3):44–60.
30. Vita A, De Peri L, Silenzi C, et al. Brain morphology in first-episode schizophrenia: a meta-analysis of quantitative magnetic resonance imaging studies. Schizophr Res 2006;82(1):75–88.
31. Velakoulis D, Wood SJ, Wong MT, et al. Hippocampal and amygdala volumes according to psychosis stage and diagnosis: a magnetic resonance imaging study of chronic schizophrenia, first-episode psychosis, and ultra-high-risk individuals. Arch Gen Psychiatry 2006;63(2):139–49.
32. Lawrie SM, Abukmeil SS. Brain abnormality in schizophrenia. A systematic and quantitative review of volumetric magnetic resonance imaging studies. Br J Psychiatry 1998;172:110–20.
33. Wright IC, Rabe-Hesketh S, Woodruff PW, et al. Meta-analysis of regional brain volumes in schizophrenia. Am J Psychiatry 2000;157(1):16–25.
34. McCarley RW, Wible CG, Frumin M, et al. MRI anatomy of schizophrenia. Biol Psychiatry 1999;45(9):1099–119.
35. Harrison PJ. The neuropathology of schizophrenia. A critical review of the data and their interpretation. Brain 1999;122(Pt 4):593–624.

36. Barkataki I, Kumari V, Das M, et al. Volumetric structural brain abnormalities in men with schizophrenia or antisocial personality disorder. Behav Brain Res 2006;169(2):239–47.
37. Crespo-Facorro B, Barbadillo L, Pelayo-Teran JM, et al. Neuropsychological functioning and brain structure in schizophrenia. Int Rev Psychiatry 2007; 19(4):325–36.
38. Cahn W, Hulshoff Pol HE, Lems EB, et al. Brain volume changes in first-episode schizophrenia: a 1-year follow-up study. Arch Gen Psychiatry 2002;59(11): 1002–10.
39. Nasrallah HA, Schwarzkopf SB, Olson SC, et al. Gender differences in schizophrenia on MRI brain scans. Schizophr Bull 1990;16(2):205–10.
40. Wexler BE, Zhu H, Bell MD, et al. Neuropsychological near normality and brain structure abnormality in schizophrenia. Am J Psychiatry 2009;166(2):189–95.
41. Ho BC, Andreasen NC, Nopoulos P, et al. Progressive structural brain abnormalities and their relationship to clinical outcome: a longitudinal magnetic resonance imaging study early in schizophrenia. Arch Gen Psychiatry 2003;60(6): 585–94.
42. Pagsberg AK, Baare WF, Raabjerg Christensen AM, et al. Structural brain abnormalities in early onset first-episode psychosis. J Neural Transm 2007;114(4): 489–98.
43. McCreadie RG, Thara R, Padmavati R, et al. Structural brain differences between never-treated patients with schizophrenia, with and without dyskinesia, and normal control subjects: a magnetic resonance imaging study. Arch Gen Psychiatry 2002;59(4):332–6.
44. Begre S, Koenig T. Cerebral disconnectivity: an early event in schizophrenia. Neuroscientist 2008;14(1):19–45.
45. Zipparo L, Whitford TJ, Redoblado Hodge MA, et al. Investigating the neuropsychological and neuroanatomical changes that occur over the first 2-3 years of illness in patients with first-episode schizophrenia. Prog Neuropsychopharmacol Biol Psychiatry 2008;32(2):531–8.
46. Kubicki M, Park H, Westin CF, et al. DTI and MTR abnormalities in schizophrenia: analysis of white matter integrity. Neuroimage 2005;26(4):1109–18.
47. Kubicki M, McCarley RW, Shenton ME. Evidence for white matter abnormalities in schizophrenia. Curr Opin Psychiatry 2005;18(2):121–34.
48. Thompson PM, Vidal C, Giedd JN, et al. Mapping adolescent brain change reveals dynamic wave of accelerated gray matter loss in very early-onset schizophrenia. Proc Natl Acad Sci U S A 2001;98(20):11650–5.
49. Gur RE, Turetsky BI, Cowell PE, et al. Temporolimbic volume reductions in schizophrenia. Arch Gen Psychiatry 2000;57(8):769–75.
50. Salgado-Pineda P, Baeza I, Perez-Gomez M, et al. Sustained attention impairment correlates to gray matter decreases in first episode neuroleptic-naïve schizophrenic patients. Neuroimage 2003;19(2 Pt 1):365–75.
51. Whitford TJ, Grieve SM, Farrow TF, et al. Progressive grey matter atrophy over the first 2-3 years of illness in first-episode schizophrenia: a tensor-based morphometry study. Neuroimage 2006;32(2):511–9.
52. McCarley RW, Salisbury DF, Hirayasu Y, et al. Association between smaller left posterior superior temporal gyrus volume on magnetic resonance imaging and smaller left temporal P300 amplitude in first-episode schizophrenia. Arch Gen Psychiatry 2002;59(4):321–31.
53. Hulshoff Pol HE, Schnack HG, Bertens MG, et al. Volume changes in gray matter in patients with schizophrenia. Am J Psychiatry 2002;159(2):244–50.

54. Molina V, Sanz J, Sarramea F, et al. Lower prefrontal gray matter volume in schizophrenia in chronic but not in first episode schizophrenia patients. Psychiatry Res 2004;131(1):45–56.
55. Nakamura M, Salisbury DF, Hirayasu Y, et al. Neocortical gray matter volume in first-episode schizophrenia and first-episode affective psychosis: a cross-sectional and longitudinal MRI study. Biol Psychiatry 2007;62(7):773–83.
56. Farrow TF, Whitford TJ, Williams LM, et al. Diagnosis-related regional gray matter loss over two years in first episode schizophrenia and bipolar disorder. Biol Psychiatry 2005;58(9):713–23.
57. van Haren NE, Hulshoff Pol HE, Schnack HG, et al. Focal gray matter changes in schizophrenia across the course of the illness: a 5-year follow-up study. Neuropsychopharmacology 2007;32(10):2057–66.
58. Saijo T, Abe T, Someya Y, et al. Ten year progressive ventricular enlargement in schizophrenia: an MRI morphometrical study. Psychiatry Clin Neurosci 2001;55(1):41–7.
59. Chua SE, Cheung C, Cheung V, et al. Cerebral grey, white matter and csf in never-medicated, first-episode schizophrenia. Schizophr Res 2007;89(1–3):12–21.
60. Douaud G, Smith S, Jenkinson M, et al. Anatomically related grey and white matter abnormalities in adolescent-onset schizophrenia. Brain 2007;130(Pt 9):2375–86.
61. Eack SM, George MM, Prasad KM, et al. Neuroanatomical substrates of foresight in schizophrenia. Schizophr Res 2008;103(1–3):62–70.
62. Weiss AP, Zalesak M, DeWitt I, et al. Impaired hippocampal function during the detection of novel words in schizophrenia. Biol Psychiatry 2004;55(7):668–75.
63. Nugent TF 3rd, Herman DH, Ordonez A, et al. Dynamic mapping of hippocampal development in childhood onset schizophrenia. Schizophr Res 2007;90(1–3):62–70.
64. Thoma RJ, Monnig M, Hanlon FM, et al. Hippocampus volume and episodic memory in schizophrenia. J Int Neuropsychol Soc 2009;15(2):182–95.
65. Shimizu M, Fujiwara H, Hirao K, et al. Structural abnormalities of the adhesio interthalamica and mediodorsal nuclei of the thalamus in schizophrenia. Schizophr Res 2008;101(1-3):331–8.
66. Gur RE, Maany V, Mozley PD, et al. Subcortical MRI volumes in neuroleptic-naïve and treated patients with schizophrenia. Am J Psychiatry 1998;155(12):1711–7.
67. Gilbert AR, Rosenberg DR, Harenski K, et al. Thalamic volumes in patients with first-episode schizophrenia. Am J Psychiatry 2001;158(4):618–24.
68. Ettinger U, Chitnis XA, Kumari V, et al. Magnetic resonance imaging of the thalamus in first-episode psychosis. Am J Psychiatry 2001;158(1):116–8.
69. Seidman LJ, Faraone SV, Goldstein JM, et al. Thalamic and amygdala-hippocampal volume reductions in first-degree relatives of patients with schizophrenia: an MRI-based morphometric analysis. Biol Psychiatry 1999;46(7):941–54.
70. Lui S, Deng W, Huang X, et al. Neuroanatomical differences between familial and sporadic schizophrenia and their parents: an optimized voxel-based morphometry study. Psychiatry Res 2009;171(2):71–81.
71. Keshavan MS, Rosenberg D, Sweeney JA, et al. Decreased caudate volume in neuroleptic-naïve psychotic patients. Am J Psychiatry 1998;155(6):774–8.
72. Shihabuddin L, Buchsbaum MS, Hazlett EA, et al. Dorsal striatal size, shape, and metabolic rate in never-medicated and previously medicated

schizophrenics performing a verbal learning task. Arch Gen Psychiatry 1998; 55(3):235–43.
73. Corson PW, Nopoulos P, Andreasen NC, et al. Caudate size in first-episode neuroleptic-naïve schizophrenic patients measured using an artificial neural network. Biol Psychiatry 1999;46(5):712–20.
74. Karlsson P, Farde L, Halldin C, et al. PET study of D(1) dopamine receptor binding in neuroleptic-naïve patients with schizophrenia. Am J Psychiatry 2002;159(5):761–7.
75. Keshavan MS, Haas GL, Kahn CE, et al. Superior temporal gyrus and the course of early schizophrenia: progressive, static, or reversible? J Psychiatr Res 1998; 32(3-4):161–7.
76. Kasparek T, Prikryl R, Schwarz D, et al. Movement sequencing abilities and basal ganglia morphology in first-episode schizophrenia. World J Biol Psychiatry 2008;30:1–11 [Epub ahead of print].
77. McDonald B, Highley JR, Walker MA, et al. Anomalous asymmetry of fusiform and parahippocampal gyrus gray matter in schizophrenia: a postmortem study. Am J Psychiatry 2000;157(1):40–7.
78. White T, Andreasen NC, Nopoulos P, et al. Gyrification abnormalities in childhood- and adolescent-onset schizophrenia. Biol Psychiatry 2003;54(4): 418–26.
79. Vogeley K, Schneider-Axmann T, Pfeiffer U, et al. Disturbed gyrification of the prefrontal region in male schizophrenic patients: a morphometric postmortem study. Am J Psychiatry 2000;157(1):34–9.
80. Joyal CC, Laakso MP, Tiihonen J, et al. A volumetric MRI study of the entorhinal cortex in first episode neuroleptic-naïve schizophrenia. Biol Psychiatry 2002; 51(12):1005–7.
81. Degreef G, Lantos G, Bogerts B, et al. Abnormalities of the septum pellucidum on MR scans in first-episode schizophrenic patients. AJNR Am J Neuroradiol 1992;13(3):835–40.
82. Keshavan MS, Jayakumar PN, Diwadkar VA, et al. Cavum septi pellucidi in first-episode patients and young relatives at risk for schizophrenia. CNS Spectr 2002;7(2):155–8.
83. Begre S, Kleinlogel H, Kiefer C, et al. White matter anisotropy related to electrophysiology of first episode schizophrenia during NoGo inhibition. Neurobiol Dis 2008;30(2):270–80.
84. Burns JK. An evolutionary theory of schizophrenia: cortical connectivity, metarepresentation, and the social brain. Behav Brain Sci 2004;27(6):831–55 [discussion: 855–85].
85. Crow TJ, Paez P, Chance SA. Callosal misconnectivity and the sex difference in psychosis. Int Rev Psychiatry 2007;19(4):449–57.
86. Friston KJ, Frith CD. Schizophrenia: a disconnection syndrome? Clin Neurosci 1995;3(2):89–97.
87. Konrad A, Vucurevic G, Musso F, et al. ErbB4 genotype predicts left frontotemporal structural connectivity in human brain. Neuropsychopharmacology 2009; 34(3):641–50.
88. Spoletini I, Cherubini A, Di Paola M, et al. Reduced fronto-temporal connectivity is associated with frontal gray matter density reduction and neuropsychological deficit in schizophrenia. Schizophr Res 2009;108(1–3):57–68.
89. Karlsgodt KH, Sun D, Jimenez AM, et al. Developmental disruptions in neural connectivity in the pathophysiology of schizophrenia. Dev Psychopathol 2008; 20(4):1297–327.

90. Koch G, Ribolsi M, Mori F, et al. Connectivity between posterior parietal cortex and ipsilateral motor cortex is altered in schizophrenia. Biol Psychiatry 2008; 64(9):815–9.
91. Konrad A, Winterer G. Disturbed structural connectivity in schizophrenia primary factor in pathology or epiphenomenon? Schizophr Bull 2008;34(1):72–92.
92. Kubicki M, Styner M, Bouix S, et al. Reduced interhemispheric connectivity in schizophrenia-tractography based segmentation of the corpus callosum. Schizophr Res 2008;106(2–3):125–31.
93. Magnotta VA, Adix ML, Caprahan A, et al. Investigating connectivity between the cerebellum and thalamus in schizophrenia using diffusion tensor tractography: a pilot study. Psychiatry Res 2008;163(3):193–200.
94. Welsh RC, Chen AC, Taylor SF. Low-frequency BOLD fluctuations demonstrate altered thalamocortical connectivity in schizophrenia. Schizophr Bull 2008 [Epub ahead of print].
95. Williams LM. Voxel-based morphometry in schizophrenia: implications for neurodevelopmental connectivity models, cognition and affect. Expert Rev Neurother 2008;8(7):1049–65.
96. Kubicki M, Westin CF, McCarley RW, et al. The application of DTI to investigate white matter abnormalities in schizophrenia. Ann N Y Acad Sci 2005;1064:134–48.
97. Wernicke K. Grundriss Der Psychiatrie Leipzig. Verlag von Georg Thieme; 1906.
98. Bleuler E. Dementia Praecox, Oder Gruppe Der Schizophrenien. Leipzig: F. Deuticke; 1911.
99. Kyriakopoulos M, Vyas NS, Barker GJ, et al. A diffusion tensor imaging study of white matter in early-onset schizophrenia. Biol Psychiatry 2008;63(5):519–23.
100. Witthaus H, Brune M, Kaufmann C, et al. White matter abnormalities in subjects at ultra high-risk for schizophrenia and first-episode schizophrenic patients. Schizophr Res 2008;102(1–3):141–9.
101. Szeszko PR, Ardekani BA, Ashtari M, et al. White matter abnormalities in first-episode schizophrenia or schizoaffective disorder: a diffusion tensor imaging study. Am J Psychiatry 2005;162(3):602–5.
102. Kumra S, Ashtari M, Cervellione KL, et al. White matter abnormalities in early-onset schizophrenia: a voxel-based diffusion tensor imaging study. J Am Acad Child Adolesc Psychiatry 2005;44(9):934–41.
103. Hao Y, Liu Z, Jiang T, et al. White matter integrity of the whole brain is disrupted in first-episode schizophrenia. Neuroreport 2006;17(1):23–6.
104. Mori T, Ohnishi T, Hashimoto R, et al. Progressive changes of white matter integrity in schizophrenia revealed by diffusion tensor imaging. Psychiatry Res 2007; 154(2):133–45.
105. Federspiel A, Begre S, Kiefer C, et al. Alterations of white matter connectivity in first episode schizophrenia. Neurobiol Dis 2006;22(3):702–9.
106. Fields RD. White matter in learning, cognition and psychiatric disorders. Trends Neurosci 2008;31(7):361–70.
107. Bartzokis G, Lu PH, Nuechterlein KH, et al. Differential effects of typical and atypical antipsychotics on brain myelination in schizophrenia. Schizophr Res 2007;93(1–3):13–22.
108. Davis KL, Stewart DG, Friedman JI, et al. White matter changes in schizophrenia: evidence for myelin-related dysfunction. Arch Gen Psychiatry 2003; 60(5):443–56.
109. Gazzaniga MS. Cerebral specialization and interhemispheric communication: does the corpus callosum enable the human condition? Brain 2000;123(Pt 7): 1293–326.

110. Bloom JS, Hynd GW. The role of the corpus callosum in interhemispheric transfer of information: excitation or inhibition? Neuropsychol Rev 2005;15(2):59–71.
111. Downhill JE Jr, Buchsbaum MS, Wei T, et al. Shape and size of the corpus callosum in schizophrenia and schizotypal personality disorder. Schizophr Res 2000;42(3):193–208.
112. Tibbo P, Nopoulos P, Arndt S, et al. Corpus callosum shape and size in male patients with schizophrenia. Biol Psychiatry 1998;44(6):405–12.
113. Venkatasubramanian G, Jayakumar PN, Gangadhar BN, et al. Measuring the corpus callosum in schizophrenia: a technique with neuroanatomical and cytoarchtectural basis. Neurol India 2003;51(2):189–92.
114. Gasparotti R, Valsecchi P, Carletti F, et al. Reduced fractional anisotropy of corpus callosum in first-contact, antipsychotic drug-naïve patients with schizophrenia. Schizophr Res 2009;108(1–3):41–8.
115. Harrison PJ. The neuropathological effects of antipsychotic drugs. Schizophr Res 1999;40(2):87–99.
116. Girgis RR, Diwadkar VA, Nutche JJ, et al. Risperidone in first-episode psychosis: a longitudinal, exploratory voxel-based morphometric study. Schizophr Res 2006;82(1):89–94.
117. Dazzan P, Morgan KD, Orr K, et al. Different effects of typical and atypical antipsychotics on grey matter in first episode psychosis: the AESOP study. Neuropsychopharmacology 2005;30(4):765–74.
118. Pariante CM, Dazzan P, Danese A, et al. Increased pituitary volume in antipsychotic-free and antipsychotic-treated patients of the AEsop first-onset psychosis study. Neuropsychopharmacology 2005;30(10):1923–31.
119. Lieberman JA, Stroup TS, McEvoy JP, et al. Effectiveness of antipsychotic drugs in patients with chronic schizophrenia. N Engl J Med 2005;353(12):1209–23.
120. Koning JP, Tenback DE, van Os J, et al. Dyskinesia and parkinsonism in antipsychotic-naïve patients with schizophrenia, first-degree relatives and healthy controls: a meta-analysis. Schizophr Bull 2008 [Epub ahead of print].
121. Mittal VA, Neumann C, Saczawa M, et al. Longitudinal progression of movement abnormalities in relation to psychotic symptoms in adolescents at high risk of schizophrenia. Arch Gen Psychiatry 2008;65(2):165–71.
122. Hoy KE, Georgiou-Karistianis N, Farrow M, et al. Neurological soft signs in schizophrenia: investigating motor overflow. World J Biol Psychiatry 2008;1:1–9 [Epub ahead of print].
123. Casey DE, Hansen TE. Spontaneous dyskinesias. In: Jeste DV, Wyatt RJ, editors. Neuropsychiatric movement disorders. Washington, DC: American Psychiatric Press; 1984. p. 68–95.
124. Gerlach J, Casey DE. Tardive dyskinesia. Acta Psychiatr Scand 1988;77(4):369–78.
125. Llorca PM, Chereau I, Bayle FJ, et al. Tardive dyskinesias and antipsychotics: a review. Eur Psychiatry 2002;17(3):129–38.
126. Fenton WS. Prevalence of spontaneous dyskinesia in schizophrenia. J Clin Psychiatry 2000;61(Suppl 4):10–4.
127. Turner TH. Schizophrenia and mental handicap: an historical review, with implications for further research. Psychol Med 1989;19(2):301–14.
128. Reiter PJ. Extrapyramidal motor-disturbances in dementia praecox. Acta Psychiatr Neurol Scand 1926;1:287–309.
129. Farran-Ridge C. Some symptoms referable to the basal ganglia occurring in dementia praecox and epidemic encephalitis. J Ment Sci 1926;72:513–23.

130. Kane JM, Smith JM. Tardive dyskinesia: prevalence and risk factors, 1959 to 1979. Arch Gen Psychiatry 1982;39(4):473–81.
131. Chatterjee A, Chakos M, Koreen A, et al. Prevalence and clinical correlates of extrapyramidal signs and spontaneous dyskinesia in never-medicated schizophrenic patients. Am J Psychiatry 1995;152(12):1724–9.
132. Gervin M, Browne S, Lane A, et al. Spontaneous abnormal involuntary movements in first-episode schizophrenia and schizophreniform disorder: baseline rate in a group of patients from an Irish catchment area. Am J Psychiatry 1998;155(9):1202–6.
133. Puri BK, Barnes TR, Chapman MJ, et al. Spontaneous dyskinesia in first episode schizophrenia. J Neurol Neurosurg Psychiatr 1999;66(1):76–8.
134. McCreadie RG, Thara R, Kamath S, et al. Abnormal movements in never-medicated Indian patients with schizophrenia. Br J Psychiatry 1996;168(2):221–6.
135. Fenton WS, Blyler CR, Wyatt RJ, et al. Prevalence of spontaneous dyskinesia in schizophrenic and non-schizophrenic psychiatric patients. Br J Psychiatry 1997;171:265–8.
136. Bai YM, Chou KH, Lin CP, et al. White matter abnormalities in schizophrenia patients with tardive dyskinesia: a diffusion tensor image study. Schizophr Res 2009;109(1–3):167–81.
137. Zai CC, Tiwari AK, Basile V, et al. Association study of tardive dyskinesia and five DRD4 polymorphisms in schizophrenia patients. Pharmacogenomics J 2009;9(3):168–74.
138. Tenback DE, van Harten PN, Slooff CJ, et al. Evidence that early extrapyramidal symptoms predict later tardive dyskinesia: a prospective analysis of 10,000 patients in the European Schizophrenia Outpatient Health Outcomes (SOHO) study. Am J Psychiatry 2006;163(8):1438–40.
139. Emsley R, Turner HJ, Schronen J, et al. A single-blind, randomized trial comparing quetiapine and haloperidol in the treatment of tardive dyskinesia. J Clin Psychiatry 2004;65(5):696–701.
140. Kopala LC, Good KP, Milliken H, et al. Treatment of a first episode of psychotic illness with quetiapine: an analysis of 2 year outcomes. Schizophr Res 2006; 81(1):29–39.
141. Morgante L, Epifanio A, Spina E, et al. Quetiapine and clozapine in parkinsonian patients with dopaminergic psychosis. Clin Neuropharmacol 2004;27(4):153–6.
142. Morgante L, Epifanio A, Spina E, et al. Quetiapine versus clozapine: a preliminary report of comparative effects on dopaminergic psychosis in patients with Parkinson's disease. Neurol Sci 2002;23(Suppl 2):S89–90.
143. Manson AJ, Schrag A, Lees AJ. Low-dose olanzapine for levodopa induced dyskinesias. Neurology 2000;55(6):795–9.
144. Carlson CD, Cavazzoni PA, Berg PH, et al. An integrated analysis of acute treatment-emergent extrapyramidal syndrome in patients with schizophrenia during olanzapine clinical trials: comparisons with placebo, haloperidol, risperidone, or clozapine. J Clin Psychiatry 2003;64(8):898–906.
145. Schooler N, Rabinowitz J, Davidson M, et al. Risperidone and haloperidol in first-episode psychosis: a long-term randomized trial. Am J Psychiatry 2005; 162(5):947–53.
146. Trimble MR. The neurology of schizophrenia. Br Med Bull 1987;43(3):587–98.
147. Mittal VA, Hasenkamp W, Sanfilipo M, et al. Relation of neurological soft signs to psychiatric symptoms in schizophrenia. Schizophr Res 2007;94(1–3):37–44.
148. Browne S, Clarke M, Gervin M, et al. Determinants of neurological dysfunction in first episode schizophrenia. Psychol Med 2000;30(6):1433–41.

149. Schroder J, Niethammer R, Geider FJ, et al. Neurological soft signs in schizophrenia. Schizophr Res 1991;6(1):25–30.
150. Madsen AL, Vorstrup S, Rubin P, et al. Neurological abnormalities in schizophrenic patients: a prospective follow-up study 5 years after first admission. Acta Psychiatr Scand 1999;100(2):119–25.
151. Thomann PA, Wustenberg T, Santos VD, et al. Neurological soft signs and brain morphology in first-episode schizophrenia. Psychol Med 2009;39(3): 371–9.
152. Dazzan P, Murray RM. Neurological soft signs in first-episode psychosis: a systematic review. Br J Psychiatry Suppl 2002;43:s50–7.
153. Keshavan MS, Sanders RD, Sweeney JA, et al. Diagnostic specificity and neuroanatomical validity of neurological abnormalities in first-episode psychoses. Am J Psychiatry 2003;160(7):1298–304.
154. Kolakowska T, Williams AO, Jambor K, et al. Schizophrenia with good and poor outcome. III: neurological 'soft' signs, cognitive impairment and their clinical significance. Br J Psychiatry 1985;146:348–57.
155. Krebs MO, Mouchet S. Neurological soft signs and schizophrenia: a review of current knowledge. Rev Neurol (Paris) 2007;163(12):1157–68.
156. Biswas P, Malhotra S, Malhotra A, et al. Comparative study of neurological soft signs in schizophrenia with onset in childhood, adolescence and adulthood. Acta Psychiatr Scand 2007;115(4):295–303.
157. Prikryl R, Ceskova E, Kasparek T, et al. Neurological soft signs and their relationship to 1-year outcome in first-episode schizophrenia. Eur Psychiatry 2007; 22(8):499–504.
158. Manschreck TC, Ames D. Neurologic features and psychopathology in schizophrenic disorders. Biol Psychiatry 1984;19(5):703–19.
159. Bottmer C, Bachmann S, Pantel J, et al. Reduced cerebellar volume and neurological soft signs in first-episode schizophrenia. Psychiatry Res 2005;140(3): 239–50.
160. Holzman PS, Solomon CM, Levin S, et al. Pursuit eye movement dysfunctions in schizophrenia. Family evidence for specificity. Arch Gen Psychiatry 1984;41(2): 136–9.
161. Bachmann S, Bottmer C, Schroder J. Neurological soft signs in first-episode schizophrenia: a follow-up study. Am J Psychiatry 2005;162(12):2337–43.
162. Lawrie SM, Byrne M, Miller P, et al. Neurodevelopmental indices and the development of psychotic symptoms in subjects at high risk of schizophrenia. Br J Psychiatry 2001;178:524–30.
163. Ismail B, Cantor-Graae E, McNeil TF. Minor physical anomalies in schizophrenic patients and their siblings. Am J Psychiatry 1998;155(12):1695–702.
164. Niethammer R, Weisbrod M, Schiesser S, et al. Genetic influence on laterality in schizophrenia? A twin study of neurological soft signs. Am J Psychiatry 2000; 157(2):272–4.
165. Prasad KM, Sanders R, Sweeney J, et al. Neurological abnormalities among offspring of persons with schizophrenia: Relation to premorbid psychopathology. Schizophr Res 2009;108(1–3):163–9.
166. Chan RC, Gottesman II. Neurological soft signs as candidate endophenotypes for schizophrenia: a shooting star or a Northern star? Neurosci Biobehav Rev 2008;32(5):957–71.
167. Schroder J, Essig M, Baudendistel K, et al. Motor dysfunction and sensorimotor cortex activation changes in schizophrenia: a study with functional magnetic resonance imaging. Neuroimage 1999;9(1):81–7.

168. Andreasen NC, O'Leary DS, Cizadlo T, et al. Schizophrenia and cognitive dysmetria: a positron-emission tomography study of dysfunctional prefrontal-thalamic-cerebellar circuitry. Proc Natl Acad Sci U S A 1996; 93(18):9985–90.
169. Boks MP, Liddle PF, Burgerhof JG, et al. Neurological soft signs discriminating mood disorders from first episode schizophrenia. Acta Psychiatr Scand 2004; 110(1):29–35.
170. Kinney DK, Yurgelun-Todd DA, Woods BT. Hard neurologic signs and psychopathology in relatives of schizophrenic patients. Psychiatry Res 1991;39(1): 45–53.
171. Griffiths TD, Sigmundsson T, Takei N, et al. Neurological abnormalities in familial and sporadic schizophrenia. Brain 1998;121(Pt 2):191–203.
172. Torrey EF. Neurological abnormalities in schizophrenic patients. Biol Psychiatry 1980;15(3):381–8.
173. Schroder J, Buchsbaum MS, Siegel BV, et al. Structural and functional correlates of subsyndromes in chronic schizophrenia. Psychopathology 1995;28(1): 38–45.
174. Nasrallah HA, Tippin J, McCalley-Whitters M, et al. Neurological differences between paranoid and nonparanoid schizophrenia: part III. neurological soft signs. J Clin Psychiatry 1982;43(8):310–2.
175. Gureje O. Neurological soft signs in Nigerian schizophrenics: a controlled study. Acta Psychiatr Scand 1988;78(4):505–9.
176. Nasrallah H, Lyskowski J, Shroeder D. Tricyclic-induced mania: differences between switchers and non-switchers. Biol Psychiatry 1982;17:271–4.
177. Schroder J, Geider FJ, Binkert M, et al. Subsyndromes in chronic schizophrenia: do their psychopathological characteristics correspond to cerebral alterations? Psychiatry Res 1992;42(3):209–20.
178. Schroder J, Buchsbaum MS, Siegel BV, et al. Cerebral metabolic activity correlates of subsyndromes in chronic schizophrenia. Schizophr Res 1996;19(1): 41–53.
179. Schroder J, Silvestri S, Bubeck B, et al. D2 dopamine receptor up-regulation, treatment response, neurological soft signs, and extrapyramidal side effects in schizophrenia: a follow-up study with ^{123}I-iodobenzamide single photon emission computed tomography in the drug-naïve state and after neuroleptic treatment. Biol Psychiatry 1998;43(9):660–5.
180. Stevens JR. An anatomy of schizophrenia? Arch Gen Psychiatry 1973;29(2): 177–89.
181. Slaghuis WL, Hawkes A, Holthouse T, et al. Eye movement and visual motion perception in schizophrenia I: apparent motion evoked smooth pursuit eye movement reveals a hidden dysfunction in smooth pursuit eye movement in schizophrenia. Exp Brain Res 2007;182(3):399–413.
182. Slaghuis WL, Holthouse T, Hawkes A, et al. Eye movement and visual motion perception in schizophrenia II: global coherent motion as a function of target velocity and stimulus density. Exp Brain Res 2007;182(3):415–26.
183. Kallimani D, Theleritis C, Evdokimidis I, et al. The effect of change in clinical state on eye movement dysfunction in schizophrenia. Eur Psychiatry 2009; 24(1):17–26.
184. Suzuki M, Takahashi S, Matsushima E, et al. Exploratory eye movement dysfunction as a discriminator for schizophrenia: a large sample study using a newly developed digital computerized system. Eur Arch Psychiatry Clin Neurosci 2009;259(3):186–94.

185. Takahashi S, Tanabe E, Yara K, et al. Impairment of exploratory eye movement in schizophrenia patients and their siblings. Psychiatry Clin Neurosci 2008;62(5): 487–93.
186. Takahashi S, Tanabe E, Sakai T, et al. Relationship between exploratory eye movement, P300, and reaction time in schizophrenia. Psychiatry Clin Neurosci 2008;62(4):396–403.
187. Calkins ME, Iacono WG, Ones DS. Eye movement dysfunction in first-degree relatives of patients with schizophrenia: a meta-analytic evaluation of candidate endophenotypes. Brain Cogn 2008;68(3):436–61.
188. Barch DM, Carter CS, Braver TS, et al. Selective deficits in prefrontal cortex function in medication-naïve patients with schizophrenia. Arch Gen Psychiatry 2001;58(3):280–8.
189. Egan MF, Goldberg TE, Kolachana BS, et al. Effect of COMT Val108/158 Met genotype on frontal lobe function and risk for schizophrenia. Proc Natl Acad Sci U S A 2001;98(12):6917–22.
190. Goldberg TE, Egan MF, Gscheidle T, et al. Executive subprocesses in working memory: relationship to catechol-O-methyltransferase Val158Met genotype and schizophrenia. Arch Gen Psychiatry 2003;60(9):889–96.
191. Perlstein WM, Carter CS, Noll DC, et al. Relation of prefrontal cortex dysfunction to working memory and symptoms in schizophrenia. Am J Psychiatry 2001; 158(7):1105–13.
192. Quintana J, Wong T, Ortiz-Portillo E, et al. Prefrontal-posterior parietal networks in schizophrenia: primary dysfunctions and secondary compensations. Biol Psychiatry 2003;53(1):12–24.
193. Weinberger DR, Egan MF, Bertolino A, et al. Prefrontal neurons and the genetics of schizophrenia. Biol Psychiatry 2001;50(11):825–44.
194. Potkin SG, Alva G, Fleming K, et al. A PET study of the pathophysiology of negative symptoms in schizophrenia. Positron emission tomography. Am J Psychiatry 2002;159(2):227–37.
195. Pennington K, Beasley CL, Dicker P, et al. Prominent synaptic and metabolic abnormalities revealed by proteomic analysis of the dorsolateral prefrontal cortex in schizophrenia and bipolar disorder. Mol Psychiatry 2008;13(12): 1102–17.
196. Smesny S, Rosburg T, Nenadic I, et al. Metabolic mapping using 2D 31P-MR spectroscopy reveals frontal and thalamic metabolic abnormalities in schizophrenia. Neuroimage 2007;35(2):729–37.
197. Glahn DC, Ragland JD, Abramoff A, et al. Beyond hypofrontality: a quantitative meta-analysis of functional neuroimaging studies of working memory in schizophrenia. Hum Brain Mapp 2005;25(1):60–9.
198. Schirmer TN, Dorflinger JM, Marlow-O'Connor M, et al. FMRI indices of auditory attention in schizophrenia. Prog Neuropsychopharmacol Biol Psychiatry 2009; 33(1):25–32.
199. Hyde TM, Weinberger DR. Seizures and schizophrenia. Schizophr Bull 1997; 23(4):611–22.
200. Marsh L, Rao V. Psychiatric complications in patients with epilepsy: a review. Epilepsy Res 2002;49(1):11–33.
201. Adachi N, Onuma T, Nishiwaki S, et al. Inter-ictal and post-ictal psychoses in frontal lobe epilepsy: a retrospective comparison with psychoses in temporal lobe epilepsy. Seizure 2000;9(5):328–35.
202. Makikyro T, Karvonen JT, Hakko H, et al. Comorbidity of hospital-treated psychiatric and physical disorders with special reference to schizophrenia: a 28 year

follow-up of the 1966 northern Finland general population birth cohort. Public Health 1998;112(4):221–8.
203. Cascella NG, Schretlen DJ, Sawa A. Schizophrenia and epilepsy: is there a shared susceptibility? Neurosci Res 2009;63(4):227–35.
204. Qin P, Xu H, Laursen TM, et al. Risk for schizophrenia and schizophrenia-like psychosis among patients with epilepsy: population based cohort study. BMJ 2005;331(7507):23.
205. Manchanda R, Freeland A, Schaefer B, et al. Auras, seizure focus, and psychiatric disorders. Neuropsychiatry Neuropsychol Behav Neurol 2000;13(1):13–9.
206. Adachi N, Hara T, Oana Y, et al. Difference in age of onset of psychosis between epilepsy and schizophrenia. Epilepsy Res 2008;78(2–3):201–6.
207. Tebartz Van Elst L, Baeumer D, Lemieux L, et al. Amygdala pathology in psychosis of epilepsy: a magnetic resonance imaging study in patients with temporal lobe epilepsy. Brain 2002;125(Pt 1):140–9.
208. Heath RG. Common characteristics of epilepsy and schizophrenia: clinical observation and depth electrode studies. 1961. Epilepsy Behav 2005;6(4): 633–45.
209. Petersen MC, Bickford G, Sem-Jacobsen CW, et al. The depth electrogram in schizophrenic patients. Proc Staff Meet Mayo Clin 1953;28(6):170–5.
210. Bob P, Palus M, Susta M, et al. EEG phase synchronization in patients with paranoid schizophrenia. Neurosci Lett 2008;447(1):73–7.
211. Lauer CJ, Krieg JC. Slow-wave sleep and ventricular size: a comparative study in schizophrenia and major depression. Biol Psychiatry 1998;44(2):121–8.
212. Lauer CJ, Schreiber W, Pollmacher T, et al. Sleep in schizophrenia: a polysomnographic study on drug-naïve patients. Neuropsychopharmacology 1997;16(1): 51–60.
213. Yang C, Winkelman JW. Clinical significance of sleep EEG abnormalities in chronic schizophrenia. Schizophr Res 2006;82(2–3):251–60.
214. Higashima M, Takeda T, Kikuchi M, et al. State-dependent changes in intrahemispheric EEG coherence for patients with acute exacerbation of schizophrenia. Psychiatry Res 2007;149(1–3):41–7.
215. Begre S, Federspiel A, Kiefer C, et al. Reduced hippocampal anisotropy related to anteriorization of alpha EEG in schizophrenia. Neuroreport 2003;14(5): 739–42.
216. Lehmann D, Faber PL, Galderisi S, et al. EEG microstate duration and syntax in acute, medication-naïve, first-episode schizophrenia: a multi-center study. Psychiatry Res 2005;138(2):141–56.
217. Koenig T, Lehmann D, Merlo MC, et al. A deviant EEG brain microstate in acute, neuroleptic-naïve schizophrenics at rest. Eur Arch Psychiatry Clin Neurosci 1999;249(4):205–11.
218. Boutros NN, Arfken C, Galderisi S, et al. The status of spectral EEG abnormality as a diagnostic test for schizophrenia. Schizophr Res 2008;99(1–3):225–37.
219. Koenig T, Lehmann D, Saito N, et al. Decreased functional connectivity of EEG theta-frequency activity in first-episode, neuroleptic-naïve patients with schizophrenia: preliminary results. Schizophr Res 2001;50(1–2):55–60.
220. Boutros NN, Torello MW, Barker BA, et al. The P50 evoked potential component and mismatch detection in normal volunteers: implications for the study of sensory gating. Psychiatry Res 1995;57(1):83–8.
221. Patterson JV, Hetrick WP, Boutros NN, et al. P50 sensory gating ratios in schizophrenics and controls: a review and data analysis. Psychiatry Res 2008;158(2): 226–47.

222. Kawasaki Y, Sumiyoshi T, Higuchi Y, et al. Voxel-based analysis of P300 electrophysiological topography associated with positive and negative symptoms of schizophrenia. Schizophr Res 2007;94(1–3):164–71.
223. Ozgurdal S, Gudlowski Y, Witthaus H, et al. Reduction of auditory event-related P300 amplitude in subjects with at-risk mental state for schizophrenia. Schizophr Res 2008;105(1–3):272–8.
224. Gonul AS, Suer C, Coburn K, et al. Effects of olanzapine on auditory P300 in schizophrenia. Prog Neuropsychopharmacol Biol Psychiatry 2003;27(1):173–7.
225. Turetsky BI, Moberg PJ, Mozley LH, et al. Memory-delineated subtypes of schizophrenia: relationship to clinical, neuroanatomical, and neurophysiological measures. Neuropsychology 2002;16(4):481–90.
226. Boutros N, Nasrallah H, Leighty R, et al. Auditory evoked potentials, clinical vs. research applications. Psychiatry Res 1997;69(2–3):183–95.
227. Jeon YW, Polich J. P300 asymmetry in schizophrenia: a meta-analysis. Psychiatry Res 2001;104(1):61–74.
228. de Wilde OM, Bour LJ, Dingemans PM, et al. P300 deficits are present in young first-episode patients with schizophrenia and not in their healthy young siblings. Clin Neurophysiol 2008;119(12):2721–6.
229. Shin KS, Kang DH, Choi JS, et al. Neuropsychological correlates of N400 anomalies in patients with schizophrenia: a preliminary report. Neurosci Lett 2008; 448(2):226–30.
230. Potvin S, Stip E, Tempier A, et al. Pain perception in schizophrenia: no changes in diffuse noxious inhibitory controls (DNIC) but a lack of pain sensitization. J Psychiatr Res 2008;42(12):1010–6.
231. Singh MK, Giles LL, Nasrallah HA. Pain insensitivity in schizophrenia: trait or state marker? J Psychiatr Pract 2006;12(2):90–102.
232. Fishbain DA. Pain insensitivity in psychosis. Ann Emerg Med 1982;11(11): 630–2.
233. Guieu R, Samuelian JC, Coulouvrat H. Objective evaluation of pain perception in patients with schizophrenia. Br J Psychiatry 1994;164(2):253–5.
234. Bender L, Schilder P. Unconditioned and conditioned reactions to pain in schizophrenia. Am J Psychiatry 1930;10:365–84.
235. Haslam J. Observations on insanity: with practical remarks on the disease. London: F. and C. Rivington; 1798.
236. Esquirol JE. Des maladies mentales. Paris: Bailliere; 1838.
237. Lieberman AL. Painless myocardial infarction in psychotic patients. Geriatrics 1955;10(12):579–80.
238. Marchand WE. Occurrence of painless myocardial infarction in psychotic patients. N Engl J Med 1955;253(2):51–5.
239. Marchand WE, Sarota B, Marble HC, et al. Occurrence of painless acute surgical disorders in psychotic patients. N Engl J Med 1959;260(12):580–5.
240. Tyler M. Somatic symptoms in schizophrenia. Schizophr Res 1995;18(1):87–8.
241. Dworkin RH. Pain insensitivity in schizophrenia: a neglected phenomenon and some implications. Schizophr Bull 1994;20(2):235–48.
242. Bonnot O, Tordjman S. Schizophrenia and pain reactivity. Presse Med 2008; 37(11):1561–8.
243. Jochum T, Letzsch A, Greiner W, et al. Influence of antipsychotic medication on pain perception in schizophrenia. Psychiatry Res 2006;142(2–3):151–6.
244. Mohamed S, Rosenheck R, Swartz M, et al. Relationship of cognition and psychopathology to functional impairment in schizophrenia. Am J Psychiatry 2008;165(8):978–87.

245. Reichenberg A, Harvey PD, Bowie CR, et al. Neuropsychological function and dysfunction in schizophrenia and psychotic affective disorders. Schizophr Bull 2008;35(5):1022–9.
246. Keefe RS, Fenton WS. How should DSM-V criteria for schizophrenia include cognitive impairment? Schizophr Bull 2007;33(4):912–20.
247. Heinrichs RW, Ammari N, Miles A, et al. Psychopathology and cognition in divergent functional outcomes in schizophrenia. Schizophr Res 2009;109(1–3):46–51.
248. Frangou S, Hadjulis M, Vourdas A. The Maudsley early onset schizophrenia study: cognitive function over a 4-year follow-up period. Schizophr Bull 2008; 34(1):52–9.
249. Waddington JL, Youssef HA. Cognitive dysfunction in chronic schizophrenia followed prospectively over 10 years and its longitudinal relationship to the emergence of tardive dyskinesia. Psychol Med 1996;26(4):681–8.
250. Szoke A, Trandafir A, Dupont ME, et al. Longitudinal studies of cognition in schizophrenia: meta-analysis. Br J Psychiatry 2008;192(4):248–57.
251. Riley EM, McGovern D, Mockler D, et al. Neuropsychological functioning in first-episode psychosis—evidence of specific deficits. Schizophr Res 2000;43(1): 47–55.
252. Reichenberg A, Harvey PD. Neuropsychological impairments in schizophrenia: integration of performance-based and brain imaging findings. Psychol Bull 2007;133(5):833–58.
253. Yoon JH, Minzenberg MJ, Ursu S, et al. Association of dorsolateral prefrontal cortex dysfunction with disrupted coordinated brain activity in schizophrenia: relationship with impaired cognition, behavioral disorganization, and global function. Am J Psychiatry 2008;165(8):1006–14.
254. Maccabe JH. Population-based cohort studies on premorbid cognitive function in schizophrenia. Epidemiol Rev 2008;30:77–83.
255. Kuperberg G, Heckers S. Schizophrenia and cognitive function. Curr Opin Neurobiol 2000;10(2):205–10.
256. Lussier I, Stip E. Memory and attention deficits in drug naïve patients with schizophrenia. Schizophr Res 2001;48(1):45–55.
257. Goldberg TE, Goldman RS, Burdick KE, et al. Cognitive improvement after treatment with second-generation antipsychotic medications in first-episode schizophrenia: is it a practice effect? Arch Gen Psychiatry 2007;64(10):1115–22.
258. Saykin AJ, Shtasel DL, Gur RE, et al. Neuropsychological deficits in neuroleptic naïve patients with first-episode schizophrenia. Arch Gen Psychiatry 1994;51(2): 124–31.
259. Bilder RM, Goldman RS, Volavka J, et al. Neurocognitive effects of clozapine, olanzapine, risperidone, and haloperidol in patients with chronic schizophrenia or schizoaffective disorder. Am J Psychiatry 2002;159(6):1018–28.
260. Holmen A, Juuhl-Langseth M, Thormodsen R, et al. Neuropsychological profile in early-onset schizophrenia-spectrum disorders: measured with the MATRICS battery. Schizophr Bull 2009;17 [Epub ahead of print]
261. Woodberry KA, Giuliano AJ, Seidman LJ. Premorbid IQ in schizophrenia: a meta-analytic review. Am J Psychiatry 2008;165(5):579–87.
262. Leeson VC, Barnes TR, Hutton SB, et al. IQ as a predictor of functional outcome in schizophrenia: a longitudinal, four-year study of first-episode psychosis. Schizophr Res 2009;107(1):55–60.
263. Ma X, Wang Q, Sham PC, et al. Neurocognitive deficits in first-episode schizophrenic patients and their first-degree relatives. Am J Med Genet B Neuropsychiatr Genet 2007;144(4):407–16.

264. Tan HY, Chen Q, Goldberg TE, et al. Catechol-O-methyltransferase Val158Met modulation of prefrontal-parietal-striatal brain systems during arithmetic and temporal transformations in working memory. J Neurosci 2007;27(49):13393–401.
265. Tan HY, Chen Q, Sust S, et al. Epistasis between catechol-O-methyltransferase and type II metabotropic glutamate receptor 3 genes on working memory brain function. Proc Natl Acad Sci U S A 2007;104(30):12536–41.
266. Censits DM, Ragland JD, Gur RC, et al. Neuropsychological evidence supporting a neurodevelopmental model of schizophrenia: a longitudinal study. Schizophr Res 1997;24(3):289–98.
267. Schuepbach D, Keshavan MS, Kmiec JA, et al. Negative symptom resolution and improvements in specific cognitive deficits after acute treatment in first-episode schizophrenia. Schizophr Res 2002;53(3):249–61.
268. Snyder PJ, Jackson CE, Piskulic D, et al. Spatial working memory and problem solving in schizophrenia: the effect of symptom stabilization with atypical antipsychotic medication. Psychiatry Res 2008;160(3):316–26.
269. Hartman M, Steketee MC, Silva S, et al. Working memory and schizophrenia: evidence for slowed encoding. Schizophr Res 2003;59(2–3):99–113.
270. Honey GD, Bullmore ET, Sharma T. De-coupling of cognitive performance and cerebral functional response during working memory in schizophrenia. Schizophr Res 2002;53(1–2):45–56.
271. Okada A. Deficits of spatial working memory in chronic schizophrenia. Schizophr Res 2002;53(1–2):75–82.
272. Tek C, Gold J, Blaxton T, et al. Visual perceptual and working memory impairments in schizophrenia. Arch Gen Psychiatry 2002;59(2):146–53.
273. Spindler KA, Sullivan EV, Menon V, et al. Deficits in multiple systems of working memory in schizophrenia. Schizophr Res 1997;27(1):1–10.
274. Zilles D, Burke S, Schneider-Axmann T, et al. Diagnosis-specific effect of familial loading on verbal working memory in schizophrenia. Eur Arch Psychiatry Clin Neurosci 2009;259(6):309–15.
275. Pae CU, Juh R, Yoo SS, et al. Verbal working memory dysfunction in schizophrenia: an FMRI investigation. Int J Neurosci 2008;118(10):1467–87.
276. Potkin SG, Turner JA, Brown GG, et al. Working memory and DLPFC inefficiency in schizophrenia: the FBIRN study. Schizophr Bull 2009;35(1):19–31.
277. Driesen NR, Leung HC, Calhoun VD, et al. Impairment of working memory maintenance and response in schizophrenia: functional magnetic resonance imaging evidence. Biol Psychiatry 2008;64(12):1026–34.
278. Forbes NF, Carrick LA, McIntosh AM, et al. Working memory in schizophrenia: a meta-analysis. Psychol Med 2009;39(6):889–905.
279. Zanello A, Curtis L, Badan Ba M, et al. Working memory impairments in first-episode psychosis and chronic schizophrenia. Psychiatry Res 2009;165(1–2):10–8.
280. Kebir O, Tabbane K. Working memory in schizophrenia: a review. Encephale 2008;34(3):289–98.
281. Meda SA, Bhattarai M, Morris NA, et al. An fMRI study of working memory in first-degree unaffected relatives of schizophrenia patients. Schizophr Res 2008;104(1–3):85–95.
282. Fuller RL, Luck SJ, Braun EL, et al. Impaired visual working memory consolidation in schizophrenia. Neuropsychology 2009;23(1):71–80.
283. Calkins ME, Gur RC, Ragland JD, et al. Face recognition memory deficits and visual object memory performance in patients with schizophrenia and their relatives. Am J Psychiatry 2005;162(10):1963–6.

284. Weiss AP, Schacter DL, Goff DC, et al. Impaired hippocampal recruitment during normal modulation of memory performance in schizophrenia. Biol Psychiatry 2003;53(1):48–55.
285. Snitz BE, Macdonald AW 3rd, Carter CS. Cognitive deficits in unaffected first-degree relatives of schizophrenia patients: a meta-analytic review of putative endophenotypes. Schizophr Bull 2006;32(1):179–94.
286. Skelley SL, Goldberg TE, Egan MF, et al. Verbal and visual memory: characterizing the clinical and intermediate phenotype in schizophrenia. Schizophr Res 2008;105(1–3):78–85.
287. Landro NI, Ueland T. Verbal memory and verbal fluency in adolescents with schizophrenia spectrum disorders. Psychiatry Clin Neurosci 2008;62(6):653–61.
288. Manschreck TC, Maher BA, Candela SF, et al. Impaired verbal memory is associated with impaired motor performance in schizophrenia: relationship to brain structure. Schizophr Res 2000;43(1):21–32.
289. Elvevag B, Weinberger DR, Goldberg TE. The phonological similarity effect in short-term memory serial recall in schizophrenia. Psychiatry Res 2002;112(1):77–81.
290. Gabrovska VS, Laws KR, Sinclair J, et al. Visual object processing in schizophrenia: evidence for an associative agnosic deficit. Schizophr Res 2003;59(2–3):277–86.
291. Perry W, Light GA, Davis H, et al. Schizophrenia patients demonstrate a dissociation on declarative and non-declarative memory tests. Schizophr Res 2000;46(2–3):167–74.
292. Ungvari GS, Xiang YT, Tang WK, et al. Prospective memory and its correlates and predictors in schizophrenia: an extension of previous findings. Arch Clin Neuropsychol 2008;23(5):613–22.
293. Wang Y, Chan RC, Hong X, et al. Prospective memory in schizophrenia: further clarification of nature of impairment. Schizophr Res 2008;105(1–3):114–24.
294. Ranganath C, Minzenberg MJ, Ragland JD. The cognitive neuroscience of memory function and dysfunction in schizophrenia. Biol Psychiatry 2008;64(1):18–25.
295. Kuperberg GR, West WC, Lakshmanan BM, et al. Functional magnetic resonance imaging reveals neuroanatomical dissociations during semantic integration in schizophrenia. Biol Psychiatry 2008;64(5):407–18.
296. Razafimandimby A, Maiza O, Herve PY, et al. Stability of functional language lateralization over time in schizophrenia patients. Schizophr Res 2007;94(1–3):197–206.
297. Nicolson R, Lenane M, Singaracharlu S, et al. Premorbid speech and language impairments in childhood-onset schizophrenia: association with risk factors. Am J Psychiatry 2000;157(5):794–800.
298. Jones P, Rodgers B, Murray R, et al. Child development risk factors for adult schizophrenia in the British 1946 birth cohort. Lancet 1994;344(8934):1398–402.
299. Done DJ, Crow TJ, Johnstone EC, et al. Childhood antecedents of schizophrenia and affective illness: social adjustment at ages 7 and 11. BMJ 1994;309(6956):699–703.
300. Marini A, Spoletini I, Rubino IA, et al. The language of schizophrenia: an analysis of micro and macrolinguistic abilities and their neuropsychological correlates. Schizophr Res 2008;105(1–3):144–55.
301. Elvevag B, Weinstock DM, Akil M, et al. A comparison of verbal fluency tasks in schizophrenic patients and normal controls. Schizophr Res 2001;51(2–3):119–26.

302. Doughty OJ, Done DJ, Lawrence VA, et al. Semantic memory impairment in schizophrenia—deficit in storage or access of knowledge? Schizophr Res 2008;105(1–3):40–8.
303. Li X, Branch CA, Bertisch HC, et al. An fMRI study of language processing in people at high genetic risk for schizophrenia. Schizophr Res 2007;91(1–3):62–72.
304. Harris JG, Minassian A, Perry W. Stability of attention deficits in schizophrenia. Schizophr Res 2007;91(1–3):107–11.
305. Liu SK, Chiu CH, Chang CJ, et al. Deficits in sustained attention in schizophrenia and affective disorders: stable versus state-dependent markers. Am J Psychiatry 2002;159(6):975–82.
306. Birkett P, Sigmundsson T, Sharma T, et al. Reaction time and sustained attention in schizophrenia and its genetic predisposition. Schizophr Res 2007;95(1–3):76–85.
307. Tsuang HC, Lin SH, Liu SK, et al. More severe sustained attention deficits in nonpsychotic siblings of multiplex schizophrenia families than in those of simplex ones. Schizophr Res 2006;87(1–3):172–80.
308. Luck SJ, Gold JM. The construct of attention in schizophrenia. Biol Psychiatry 2008;64(1):34–9.
309. Fuller RL, Luck SJ, Braun EL, et al. Impaired control of visual attention in schizophrenia. J Abnorm Psychol 2006;115(2):266–75.
310. Gur RE, Turetsky BI, Loughead J, et al. Visual attention circuitry in schizophrenia investigated with oddball event-related functional magnetic resonance imaging. Am J Psychiatry 2007;164(3):442–9.
311. O'Grada C, Barry S, McGlade N, et al. Does the ability to sustain attention underlie symptom severity in schizophrenia? Schizophr Res 2009;107(2–3):319–23.
312. Kerns JG, Nuechterlein KH, Braver TS, et al. Executive functioning component mechanisms and schizophrenia. Biol Psychiatry 2008;64(1):26–33.
313. Rusch N, Spoletini I, Wilke M, et al. Prefrontal-thalamic-cerebellar gray matter networks and executive functioning in schizophrenia. Schizophr Res 2007;93(1–3):79–89.
314. Szeszko PR, Strous RD, Goldman RS, et al. Neuropsychological correlates of hippocampal volumes in patients experiencing a first episode of schizophrenia. Am J Psychiatry 2002;159(2):217–26.
315. Mortimer AM. Cognitive function in schizophrenia—do neuroleptics make a difference? Pharmacol Biochem Behav 1997;56(4):789–95.
316. Heinrichs RW, Zakzanis KK. Neurocognitive deficit in schizophrenia: a quantitative review of the evidence. Neuropsychology 1998;12(3):426–45.
317. Cuesta MJ, Peralta V, Zarzuela A. Effects of olanzapine and other antipsychotics on cognitive function in chronic schizophrenia: a longitudinal study. Schizophr Res 2001;48(1):17–28.
318. Pallanti S, Quercioli L, Pazzagli A. Effects of clozapine on awareness of illness and cognition in schizophrenia. Psychiatry Res 1999;86(3):239–49.
319. Purdon SE, Jones BD, Stip E, et al. Neuropsychological change in early phase schizophrenia during 12 months of treatment with olanzapine, risperidone, or haloperidol. The Canadian Collaborative Group for research in schizophrenia. Arch Gen Psychiatry 2000;57(3):249–58.
320. Purdon SE, Malla A, Labelle A, et al. Neuropsychological change in patients with schizophrenia after treatment with quetiapine or haloperidol. J Psychiatry Neurosci 2001;26(2):137–49.

321. Smith RC, Infante M, Singh A, et al. The effects of olanzapine on neurocognitive functioning in medication-refractory schizophrenia. Int J Neuropsychopharmacol 2001;4(3):239–50.
322. Velligan DI, Newcomer J, Pultz J, et al. Does cognitive function improve with quetiapine in comparison to haloperidol? Schizophr Res 2002;53(3):239–48.
323. Velligan DI, Prihoda TJ, Sui D, et al. The effectiveness of quetiapine versus conventional antipsychotics in improving cognitive and functional outcomes in standard treatment settings. J Clin Psychiatry 2003;64(5):524–31.
324. Woodward ND, Purdon SE, Meltzer HY, et al. A meta-analysis of neuropsychological change to clozapine, olanzapine, quetiapine, and risperidone in schizophrenia. Int J Neuropsychopharmacol 2005;8(3):457–72.
325. Keefe RS, Silva SG, Perkins DO, et al. The effects of atypical antipsychotic drugs on neurocognitive impairment in schizophrenia: a review and meta-analysis. Schizophr Bull 1999;25(2):201–22.
326. Davidson M, Galderisi S, Weiser M, et al. Cognitive effects of antipsychotic drugs in first-episode schizophrenia and schizophreniform disorder: a randomized, open-label clinical trial (EUFEST). Am J Psychiatry 2009;166(6):675–82.
327. Gallhofer B, Jaanson P, Mittoux A, et al. Course of recovery of cognitive impairment in patients with schizophrenia: a randomised double-blind study comparing sertindole and haloperidol. Pharmacopsychiatry 2007;40(6):275–86.
328. Houthoofd SA, Morrens M, Sabbe BG. Cognitive and psychomotor effects of risperidone in schizophrenia and schizoaffective disorder. Clin Ther 2008;30(9):1565–89.
329. Good KP, Kiss I, Buiteman C, et al. Improvement in cognitive functioning in patients with first-episode psychosis during treatment with quetiapine: an interim analysis. Br J Psychiatry Suppl 2002;43:s45–9.
330. Harvey PD, Sacchetti E, Galluzzo A, et al. A randomized double-blind comparison of ziprasidone vs. clozapine for cognition in patients with schizophrenia selected for resistance or intolerance to previous treatment. Schizophr Res 2008;105(1–3):138–43.
331. Mohamed S, Paulsen JS, O'Leary D, et al. Generalized cognitive deficits in schizophrenia: a study of first-episode patients. Arch Gen Psychiatry 1999;56(8):749–54.
332. Galletly C. Recent advances in treating cognitive impairment in schizophrenia. Psychopharmacology (Berl) 2009;202(1–3):259–73.
333. Remillard S, Pourcher E, Cohen H. Long-term effects of risperidone versus haloperidol on verbal memory, attention, and symptomatology in schizophrenia. J Int Neuropsychol Soc 2008;14(1):110–8.
334. Akdede BB, Anil Yagcioglu AE, Alptekin K, et al. A double-blind study of combination of clozapine with risperidone in patients with schizophrenia: effects on cognition. J Clin Psychiatry 2006;67(12):1912–9.
335. Elie D, Poirier M, Chianetta J, et al. Cognitive effects of antipsychotic dosage and polypharmacy: a study with the BACS in patients with schizophrenia and schizoaffective disorder. J Psychopharmacol 2009;22 [Epub ahead of print].
336. Buchanan RW, Freedman R, Javitt DC, et al. Recent advances in the development of novel pharmacological agents for the treatment of cognitive impairments in schizophrenia. Schizophr Bull 2007;33(5):1120–30.
337. Barr RS, Culhane MA, Jubelt LE, et al. The effects of transdermal nicotine on cognition in nonsmokers with schizophrenia and nonpsychiatric controls. Neuropsychopharmacology 2008;33(3):480–90.

338. Harvey PD, Cornblatt BA. Pharmacological treatment of cognition in schizophrenia: an idea whose method has come. Am J Psychiatry 2008;165(2):163–5.
339. Nuechterlein KH, Green MF, Kern RS, et al. The MATRICS consensus cognitive battery, part 1: test selection, reliability, and validity. Am J Psychiatry 2008;165(2):203–13.
340. Sergi MJ, Rassovsky Y, Widmark C, et al. Social cognition in schizophrenia: relationships with neurocognition and negative symptoms. Schizophr Res 2007;90(1–3):316–24.
341. Sergi MJ, Rassovsky Y, Nuechterlein KH, et al. Social perception as a mediator of the influence of early visual processing on functional status in schizophrenia. Am J Psychiatry 2006;163(3):448–54.

Management of Schizophrenia with Medical Disorders: Cardiovascular, Pulmonary, and Gastrointestinal

Delmar D. Short, MD[a,b,*], Joanne M. Hawley, PharmD[a,c], Maureen F. McCarthy, MD[a,d]

KEYWORDS

• Atypical antipsychotic • QT prolongation • Anticholinergic

Medical illnesses are particularly common in patients who have schizophrenia and pose challenges for the treatment of these patients in our health care systems, specifically in choosing the most appropriate antipsychotic medications. Patients who have schizophrenia have up to a 20% shorter life span than the general population, with the leading cause of death being cardiovascular disease.[1] A recent review[2] noted that there may be a 15-year decrease in life expectancy in patients who have schizophrenia compared with the general population. Patients who have schizophrenia have increased prevalence of the metabolic syndrome, which includes obesity, insulin resistance, diabetes, dyslipidemia, and hypertension (discussed in another article of this publication). The higher rates of morbidity and mortality in patients who have schizophrenia result in significant problems for these individuals and a high socioeconomic cost.[3] Patients who have schizophrenia also face barriers to receiving prompt and appropriate medical health care.[3] These barriers include difficulties in negotiating

[a] Mental Health Service Line (116A), Department of Veterans Affairs Medical Center, 1970 Roanoke Boulevard, Salem, VA 24153, USA
[b] Department of Psychiatry, Virginia Tech Carilion School of Medicine, PO Box 13727, Roanoke, VA 24036, USA
[c] Edward C Via Virginia College of Osteopathic Medicine, 2265 Kraft Drive, Blacksburg, VA 24060
[d] Department of Psychiatric Medicine, University of Virginia School of Medicine, PO Box 800623, Charlottesville, VA 22908, USA
* Corresponding author. Mental Health Service Line (116A), Department of Veterans Affairs Medical Center, 1970 Roanoke Boulevard, Salem, VA 24153.
E-mail address: Delmar.Short@va.gov (D.D. Short).

Psychiatr Clin N Am 32 (2009) 759–773
doi:10.1016/j.psc.2009.09.005
0193-953X/09/$ – see front matter. Published by Elsevier Inc.

the health care system. Also, primary care doctors often do not have sufficient time to deal with their multiple complex issues and communication problems.

According to Newcomer,[1] "Considerable evidence indicates that mentally ill patients often do not receive adequate recognition of, monitoring of, or care for their medical illnesses." He continues to note that there is a critical need for psychiatrists and primary care professionals to increase their awareness of the physical health problems of persons who have mental illness, especially as it relates to metabolic adverse events associated with psychiatric medications (discussed elsewhere in this publication). Kane and colleagues[4] did a survey that included 60 questions with 994 options to an expert panel. These experts stressed the importance of monitoring for health problems, especially obesity, diabetes, cardiovascular problems, HIV risk behaviors, medical complications of substance abuse, heavy smoking and its effects, hypertension, and amenorrhea in patients being treated with antipsychotics. This problem needs increased attention by psychiatrists and primary care professionals. Establishment of comprehensive programs of care that can address this need is recommended.[3]

Because the authors have had a major focus in affiliation with University of Virginia at the Salem VA Medical Center, and some of our psychiatrists have also been trained in internal medicine, they developed a primary care psychiatry clinic in 1996. This clinic was under the supervision of double-boarded psychiatrists, with residents in the authors' general psychiatry and medicine-psychiatry residencies seeing patients under supervision. The authors showed a significant cost savings as a result of this model primarily because of decreased costs of subsequent inpatient psychiatric care.[5] This differs from a major current focus in the VA at this time in having consultative-collaborative sorts of models or co-located models of mental health in primary care. That model addresses a larger population of patients who have less severe mental illnesses that are able to access care for their medical illnesses through primary care clinics. Although this is also an important issue, it is not the focus of this article.

The prevalence of diabetes (discussed elsewhere in this publication), lung disease, and liver problems are particularly increased[6] in patients who have serious mental illness. The odds of having respiratory illnesses are also increased in seriously mentally ill patient groups, even after controlling for smoking.[6] Patients who have schizophrenia and other mental illnesses have several risk factors that are preventable, including smoking, high alcohol consumption, poor diet, and lack of exercise.[7] This comorbidity accounts for 60% of premature deaths not related to suicide.[7] The causes of high rates of physical illness seem to be varied, including shared vulnerability, genetic factors, and rates of smoking.

Cardiovascular risk factors are becoming of particular concern with the newer atypical antipsychotics.[8] Other authors[9] suggest routine assessment in monitoring the physical health needs of patients who have serious mental illness. These authors[9] note the odds ratio for eight medical disorders in Medicaid beneficiaries who have psychiatric disorders compared with those without psychiatric disorders. Diabetes, hypertension, heart disease, asthma, gastrointestinal illnesses, cancer, acute respiratory disorders, and skin infections are all increased relative to the comparison group.

Some differences of opinion exist regarding whether these results would be the same if the data were adjusted for various health and lifestyle issues. For example, when controlling for smoking, the debate is whether certain illnesses (eg, cancer) remain elevated. Compared with those without a mental illness, those with a serious mental illness have more than twice the likelihood of smoking cigarettes and a 50% increase in the likelihood of being overweight or obese.[10] "Various biological, iatrogenic, and social factors" may lead to these increased risks.[10] The same preventive approaches developed for other patients are likely to be effective in patients who have serious mental disorders, although we may need to specifically tailor our approach for this population.[10] One study demonstrated long-term effectiveness of nicotine-patch therapy in patients who had schizophrenia.[11] Research in the United Kingdom also showed that subjects who had serious mental illness had an increased risk for death from cardiovascular disease, but results regarding cancer mortality were unclear, especially when controlled for other factors, such as smoking.[12] When comparing cancer deaths, and in particular, respiratory tumors, 50- to 75-year-old subjects had an increased risk that lost statistical significance after controlling for smoking and social deprivation. The increased hazard ratio for coronary heart disease was elevated even after controlling for other risk factors. A higher prescribed dose of antipsychotics predicted greater risk for mortality from coronary heart disease and stroke.[12] In at least one study,[13] there was a decreased risk for prostate cancer in subjects who had schizophrenia, but other rates of cancer were elevated. Another study[14] found that, after adjustments for other risk factors, subjects who had serious mental illness were no more or less likely to develop a malignancy than those who did not have a serious mental illness. Subjects who had mental disorders did develop cancers at younger ages and had increased rates for primary central nervous system tumors in women and men, and in respiratory cancers in men and women. This study determined the odds of respiratory tumors are likely the results of increased rates of smoking.[14] In another review, subjects who had schizophrenia had an increased risk for having one or more chronic conditions compared with controls, especially hyperthyroidism, chronic obstructive pulmonary disease, diabetes with complications, hepatitis C, fluid and electrolyte disorders, and nicotine abuse/dependence.[15]

Understanding the differentiation of delirium and dementia from schizophrenia, and several medical illnesses that present with psychiatric symptoms or psychotic symptoms in the absence of delirium, is important. Illnesses that commonly need to be ruled out that may coexist with schizophrenia or may contribute to psychotic symptoms in the absence of schizophrenia include neoplasms, cerebrovascular disease, Huntington's disease, multiple sclerosis, epilepsy, migraine, central nervous system infections, endocrine disorders, metabolic conditions, fluid or electrolyte imbalances, hepatic or renal diseases, and autoimmune disorders with CNS involvement.[16] Numerous medications should be considered as potential causes of psychotic symptoms, especially with atypical presentations in later life.

Often psychotropic medications are removed when patients who have schizophrenia become seriously medically ill. After reduction or discontinuation of psychotropic medications, when patients become acutely medically ill, we sometimes see an exacerbation of psychiatric symptoms if the medications are not reinstated or increased once patients are medically stable.

A common issue, and one of consultation liaison psychiatry's major contributions, is for consultation-liaison psychiatrists and those treating patients who have schizophrenia with co-morbid medical illness to determine which medications are safest in what medical conditions. A significant concern 15 to 20 years ago was the relative anticholinergic activity and sedation of the older antipsychotics, but of especially serious concern was QRS and QTc prolongation. Thioridazine (Mellaril) and mesoridazine (Serentil) were particularly problematic in delaying cardiac conduction. Many years ago, the authors saw one case of torsades de pointe in a patient that was given too much mesoridazine (Mesoridazine [Serentil] has since been pulled from the market). The anticholinergic activities of the lower potency antipsychotics, such as chlorpromazine (Thorazine) and thioridazine (Mellaril), tend to cause worsening cognition, (particularly in elderly patients), constipation and urinary retention, and concerns about narrow angle glaucoma. Haloperidol (Haldol) was, and still is, a favorite of consultation-liaison psychiatrists because of its low anticholinergic activity and safety in several medical conditions. Most of the remainder of this article looks at the novel, newer, or atypical antipsychotics, comparing them with each other and with older antipsychotics in their anticholinergic effects and their cardiac side effects. The authors look at their relative safety in pulmonary and gastrointestinal disease.

CARDIOVASCULAR

The authors begin with the issue of cardiovascular side effects of the newer antipsychotic agents. Cardiac conduction has been an issue for psychiatrists for a long time, especially when the length of the QRS interval on the ECG is over 110 milliseconds or the QTc interval is over 440 milliseconds or 450 milliseconds. A QRS interval greater than 120 milliseconds suggests first degree heart block, right or left bundle branch block, or an intraventricular conduction defect.[17,18] Prolongation of the QT interval can point to hypokalemia, myocardial disease, or a drug effect. The authors have long been concerned about tricyclic antidepressants and medications, such as thioridazine and formerly mesoridazine. Pacher and Kecskemeti[19] note that the cardiovascular toxicity of older neuroleptics is well established. These drugs inhibit cardiovascular sodium, calcium, and potassium channels, sometimes leading to life-threatening arrhythmias. There have been an increased number of case reports demonstrating that the use of the newer antipsychotics can also be associated with cases of arrhythmias, prolonged QTc intervals, and orthostatic hypotension, even in patients lacking cardiovascular disorders.[19] These same authors[19] further note that these medicines show marked cardiovascular effects in different mammalian and human cardiovascular preparations by inhibiting these same cardiac and vascular channels. In addition to QT prolongation and concomitant ventricular arrhythmias, autonomic dysfunction causing low heart rate variability may lead to malignant arrhythmias.[20] One study[21] compared QTc prolongation between several antipsychotics, and found the greatest interval change in the thioridazine group compared with haloperidol, ziprasidone, quetiapine, olanzapine, and risperidone. A recent and comprehensive review of Medicaid enrollees in Tennessee[22] found that current (but not former) users of typical and atypical antipsychotics had a similar dose-related increased risk for sudden cardiac death. The adjusted incidence-rate ratios were approximately doubled and also approximately doubled between low-dose and high-dose use.

In a totally different way of looking at antipsychotics and overall heart disease risk, Daumit and colleagues[23] used Clinical Antipsychotic Trials of Intervention Effectiveness (CATIE) data to estimate 10-year coronary heart disease risk based on cholesterol, blood pressure, and diabetes risk differences among the antipsychotics olanzapine, perphenazine, quetiapine, risperidone, and ziprasidone. They found the risk estimates were highest for olanzapine and quetiapine. There was actually decreased risk of 0.6% for risperidone and ziprasidone and 0.5% for perphenazine.

Schizophrenia itself increases the risk for developing cardiac disease, according to a study by Gegenava and Kavtaradze.[24] Risk factors from their study included the following: elevated levels of triglycerides and low-density lipoprotein cholesterol (LDL-C); smoking; lack of exercise; psychosocial factors, such as depression, social isolation, lack of social support; and low socioeconomic status. Glassman[25] notes that psychiatric populations are at high risk for cardiovascular disease and that some atypical antipsychotics may be associated with cardiovascular adverse events unrelated to QT prolongation. Glassman states that although there has been concern about QT prolongation, like there was with mesoridazine, evidence suggests that even though atypical antipsychotics may increase the QT interval, prolongation does not seem to result in torsades de pointes, as observed with some conventional antipsychotics. Available data did not support the occurrence of torsades de pointes with any of the available newer antipsychotic drugs, including ziprasidone (Geodon). On the other hand, some newer or atypical antipsychotic drugs have either been withdrawn from clinical use or have been delayed in reaching the marketplace because of concerns about QTc interval prolongation.[26] Vieweg[26] notes that QTc interval prolongation serves as a surrogate marker for the potentially life-threatening arrhythmia, torsades de pointes. He notes that even though there is no evidence that proves that the new generation of antipsychotic drugs produces torsades de pointes, the absence of such evidence is not proof that new antipsychotic drugs do not cause this. Many times throughout psychiatry and the history of medicine, we have only discovered problems after a considerable period of time. For example, it was not until the 1980s that mesoridazine was known to cause torsades de pointes. Vieweg[26] further notes that there is no specific consultative or laboratory intervention necessary before administrating a new generation antipsychotic drug. However, when risk factors are present those risk factors should cause the clinician to be cautious and perform an ECG.

Additional mechanisms by which antipsychotic medications can influence cardiovascular function include the following: receptor blockade, conduction disturbance, delayed ventricular repolarization (prolonged QTc interval), left ventricular dysfunction, sinus node abnormalities, myocarditis, postural hypotension, polydipsia, hyponatremia syndrome, weight gain, and glucose intolerance.[27] QTc prolongation is of particular concern, as this arrhythmia can lead to fatal ventricular tachyarrhythmia (torsades de pointes) and is unpredictable and difficult to manage.[27] Ziprasidone has been of particular concern, among the novel antipsychotics, in its prolongation of the QTc interval.[28] Although there have been no reports of arrhythmia or sudden death with ziprasidone, some caution is probably reasonable.[28] Ziprasidone should probably be avoided in patients who have some types of cardiac disease or uncontrolled electrolyte disturbance. Ziprasidone should be avoided, if possible, whenever patients are already on a medicine that prolongs the QT interval. When cross-tapering, there should be some caution about high total load of antipsychotics when both drugs prolong the QT interval. Under most clinical circumstances, ziprasidone may be safely used without EKG monitoring or other specific special precautions. Ziprasidone tends to have a more favorable effect on body weight and glucose than most other novel antipsychotics.[28]

Alternatively, olanzapine does not appear to prolong QTc significantly.[26] These reviewers[29] looked at ECG recordings in 2700 subjects from four randomized, controlled clinical trials. The results showed that the incidence of a maximum QTc greater than or equal to 450 milliseconds during treatment was approximately equal to the incidence at baseline. These authors[29] conclude that when olanzapine is clinically administered to patients who have schizophrenia, it does not appear to contribute to QTc prolongation resulting in potentially fatal ventricular arrhythmias. Likewise, in another review,[30] olanzapine did not contribute significantly to QTc prolongation that could result in potentially fatal ventricular arrhythmias.

Sertindole (Serlect), an atypical antipsychotic, was voluntarily suspended in the European Union in 1998 following concerns over reports of serious cardiac dysrythmias, and sudden unexpected deaths.[31] In contrast, the incidence of prolonged QTc from haloperidol or droperidol is low.[32] (However, see information below regarding recent US Food and Drug Administration [FDA] warning.) Most of the cases of conduction disturbance from these medicines occurred in critically ill patients who had a history of cardiovascular disease prescribed more than 50 mg per day. This usually occurred in intensive care settings with high doses of parenteral haloperidol. Prolonged QT interval with torsades de pointes has been described during a high rate of infusion of haloperidol (40 mg/hr).[33] These authors[33] recommend assessing a baseline QTc interval and measuring serum magnesium and potassium concentrations in patients who are critically ill. They further note that when a baseline QTc interval is more than 440 milliseconds, or when patients are receiving other drugs that may prolong the QTc or when they have electrolyte disturbances, haloperidol or droperidol should be used with caution. Patients who are critically ill and receiving droperidol or haloperidol should have ECG monitoring, and if the QTc interval lengthens by 25% or more, the haloperidol should be discontinued or the dosage should be reduced.[33] The FDA and the manufacturer issued a warning in September 2007 about QT prolongation and torsades de pointes in patients treated with intravenous haloperidol given at higher doses than recommended.

Clozapine (Clozaril) has been associated with premature ventricular contractions at a frequency of less than 1%.(Product information on Clozaril 2008). Several patients have experienced ischemic changes, myocardial infarction, and sudden death with clozapine (Product information on Clozaril 2008). Also, post-marketing evaluation revealed cases of myocarditis, pericarditis, or pericardial effusions. Determination of causality was complicated by the preexistence of serious cardiac disease. (Product information Clozaril 2008). Hypotension and syncope occurred in more than 5% of patients, tachycardia in almost 25% of patients, and hypertension and chest pain in 1% to 4%. Clozapine has also induced orthostatic hypotension severe enough to cause collapse and respiratory arrest (Product information Clozaril 2008).

QRS prolongation and QTc prolongation, sometimes resulting in death, have been reported in patients taking risperidone.[34] On the other hand,(Product information Risperdal Consta long acting intramuscular (IM) injection 2009) there were no significant differences in the QTc intervals between IM risperidone and placebo.

With quetiapine (Seroquel), an increase in heart rate of about nine beats per minute has been determined during a 6-week study.[35] More than 20% of subjects receiving 100 to 200 mg of quetiapine daily showed either an increase in heart rate of 20 or more beats per minute or elevations of 30 mm/mercury or more in systolic blood pressure.[36] Orthostatic hypotension has been observed in 4% to 7% of subjects receiving quetiapine in clinical trials (Product information Seroquel 2009).

With paliperidone (Invega), QTc intervals have been prolonged in about 3% to 5% of subjects compared with 3% of placebo-treated subjects. In a study of 850 subjects, change in QTc interval exceeding 60 milliseconds occurred in only one subject taking a 12 mg dosage. None of the subjects had a QTc interval exceeding 500 milliseconds (Product information Invega 2009). Orthostatic hypotension occurred in 1to 4% (Product information Invega 2009).

With aripiprazole (Abilify), QTc prolongation has been rarely observed (Product information Abilify 2008). The incidence of orthostatic hypotension is 0.7% to 1.9%. However, this was not significantly different from placebo, which occurred in about 0 .5 to 1.0% (Product information Abilify 2008).

The 2006 American Psychiatric Association (APA) Practice Guidelines for the Treatment of Schizophrenia[37] note that patients who have prolonged QTc, bradycardia, certain electrolyte disturbances, heart failure, or recent myocardial infarction (MI), and patients who are already taking medications that prolong QT intervals, should not be treated with an antipsychotic that further prolongs the QT interval. These antipsychotics include thioridazine, droperidol (Inapsine), ziprasidone, and possibly pimozide (Orap).

The 2006 APA Practice Guideline table[38] suggests that the relative risks for QTc prolongation are as follows: worse for thioridazine, ziprasidone, and risperidone (**Table 1**). Currently, there is very little known risk for QTc prolongation for perphenazine (Trilafon), clozapine, olanzapine, quetiapine, aripiprazole, and haloperidol (except in high doses in the critically ill and given parentally). Therefore, in practice, the better choices when there is concern about worsening QT prolongation, or when patients are taking other medicines that prolong QT, would be haloperidol, aripiprazole, quetiapine, olanzapine, and clozapine. Thioridazine should definitely be avoided.

The FDA and the manufacturer issued a warning in September 2007 about QT prolongation and torsades de pointes in patients treated with haloperidol when given intravenously (IV) and at higher doses than recommended.

This same table also gives relative hypotension rates with clozapine, thioridazine and quetiapine, perphenazine, risperidone and olanzapine, ziprasidone, aripiprazole, and haloperidol (see **Table 1**).

GASTROINTESTINAL

Anticholinergic adverse effects, which include not only gastrointestinal side effects but also urinary, cardiovascular, vision, and cognitive side effects, have long been a concern with the use of psychotropic medications, including antipsychotic medications, and can be especially problematic in the medically ill or elderly. The lower-potency older antipsychotics have long been known to have higher rates of

Table 1
Relative risk of antipsychotics in patients who have cardiovascular, pulmonary, or gastrointestinal issues

	QTC Prolongation	Orthostatic Hypotension	Liver Enzymes Elevation	Anticho-linergic	Respiratory Depression
Thioridazine	+++	++		++	++
Chlorpromazine	0	++	+++++ Contra-indicated	++	++
Perphenazine	0	+		0	
Haloperidol	High dose IV is only concern	0	Near 0	0	
Clozapine	0	+++	+++	+++	+++
Olanzapine	0	+	++	++	+
Quetiapine	0	++	+	0	?+
Risperidone	+	+	+	0	
Ziprasidone	++	0		0	
Aripiprazole	0	0		0	

Missing information in table denotes insufficient data.

Data from Product Information from Clozaril 2008, Zyprexo 2004, Seroquel 2009, Risperdal 2006, and Geodon 2006 and from Lehman AF, Leiberman JA, Dixon LB, et al. Practice Guidelines for the Treatment of Patients with Schizophrenia. In: Quick CM, Adams DC, Bowden CL, et al, editors. APA Practice Guidelines for the treatment of psychiatric disorders. 2nd edition. p. 616; Lehman AF, Leiberman JA, Dixon LB, et al. Practice Guidelines for the Treatment of Patients with Schizophrenia. In: Quick CM, Adams DC, Bowden CL, editors. APA Practice Guidelines for the treatment of psychiatric disorders. 2nd edition. p. 592.

anticholinergic effects. Serum anticholinergic levels (using a radioreceptor binding assay) were determined in 12 subjects receiving olanzapine and 12 subjects receiving clozapine.[39] They evaluated anticholinergic effects among subjects who had schizophrenia and other psychotic disorders. Subjects treated with olanzapine had serum anticholinergic levels that were only approximately 20% of the subjects treated with clozapine. Clinical evaluations also showed that subjects treated with clozapine experienced more frequent and severe anticholinergic side effects. These side effects included constipation and urinary retention, but not dry mouth. With olanzapine, 9% to 11% of subjects experienced constipation (Product information Zyprexa 2004), which appears to be dose related. In comparison, constipation occurred in 14% of subjects on clozapine therapy. Older patients may be particularly susceptible to the anticholinergic effects of clozapine. Fecal impaction has also been reported (Product information Clozaril 2002). This usually occurs when the dose exceeds 150 mg. Adverse effects may disappear over time. Urinary retention occurred in 1% of subjects during clozapine therapy, and again, elderly patients are particularly susceptible (Product information Clozaril 2002). With risperidone, constipation has occurred in 5% to 21% of subjects in clinical trials (Product information Risperdal 2006). Anticholinergic activity with quetiapine appears to be dose related and dry mouth occurs in 8% to 17%. Constipation has also been reported in clinical trials.[37] Constipation with Abilify has occurred in 11% (Product information Abilify Oral Tablets and Oral Solutions 2006), compared with 7% of subjects receiving placebo. According to the 2006 APA Practice Guidelines,[39] anticholinergic side effects for the antipsychotics are in this order: clozapine, thioridazine and olanzapine, perphenazine, haloperidol, risperidone, quetiapine, ziprasidone, and aripiprazole (see **Table 1**).

Liver disease is another common area that the authors encounter in consultation-liaison psychiatry and in the treatment of patients who are seriously mentally ill. If patients have liver disease, we are concerned about what medications we are going to use. Among the more than 1000 drugs noted to have hepatic side effects, 16% were neuropsychiatric drugs.[40] Hepatic enzyme elevations occur frequently with phenothiazine drugs at about 20%, but also with other classes of antipsychotics. Clinical hepatitis has been rarely described with neuroleptic drugs, with rates of phenothiazine agents at 0.1% to 1.0% and with haloperidol at 0.002%.[40] Dumartier and colleagues[40] reviewed available atypical antipsychotic drugs in France, including clozapine, olanzapine, and risperidone. They found the frequency of hepatic problems, in general, was very low. In a study of clozapine versus haloperidol,[40] 37.3% of subjects treated with clozapine showed a significant alanine aminotransferase (ALT) increase compared with 16.6% seen in subjects treated with haloperidol. Hepatic injuries usually occurred within the first weeks of treatment, but this varied considerably. Cases reported were reversible after the atypical antipsychotic drug was withdrawn, except with one subject treated with clozapine who developed a form of irreversible hepatitis after 8 weeks on clozapine. Re-challenge with clozapine after a first episode was done in three subjects and one developed a new hepatic disorder. Re-challenge may be done, but only with special care, if the agent is thought to be indispensable after a first episode of isolated hepatic enzyme elevation. However, with clinical hepatotoxicity, re-challenge is inadvisable according to Dumortier and colleagues[40] In the absence of risk factors, these authors[40] advise that systematic and regular checking of hepatic enzymes does not seem necessary. Olanzapine in particular may result rarely in hepatotoxicity, such as a report of a tenfold increase in liver enzyme levels during the third year of olanzapine treatment that returned to normal 3 weeks after olanzapine discontinuation.[41] Clinicians should be aware of hepatotoxic effects of atypical antipsychotics and monitor liver enzyme levels when there are clinical concerns.[41] The incidence of elevated liver function tests with risperidone is estimated to be 0.1 to 1% (Product information Risperdal 2006). Quetiapine has also had transient, reversible elevations in serum transaminases, primarily ALT. Peak elevations are usually seen between 7 and 21 days after initiation of treatment, and most patients are able to continue therapy with a return to near normal values (Product information Seroquel 2004). Almost all psychotropics are metabolized by Phase I oxidation in the liver, with the exceptions of lithium (Eskalith), gabapentin (Neurontin), lorazepam (Ativan), oxazepam (Serax), and temazepam (Restoril).[42] Wyszynski and colleagues[42] note that there is accumulating experience on the safety of atypical antipsychotics in liver failure. However, their recommendation is to start low and go slow in all patients who are medically ill, especially those with liver disease. Chlorpromazine is contraindicated because of its tendency to exacerbate hepatotoxicity.[43] Haloperidol, a high clearance drug with significant first pass metabolism, is used frequently in patients who have liver disease.

For patients who have liver disease, the following antipsychotics are listed in order of descending risk and tendency to elevate liver enzymes: chlorpromazine (contraindicated), clozapine, olanzapine, risperidone and quetiapine, and haloperidol (see **Table 1**).

PULMONARY

Another concern, especially of consultation-liaison psychiatry, is respiratory suppression in patients who have already compromised respiratory function. Respiratory suppression can be a serious side effect and a danger in patients who have impaired pulmonary function.[44] Sleep apnea is also a concern. Antipsychotics, when coadministered with other drugs that have similar respiratory effects (eg, benzodiazepines, barbiturates, or opiates) may exacerbate the problem of respiratory depression.[44] Concurrent use of benzodiazepines with clozapine has possibly resulted in increased risks for collapse, respiratory arrest, or cardiac arrest (Product information Clozaril 2005).

Some of the concerns about increased mortality in elderly patients who have dementia being given atypical antipsychotics may have been related to concomitant use of benzodiazepine in the presence of pulmonary conditions (Product information Zyprexa 2004). Respiratory failure was described in a 92-year-old woman, with chronic obstructive pulmonary disease (COPD) admitted to the hospital with pneumonia after being given quetiapine.[44] Quetiapine has generally been very safe, even in the elderly.[44] Pulmonary embolism has been reported in patients on olanzapine, and at least six cases of venous thrombosis have been reported in patients treated with clozapine (Product information Clozaril 2002). Benzodiazepines and sedative-hypnotics, if used as adjuncts in schizophrenia, have been implicated in worsening or precipitating sleep apnea in patients who have COPD.[45] However, their use does allow lowering the dosage of antipsychotics in agitated patients (see **Table 1**).

EMERGENCY USE OF ANTIPSYCHOTICS IN THE SETTING OF POTENTIAL COMORBID MEDICAL ILLNESS

Another medical-psychiatry interface issue frequently encountered is the issue of needing to control agitation in the emergency room when there is uncertainty about medical conditions. Some of the newer atypical antipsychotics seem to provide a safe and reasonable choice for such patients[46] and may have fewer short-term side effects than older antipsychotic agents. Available antipsychotic medications

Table 2
Significant pharmacokinetic drug interactions involving antipsychotics

Antipsychotic	Interacting Drug	Pharmacokinetic Result on the Antipsychotic	Mechanism	To Avoid Toxicity or Maintain Efficacy
Aripiprazole	Carbamazepine	↓AUC 70%	3A4 induction	Double AP dose
	Ketoconazole	↑AUC 65%	3A4 inhibition	Half AP dose
	Quinidine	↑AUC 35%	2D6inhibition	Half AP dose
Haloperidol	Aripiprazole	↓D2 binding	Aripiprazole displaces haldol and all other AP	Possible decompensation during crossover titrations
	Carbamazepine	↑Clearance	1A2, 3A4 induction	↑AP dose
	Fluvoxamine	↑Cp	1A2, 3A4 inhibition	↓AP dose
	Phenytoin	↓Cp	3A4 induction	↑AP dose
Olanzapine	Carbamazepine	↑Clearance 50%	1A2 induction	↑AP dose
	Fluvoxamine	↑AUC 50% FS & 110% MNS	1A2 inhibition	↓AP dose
Perphenazine	Aripiprazole	↓D2 binding	aripiprazole displaces *all other* AP	Possible decompensation during crossover titrations
	Bupropion paroxetine citalopram duloxetine escitalopram	↓Clearance	2D6 inhibition	Reevaluate AP dose

Quetiapine	Phenytoin	↑ Clearance 5 fold	3A4 induction	↑ AP dose
	Carbamazepine	↓ Cp quetiapine ↑Cp CBZ 10,11 epoxide	3A4 induction; unknown	↑ AP dose; may see CBZ toxicity (ataxia, sedation, diplopia)
	Thioridazine	↑ Quetiapine clearance 65%		Avoid this combination
	Ketoconazole	↑ Cp 335%	3A4 inhibition	Reevaluate AP dose
	Lorazepam	↓ Lorazepam clearance 20%		Clinically significant; reevaluate lorazepam dose
Risperidone	Fluoxetine, paroxetine	↑ Cp 2.5 fold ↑ Cp 3–9 fold	2D6 inhibition	Reevaluate AP dose
	Carbamazepine	↓ Cp 50%	3A4 induction	Double AP dose
	Phenytoin	↓ Cp	3A4 induction	↑ AP dose
	Verapamil	↑ AUC 2 fold	PGP inhibition	Reevaluate AP dose
Ziprasidone	Ketoconazole	↑ AUC 35%	3A4 inhibition	Reevaluate AP dose
	Carbamazepine	↓ AUC 35%	3A4 induction	↑ AP dose

Abbreviations: AP, antipsychotic; AUC, area under the concentration-time curve; CBZ, Carbamazepine; Cp, plasma concentration; FS, female smokers; MNS, male non-smokers; PGP, p-glycoprotein reverse transporter.

Data from Citrome L, Macher JP, Salazar DE, et al. Pharmacokinetics of aripiprazole and concomitant carbamazepine. J Clin Psychopharmacology 2007;27:279–83, and Sandson NB, Armstrong SC, Cozza KL. An overview of psychotropic drug-drug interactions. Psychosomatics 2005;46:464–94.

that can be given IM in emergency management include ziprasidone and olanzapine. Risperidone or olanzapine may be given as a rapidly dissolvable tablet[46] and risperidone is available in a liquid formulation.

DRUG INTERACTIONS OF SELECTED ATYPICAL ANTIPSYCHOTICS AND HALOPERIDOL AND PERPHENAZINE

The existence of comorbid conditions leads to the use of multiple drugs. As the number of drugs taken concurrently increases, so does the potential for harmful drug interactions and increased morbidity. Drug interactions can be classified into two general categories: pharmacodynamic or pharmacokinetic.[47] Pharmacodynamic interactions reflect added or opposing pharmacologic effects. In contrast, pharmacokinetic interactions reflect a change in the object drug concentration or passage time through the body. The majority of interactions involving antipsychotics as the precipitating agent are of the pharmacodynamic nature.

Additive pharmacodynamic effects may lead to adverse events when other drugs with similar receptor occupancy are combined with antipsychotics. Examples include hypotension with other antihypertensive agents, sedation with other central nervous system depressants, and anticholinergic effects with agents that may be used for treating parkinsonian tremors. The use of some of the fluoroquinolone antibiotics, such as gatifloxacin (Tequin), moxifloxacin (Avelox), and class IA and III anti-arrhythmics in combination with ziprasidone, is not recommended because of additive potential for QTc prolongation.(Product information Geodon November 2006) Lastly, serotonin syndrome is another example of a pharmacodynamic interaction.[48]

Some of the significant pharmacokinetic drug interactions involving antipsychotics are listed in **Table 2**.

In summary, medical illnesses are particularly common in patients who have schizophrenia and pose challenges for the treatment of these patients in our health care system. We should be monitoring for the following health problems in patients who have schizophrenia: obesity, diabetes, hyperlipidemia, hypertension, cardiovascular problems, HIV risk behaviors, medical complications of substance abuse, heavy smoking and its effects, and amenorrhea. A major task for consultation-liaison psychiatry and others is to determine which medications are safest in which medical condition. There is no specific laboratory or other study required before urgently administering an atypical or newer generation antipsychotic drug. (Obtaining baseline labs, such as glucose and lipids, weight, and blood pressure are discussed in another article.) However, when cardiovascular risk factors are present, it is prudent to obtain an ECG. In patients who are critically ill, a baseline ECG to check for the QTc interval should be obtained and serum magnesium and potassium concentrations should be measured. Patients who have prolonged QTc, bradycardia, certain electrolyte disturbances, heart failure, or recent MI, and those who are taking other drugs that prolong QT intervals, should not be treated with antipsychotic drugs that further prolong the QT interval. Antipsychotics to avoid include: thioridazine, droperidol, and ziprasidone, and possibly pimozide. Relative risks in descending order of concern are as follows: thioridazine, ziprasidone, risperidone, perphenazine, haloperidol (except in the critically ill when given parentally in high doses), clozapine, olanzapine, quetiapine, and aripiprazole (see **Table 1**).

Another significant cardiovascular risk factor with psychotropic medications is hypotension, especially orthostatic hypotension. The relative incidence in descending order is clozapine, thioridazine and quetiapine, perphenazine, risperidone and olanzapine, ziprasidone, aripiprazole, and haloperidol (see **Table 1**).

Anticholinergic effects are also important in the elderly and in the medically ill and can cause worsening cognition, urinary retention, constipation, and blurred vision. The antipsychotics are listed from most to least anticholinergic: clozapine, thioridazine and olanzapine, perphenazine, haloperidol, risperidone, quetiapine, ziprasidone, and aripiprazole (see **Table 1**). For patients who have liver disease, the antipsychotics are listed in order of descending risk and tendency to elevate liver enzymes: chlorpromazine (contraindicated), clozapine, olanzapine, risperidone and quetiapine, and haloperidol (see **Table 1**).

ACKNOWLEDGEMENTS

Special Acknowledgement to Kimberly Stadtmueller, CPhT, for assistance with editing and preparation of this article.

REFERENCES

1. Newcomer JW. Metabolic considerations in the use of antipsychotic medications: a review of recent evidence. J Clin Psychiatry 2007;68(Suppl 1):20–7.
2. Hennekens CH, Hennekens AR, Hollar D, et al. Schizophrenia and increased risks of cardiovascular disease. Am Heart J 2005;150(6):1115–21.
3. Muir-Cochrane E. Medical co-morbidity risk factors and barriers to care for people with schizophrenia. J Psychiatr Ment Health Nurs 2006;13(4):447–52.
4. Kane JM, Leucht S, Carpenter D, et al. The expert consensus guideline series. Optimizing pharmacologic treatment of psychotic disorders. Introduction: methods, commentary and summary. J Clin Psychiatry 2003;64(Suppl 12):5–19.
5. Felker B, Yazel JJ, Short D. Mortality and medical comorbidity among psychiatric patients: a review. Psychiatr Serv 1996;47(12):1356–63.
6. Sokal J, Messias E, Dickerson FB, et al. Comorbidity of medical illnesses among adults with serious mental illness who are receiving community psychiatric services. J Nerv Ment Dis 2004;192(6):421–7.
7. Lambert TJ, Velakoulis D, Pantelis C. Medical comorbidity and schizophrenia. Med J Aust 2003;178(Suppl):S67–70.
8. Mitchell AJ, Malone D. Physical health and schizophrenia. Curr Opin Psychiatry 2006;19(4):432–7.
9. Dickey B, Normand SL, Weiss RD, et al. Medical morbidity, mental illness, and substance use disorders. Psychiatr Serv 2002;53(7):861–7.
10. Compton MT, Daumit GL, Druss BG. Cigarette smoking and overweight/obesity among individuals with serious mental illnesses; a preventive perspective. Harv Rev Psychiatry 2006;14(4):212–22.
11. Chou KR, Chen R, Lee JF, et al. The effectiveness of nicotine-patch therapy for smoking cessation in patients with schizophrenia. Int J Nurs Stud 2004;41(3): 321–30.
12. Osborn DP, Levy G, Nazareth I, et al. Relative risk of cardiovascular and cancer mortality in people with severe mental illness from the United Kingdom's General Practice Research Database. Arch Gen Psychiatry 2007;64(2):242–9.
13. Mortensen PB. Neuroleptic medication and reduced risk of prostate cancer in schizophrenic patients. Acta Psychiatr Scand 1992;85(5):390–3.
14. Carney CP, Woolson RF, Jones L, et al. Occurrence of cancer among people with mental health claims in an insured population. Psychosom Med 2004;66(5): 735–43.

15. Carney CP, Jones L, Woolson RF. Medical comorbidity in women and men with schizophrenia: a population-based controlled study. J Gen Intern Med 2006; 21(11):1133–7.
16. Andreasen NC, Kane JM, Keith S, et al. Schizophrenia and other psychotic disorders. In: First MB, Ross R, editors. Diagnostic and Statistical Manual Text Revised tDSM-IV-TR. Washington, DC: American Psychiatric Association; 2000. p. 336.
17. Preskorn SH, Irwin HA. Toxicity of tricyclic antidepressants: kinetics, mechanism, intervention. J Clin Psychiatry 1982;43:151–6.
18. Roose SP, Glassman AH, Giardina EGV, et al. Tricyclic antidepressants in depressed patients with cardiac conduction disease. Arch Gen Psychiatry 1987b;44:273–5.
19. Pacher P, Kecskemeti V. Cardiovascular side effects of new antidepressants and antipsychotics: new drugs, old concerns? Curr Pharm Des 2004;10(20):2463–75.
20. Koponen H, Alaräisänen A, Saari K, et al. Schizophrenia and sudden cardiac death: a review. Nord J Psychiatry 2008;62(5):342–5.
21. Harrigan EP, Miceli JJ, Anziano R, et al. A randomized evaluation of the effects of six antipsychotic agents on QTc, in the absence and presence of metabolic inhibition. J Clin Psychopharmacol 2004;24(1):62–9.
22. Ray WA, Chung CP, Murray KT, et al. Atypical antipsychotic drugs and the risk of sudden cardiac death. N Engl J Med 2009;360(3):225–35.
23. Daumit G, Goft D, Meyer J, et al. Antipsychotic effects on estimated 10 year coronary heart disease risk in the CATIE schizophrenia study. Schizophr Res 2008; 105(1–3):175–87.
24. Gegenava M, Kavtaradze G. Risk factors for coronary heart disease in patients with schizophrenia. Georgian Med News 2006;134:55–8.
25. Glassman AH. Schizophrenia, antipsychotic drugs, and cardiovascular disease. J Clin Psychiatry 2005;66(Suppl 6):5–10.
26. Vieweg WV. New generation antipsychotic drugs in QTc interval prolongation. Prim Care Companion J Clin Psychiatry 2003;5(5):205–15.
27. Ames D, Camm J, Cook P, et al. Minimizing the risk associated with QTc prolongation in people with schizophrenia. A consensus statement by the Cardiac Safety and Schizophrenia Group. Encephale 2002;28(6 pt 1):552–62.
28. Taylor D. Ziprasidone in the management of schizophrenia: the QT interval issue in context. CNS Drugs 2003;17(6):423–30.
29. Czekalla J, Beasley CM Jr, Dellva MA, et al. Analysis of the QTc interval during the olanzapine treatment of patients with schizophrenia in related psychosis. J Clin Psychiatry 2001;62(3):191–8.
30. Czekalla J, Kollack-Walker S, Beasley CM Jr. Cardiac safety perimeters of olanzapine: comparison with other atypical and typical antipsychotics. J Clin Psychiatry 2001;62(Suppl 2):35–40.
31. Wilton LD, Heeley EL, Pickering RM, et al. Comparative study of the mortality rates in cardiac dysrythmias in post-marketing surveillance studies of sertindole and two other atypical antipsychotic drugs, risperidone and olanzapine. J Psychopharmacol 2001;15(2):120–6.
32. Lawrence KR, Nasraway SA. Conduction disturbances associated with administration of butyrophenone antipsychotics in the critically ill: a review of the literature. Pharmacotherapy 1997;17(3):531–7.
33. Riker RR, Fraser GL, Cos PM. Continuous infusion of haloperidol controls agitation in critically ill patients. Crit Care Med 1994;22(3):433–40.
34. Ravin DS, Levenson JW. Fatal cardiac event following initiation of risperidone therapy. Ann Pharmacother 1997;31(7–8):867–70.

35. Borison RL, Arvanitis LA, Miller BG. ICI 204,636, an atypical antipsychotic: efficacy and safety in a multicenter, placebo-controlled trial in patients with schizophrenia. U.S. SEROQUEL Study Group. J Clin Psychopharmacol 1996;16(2): 158–69.
36. Garver DL. Review of quetiapine side effects. J Clin Psychiatry 2000;61(Suppl 8): 31–3 [discussion: 34–5].
37. Lehman AF, Leiberman JA, Dixon LB, et al. Practice Guidelines for the Treatment of Patients with Schizophrenia. In: Quick CM, Adams DC, Bowden CL, et al, editors. APA Practice Guidelines for the treatment of psychiatric disorders. 2nd edition. p. 616.
38. Lehman AF, Leiberman JA, Dixon LB, et al. Practice Guidelines for the Treatment of Patients with Schizophrenia. In: Quick CM, Adams DC, Bowden CL, editors. APA Practice Guidelines for the treatment of psychiatric disorders. 2nd edition. p. 592.
39. Chengappa KN, Pollock BG, Parepally H, et al. Anticholinergic differences among patients receiving standard clinical doses of olanzapine or clozapine. J Clin Psychopharmacol 2002;20(3):311–6.
40. Dumortier G, Cabaret W, Stamatiadis L, et al. Hepatic tolerance of atypical antipsychotic drugs. Encephale 2002;28(6 Pt 1):542–51.
41. Ozcanli T, Erdogan A, Ozdemir S, et al. Severe liver enzyme elevations after three years of olanzapine treatment: A case report and review of olanzapine associated hepatotoxicity. Prog Neuropsychopharmacol Biol Psychiatry 30, 2006;30(6): 1163–6. Epub 2006 Apr 24.
42. Wyszynski AA. The patient with hepatic disease alcohol dependence and altered mental status. In: Wyszynski AA, Wyszynski B, editors. Manual of psychiatric care for the medically ill. Washington, DC: American Psychiatric Publishing, Inc; 2005. p. 40–6.
43. Siris SG, Rifkin A. The problem of psychopharmacotherapy in the medically Ill. Psychiatr Clin North Am 1981;4(2):379–90.
44. Jabeen S, Polli SI, Gerber DR. Acute respiratory failure with a single dose of quetiapine fumarate. Ann Pharmacother 2006;40(3):559–62.
45. Cohn MA, Morris DD, Juan D. Effects of estazolam and flurazepam on cardiopulmonary function in patients with chronic obstructive pulmonary disease. Drug Saf 1992;7:152–8.
46. Rund DA, Ewing JD, Mitzel K, et al. The use of intramuscular benzodiazepines and antipsychotic agents in the treatment of acute agitation or violence in the emergency department. J Emerg Med 2006;31(3):317–24.
47. Devane CL. Drug interactions. In: Stein D, Lerer B, Sthl S, editors. Evidence based psychopharmacology. New York: Cambridge Univeristy Press; 2005. p. 320–37.
48. Boyer EW, Shannon M. The serotonin syndrome. N Engl J Med 2005;352: 1112–20.

Management of Schizophrenia with Obesity, Metabolic, and Endocrinological Disorders

Palmiero Monteleone, MD*, Vassilis Martiadis, MD, Mario Maj, MD, PhD

KEYWORDS

- Schizophrenia • Obesity • Diabetes
- Metabolic syndrome • Hyperprolactinemia

In a meta-analysis of 152 mortality studies, patients with schizophrenia presented a twofold greater risk of premature death from medical causes compared with the general population, having a life expectancy that is approximately 20% shorter.[1] Recent data from the United States public health sector confirm that cardiovascular diseases (CVD) are the leading cause of death in people with major mental illness.[2] Key risk factors for CVD include obesity, dyslipidemia, hypertension, physical inactivity, smoking, hyperglycemia, and diabetes, which are all more prevalent in patients with schizophrenia compared with the general population.[3] Obesity, dyslipidemia, hyperglycemia, and diabetes can be caused or exacerbated by the use of psychotropic medications, namely antipsychotic (AP) drugs, which may also induce endocrine alterations. This article reviews the literature on the prevalence of obesity, metabolic disturbances, and endocrinological disturbances in people with schizophrenia, focusing especially on the impact that APs have on these conditions, and discusses their possible management and prevention.

OBESITY AND WEIGHT GAIN IN SCHIZOPHRENIA

According to World Health Organization (WHO) criteria,[4] a body mass index (BMI, calculated as weight in kilograms divided by the square of height in meters) between 18.5 and 24.9 kg/m^2 is normal; BMIs from 25 to 29.9 kg/m^2 and greater than or equal to 30 kg/m^2 define overweight and obesity, respectively, although thresholds vary with ethnicity (eg, Asians). Obesity and overweight have become a major clinical focus

Department of Psychiatry, University of Naples SUN, Naples, Largo Madonna delle Grazie, 80138, Napoli, Italy
* Corresponding author.
E-mail address: monteri@tin.it (P. Monteleone).

Psychiatr Clin N Am 32 (2009) 775–794
doi:10.1016/j.psc.2009.08.003

based on their inclusion among the cardiovascular risk factors,[5,6] and because they are independent risk factors for morbidity and mortality, being the most important risk factors for developing diabetes, hypertension,[7] respiratory problems, and some forms of cancer.[8]

There is evidence that patients with schizophrenia have an increased prevalence of obesity or overweight compared with the general population.[9] Several factors are likely to predispose an individual to body weight (BW) gain, including lack of exercise, high-fat diet, increasing age, genetic factors, and a family history of obesity. Lifestyle issues are particularly pertinent to patients with schizophrenia, as this disorder is commonly associated with poor dietary conditions and reduced physical activity. Moreover, weight gain is a well-established side effect of first-generation APs (FGA) and second-generation APs (SGA).[10]

Recent studies quantify the incidence of weight gain in patients treated with APs as approximately 80%.[11] Some investigators describe this adverse effect as the most difficult to cope with,[12] and several studies report that it can adversely affect clinical outcome and quality of life of schizophrenic patients. In fact, overweight and obesity may increase stigma and social discrimination, and may negatively influence self-esteem, with a negative impact on treatment compliance (threefold enhanced risk of drug treatment discontinuation in patients experiencing AP-induced overweight or obesity) and consequent increasing risk of relapse.[13] An estimate of treatment-emergent weight gain for specific APs has been provided by the meta-analysis of Allison and colleagues,[14] including 81 studies evaluating BW changes after 10 weeks of treatment with standard doses of FGA and SGA. In this meta-analysis, clozapine and olanzapine were associated with a mean weight gain of 4.45 and 4.15 kg, respectively; thioridazine, sertindole, chlorpromazine, and risperidone were shown to induce moderate weight gain (ranging from 3.19 kg to 2.10 kg), whereas haloperidol, aripiprazole, fluphenazine, and ziprasidone were associated with low/very low weight gain (range: 1.08–0.04 kg).

Short-term data have been confirmed in long-term studies. The Clinical Antipsychotic Trials in Intervention Effectiveness (CATIE) study, funded by the National Institute of Mental Health, examined 1493 patients diagnosed with chronic schizophrenia and treated with risperidone, olanzapine, quetiapine, ziprasidone, or perphenazine for up to 18 months.[15] Average weight gain was 4.3 kg in the olanzapine group, compared with 0.36 kg for risperidone, 0.50 kg for quetiapine, −0.73 kg for ziprasidone, and −0.91 kg for perphenazine. In particular, overall weight gain, weight gain × month, and the percentage of patients who gained more than 7% of their baseline BW (considered as the cutoff for clinically meaningful weight gain)[14] were greatest in the olanzapine group. These data are consistent with the preliminary findings of the Intercontinental Schizophrenia Outpatients Health Outcome study, a prospective, observational study including almost 5000 schizophrenic patients being treated with risperidone, olanzapine, quetiapine, or haloperidol for 3 years. Weight gain at 12 months was greater with olanzapine (3.4 kg), followed by risperidone and haloperidol (2.2 kg), and by quetiapine (1.9 kg).[16] Finally, in the Comparison of Atypicals in First-Episode Psychosis study, a 52-week double-blind study in first-episode psychotic patients, the percentages of subjects who gained more than 7% of their baseline BW were 80% for olanzapine, 57.6% for risperidone, and 50% for quetiapine.[17]

A recent review by Brecher and colleagues[18] provided information on the magnitude and pattern of weight changes in patients treated with quetiapine for up to 2 years through a retrospective analysis of quetiapine controlled trials, open-label studies and the corresponding open-label extension phases. Data showed that most of the patients (>60%) gained weight within the first 12 weeks of treatment with quetiapine;

some patients (4%) gained weight between 6 and 12 months and only 1% between 1 and 2 years; 37% of patients gained 7% or more of their baseline BW within 52 weeks of quetiapine treatment. It must be underlined that patients in the lower baseline BMI categories gained the most. McEvoy and colleagues[19] compared the efficacy and tolerability of quetiapine to olanzapine and risperidone in a double-blind multicenter study, and found that olanzapine was associated with the greatest increases in BW and related measures. In particular, at week 52, 80% of patients in the olanzapine group gained 7% or more of their baseline weight, compared with 50% and 58% of the quetiapine and risperidone groups, respectively. In female patients, risperidone was associated with greater BW and BMI increases than quetiapine.

A randomized, open-label study performed in 98 centers in 12 European countries, including 555 community treated patients with a diagnosis of schizophrenia over a 26-week period,[20] showed that patients treated with aripiprazole experienced decreased weight and improved weight-related quality of life compared with patients treated with standard of care (SOC) (ie, olanzapine, quetiapine, or risperidone based on the investigator's judgment of the optimal treatment of the patient and the patient's prior response to AP medication). In particular, more than one-quarter (26.5%) of aripiprazole participants lost at least 5% of their baseline BW, compared with 10.9% of SOC participants. In contrast, 27.9% of SOC patients gained at least 5% of their baseline weight, compared with only 11.7% of aripiprazole participants. Patients receiving aripiprazole reported significantly greater improvements in physical function, self-esteem, sexual life, and Impact of Weight on Quality of Life-Lite (a 31-item self-report rating scale evaluating changes in weight-related quality of life) total score than those receiving SOC. These data are consistent with previous findings showing that aripiprazole causes little or no weight gain compared with placebo, haloperidol, risperidone, and olanzapine.[21–24]

Most of the above studies were conducted in chronic patients previously exposed to other APs, or in mixed samples of first-episode and chronic patients. The use of patient samples with long-term previous exposure to APs with an acknowledged potential to induce weight gain, and the effect of a chronic illness on lifestyle, could have underestimated the real dimensions of AP-induced weight gain. Moreover, young patients with first-episode psychoses (FEP) are particularly vulnerable to experiencing physical adverse effects related to APs, and display BMI values lower than chronic patients and not significantly different from healthy values. Therefore, FEP patients could experience AP-induced BW gains significantly greater than those of patients who had already been exposed to AP medications. This issue has been addressed in a recent meta-analysis by Alvarez-Jimenez and colleagues,[25] who reviewed 51 randomized controlled trials (RCTs) comparing olanzapine, risperidone, or haloperidol with either placebo or an active comparator in adults ranging from 15 to 65 years old, diagnosed with psychotic disorders. The studies were divided into subgroups according to the duration of the trial (short-term vs long-term trial, 9 months being the cutoff time) and the phase of the illness (FEP vs chronic patients).

In studies on patients with chronic psychotic disorders with follow-up periods ranging from 6 to 28 weeks (short-term trials), olanzapine-induced weight gain was estimated to range from 1.80 to 5.40 kg, risperidone-induced weight gain from 1.0 to 2.30 kg and haloperidol-induced weight gain from 0.01 to 1.40 kg. The proportion of patients experiencing weight gain of greater than or equal to 7% of the baseline value was reported to range from 13.6% to 68.0% in patients receiving olanzapine, from 9% to 34.0% in patients treated with risperidone, and from 3% to 10% in patients treated with haloperidol. However, the populations studied seem to be characterized by subjects who had already experienced weight gain, because they included mainly chronic patients who had already undergone pharmacological treatments and hospitalizations. In the studies in which the patients' baseline BMI was reported, it appeared to be in the overweight range or at obese levels; therefore, the magnitude of weight gain reported may have been underestimated.

Clinical trials in chronic patients with follow-up periods ranging from 12 to 18 months (long-term trials) reported an average weight gain ranging from 2.0 to 6.2 kg for olanzapine, from 0.4 to 3.9 kg for risperidone, and from −0.7 to 0.4 kg for haloperidol. One long-term trial found no significant difference in absolute weight gain between olanzapine and risperidone after a 1-year follow-up period.[26] In this study, olanzapine was associated with a rapid but self-limited weight gain after treatment onset, whereas risperidone showed a slow but continuous weight increase resulting in similar absolute weight gains. When study participants were categorized according to a weight increase of greater than or equal to 7% of the baseline value, the percentage of patients with a clinically significant weight gain was higher with olanzapine than with risperidone (40.7% vs 17.3%). This finding illustrates the importance of assessing the percentage of weight gain rather than absolute weight changes.

Short-term RCTs on young FEP patients reported weight gains ranging from 7.1 to 9.2 kg for olanzapine, from 4.0 to 5.6 kg for risperidone, and from 2.6 to 3.8 kg for haloperidol. These data are similar to the weight gain profiles observed in patients with chronic psychotic disorders in which the AP-induced weight gain seems to be 3 to 4 times less severe. The same difference characterizes data for the proportion of patients experiencing clinically significant weight gain. Long-term follow-up RCTs performed with young patients estimated olanzapine-induced weight gain ranging from 10.2 to 15.4 kg, whereas risperidone- and haloperidol-associated weight gain were reported to range from 6.6 to 8.9 kg, and from 4.0 to 9.7 kg, respectively. Again, these data substantially exceed the findings reported by studies on chronic populations. In summary, weight gain was three- to fourfold greater in studies that included young individuals with limited previous exposure to AP drugs in short-term studies and long-term trials. The same disparity was observed regarding the proportion of patients experiencing clinically significant weight gain.

The mechanisms underlying AP-induced weight gain are not fully understood. The occupancy of serotonergic, histaminergic, muscarinic, and other receptors more or less directly involved in the modulation of food intake and energy expenditure has been suggested as the primary mechanism for AP-induced weight gain, and the different pharmacodynamic profile of APs on those receptors has been invoked as the key factor for the different weight gain liabilities of AP drugs.[27–30] Nonetheless, it is uncontroversial that not all the patients started on AP medication undergo BW increase, which suggests a role for individual genetic and nongenetic factors. Genetic association studies support a consistent role for the -759C/T polymorphism of the 5HT2C receptor gene in AP-induced weight gain; other interesting candidates genes include the adrenergic α2a receptor, leptin, the guanine nucleotide binding protein-3, and the synaptosomal-associated protein 25kDa genes, whereas results from linkage studies point to the chromosome 12p24 region, which includes the gene of the promelanin-concentrating hormone, a substance directly involved in the regulation of energy homeostasis.[31]

In terms of prediction of AP-induced weight gain, no definitive clinical or biological variables have been identified. The most consistent findings revealed that patients with lower BMIs before starting AP treatment are at higher risk of weight gain.[14,17,22–25,32] Similarly, early and rapid weight gain has been reported to be a strong predictor for long-term weight gain with olanzapine.[26] In a small study, higher serum leptin levels in the first 2 weeks of clozapine treatment negatively correlated with patients' weight gain after 6 and 8 months of therapy.[33] These findings need to be confirmed.

In summary, patients with schizophrenia are characterized by an increased incidence of overweight/obesity, and may experience further weight gain as a consequence of treatment with AP medications. The various APs differ in their liability to induce weight gain, and young patients with FEP and lower BMI before starting AP treatment seem to be particularly susceptible to this side effect.

DIABETES

Diabetes is a worldwide growing health problem. It is associated with increased mortality and morbidity due to CVD, hypertension, and stroke. Diagnostic criteria for diabetes and prediabetes (a condition characterized by impaired fasting glucose [IFG] or impaired glucose tolerance [IGT], whereby relevant glucose measures are not high enough to meet the criteria for diabetes, but are still associated with increased risk of adverse medical outcomes) are shown in **Table 1**.[34,35]

The association between diabetes and schizophrenia has been recognized for more than a century.[36] Reports of abnormal glucose regulation among schizophrenic patients predate the introduction of AP therapy,[37] suggesting that patients with psychotic disorders may have an elevated risk for disturbances in glucose regulation, independent of any adverse medication effect. Three large chart reviews confirmed increased rates of diabetes in patients with schizophrenia compared with the general population.[38–40] Recently, an increased frequency of IFG was reported in 26 drug-naive, first-episode schizophrenic patients.[41] Furthermore, Ryan and colleagues[42] observed that first-episode, drug-naive patients with schizophrenia had statistically significantly higher levels of intra-abdominal fat than age- and BMI-matched healthy controls, suggesting that schizophrenia may be associated with changes in adiposity that could increase the risk for insulin resistance, hyperglycemia, and dyslipidemia compared with the general population. In summary, the recent literature is consistent in showing a prevalence rate of diabetes of about 15% in patients with schizophrenia, or an increased diabetes risk of two- to threefold compared with the general population.[43]

The mechanisms that underlie the increased prevalence of diabetes in schizophrenia include genetic and environmental factors, because much of the increased risk can be ascribed to traditional diabetic risk factors, such as family history (up

Table 1
Diagnostic criteria for diabetes, IFG, and IGT

Diabetes (American Diabetic Association 1997)		
	FPG ≥126 mg/dL 2-HPG ≥220 mg/dL Symptoms of diabetes plus random PG ≥200 mg/dL	
"Pre-diabetes" (American Diabetic Association 2004)		
	FPG (mg/dL)	2-HPG (mg/dL)
Desirable values	<100	<140
IFG	—	140–199
IGT	100–125	—
Diabetes	≥120	≥200

Abbreviations: FPG, fasting plasma glucose; 2-HPG, 2-hour postload plasma glucose; PG, plasma glucose.

to 50% of schizophrenic patients have a family history of type 2 diabetes), physical inactivity, and poor diet. Moreover, it is now widely accepted that AP medications have the potential to induce or favor glycemic dysregulation. The first report of a link between AP and diabetes was published in the 1950s,[36] and during the 1960s a general acceptance that AP drugs could cause diabetes led to the introduction of the term "phenothiazine diabetes." The issue was forgotten until the observation that SGA may be associated with a higher risk of IGT and diabetes than FGA.[44–46] Case reports, case series, and retrospective studies based on the analysis of existing databases suggested that SGA have a significantly increased risk of new-onset diabetes compared with FGA. Differences also seem to exist among the SGA, with clozapine and olanzapine associated with the greatest risk of treatment-emergent hyperglycemia and onset of type 2 diabetes; risperidone and quetiapine seem to pose a lower risk for glucose dysregulation, whereas ziprasidone and aripiprazole seem to be associated with the lowest risk of hyperglycemia.[47] However, Haddad and Sharma,[48] in his review of retrospective studies, concluded that patients with schizophrenia treated with APs do have a risk of type 2 diabetes greater than patients not taking these drugs, but differences among the various APs are not epidemiologically relevant. Similar conclusions were reached by other investigators,[49,50] but not by Newcomer and Haupt,[46] who recently conducted a meta-analytical review, that included 14 retrospective analyses of existing databases. This review indicated that clozapine was consistently associated with increased risk for diabetes; olanzapine was also associated with increased risk for diabetes compared with FGA and no-AP treatment. Neither risperidone or quetiapine was associated with an increased diabetes risk.

Retrospective studies have methodological limitations as they do not adequately control for confounding risk factors for diabetes, and this may explain literature discrepancies. Prospective studies, accounting for potential confounders, are more appropriate for investigating the true association between APs and diabetes. In the CATIE study, olanzapine, compared with perphenazine, risperidone, quetiapine, and ziprasidone, was associated with greater increases in glycated hemoglobin, and in some cases required the addiction of glucose-lowering agents.[51] In that study, ziprasidone was the only compound associated with metabolic improvement. A prospective open-label nonrandomized study compared the effects of 6 APs on the development of metabolic syndrome, dysglycemia (IFG/IGT), or diabetes in 238 schizophrenic patients who underwent a systematic fasting metabolic evaluation and an oral glucose tolerance test (OGTT) before and after 3 months of AP treatment.[52] Aripiprazole was the only AP that was associated with no weight gain, improved glucose tolerance, and reduced incidence of metabolic syndrome, including reversal of diabetes occurring with previous treatment with other SGA.[52,53] Clozapine and olanzapine were associated with the greatest risk of weight gain and glucose alterations (including new-onset diabetes); risperidone, quetiapine, and amisulpride demonstrated an intermediate risk profile of weight gain, glucose metabolism abnormalities, and metabolic syndrome.[52] Similarly, a 24-week multicenter, open-label randomized prospective study compared changes in glucose metabolism in patients with schizophrenia receiving initial exposure to olanzapine, quetiapine, and risperidone, and found that glucose tolerance was significantly impaired during 6 months of treatment with olanzapine and risperidone, but not quetiapine. These differential changes were largely explained by modifications in insulin sensitivity.[54]

A recent systematic review and meta-analysis,[50] including 4 retrospective cohort studies and 7 prospective studies, concluded that SGA (excluding aripiprazole, ziprasidone, and amisulpride for which there were insufficient data to be included in the analysis) were associated with a 30% increased risk of diabetes compared with FGA in people with schizophrenia, but they were unable to find sufficient evidence to differentiate the risk associated with individual APs. Finally, 2 prospective studies on drug-naive, first-episode schizophrenic patients (which overcame the confounding effect of prior AP exposure) have been conducted. The first, including 160 Chinese patients who were randomized to a 12-month treatment with clozapine or chlorpromazine, found no incident case of diabetes and no between-group differences in fasting blood glucose.[55] The second study was performed on medication-naive Indian patients with schizophrenia who were randomized to receive olanzapine, risperidone, or haloperidol, compared with a matched healthy control group. The results of this study revealed that patients with schizophrenia, especially male subjects, had glycemic abnormalities before the initiation of any AP treatment, which confirms that schizophrenia itself has a higher risk of development of type 2 diabetes. Furthermore, the diabetogenic effect of FGA and SGA was confirmed, with olanzapine showing the most diabetogenic potential followed by risperidone and haloperidol.[56]

New-onset diabetes during AP therapy has also been associated with diabetic ketoacidosis as the presenting symptom, and in several cases this was fatal.[57] Most of the diabetic ketoacidoses have been observed with clozapine, olanzapine, and risperidone, whereas there is little evidence of diabetic ketoacidosis with ziprasidone and aripiprazole. Patients diagnosed with diabetic ketoacidosis were younger, less overweight at baseline, and included a higher proportion of women. The pathophysiology is likely to be complex, but, as the metabolic disorder is reversible after withdrawal of the drug, a functional defect rather than a β-cell destruction should be implicated.

Factors likely involved in the AP-induced glucose dysregulation include the pharmacodynamic profile of the drug, the underlying psychiatric disease, with its lifestyle changes, and the individual's genetic predisposition in weight maintenance, insulin resistance, and pancreatic function. In general, the rank order of risk observed for the SGA suggests that the differing weight gain liability of these agents contributes to the relative risk of insulin resistance and hyperglycemia.[10] This would be consistent with the observation that, in nonpsychiatric samples, the risk for adverse metabolic changes tends to increase with increasing adiposity.[47] However, evidence has been provided that weight gain or obesity may not be determinant factors in up to one-quarter of cases of new-onset diabetes occurring during AP treatment. In agreement with this observation, clozapine and olanzapine were suggested to have direct effects on glucose regulation by inducing insulin resistance, directly or via changes in BW and fat disposition, or limiting the capacity of β-cells to secrete an appropriate amount of insulin.[10,58,59] Experimental data demonstrate that low concentrations of clozapine and olanzapine can markedly and selectively impair cholinergic-stimulated insulin secretion by blocking muscarinic M2 receptors.[60]

In conclusion, according to Holt and Peveler,[61] it seems that the occurrence of diabetes in people with schizophrenia is largely due to traditional diabetes risk factors; schizophrenia itself is associated with a two- to threefold increased risk; any AP treatment may increase the diabetes risk up to 10%, and SGA versus FGA are endowed with less than a 2% increase of that risk, with some small differences among the various medications.

DYSLIPIDEMIA

Dyslipidemia can be defined as an alteration of 1 or more plasma lipids according to values defined by the National Cholesterol Education Program.[62] The incidence of dyslipidemia in patients with schizophrenia has been less studied than diabetes and obesity. A lifestyle survey, showing higher levels of obesity, reduced levels of exercise, and poor diets among schizophrenic individuals predicted an increased prevalence of dyslipidemia in this group compared with the general population.[63] The clinical significance of lipid changes is considerable because of their association with CVD, combined with the fact that individuals with schizophrenia are more likely to go undiagnosed[64] and, therefore, are less likely to receive treatment.[65] Furthermore, AP medications seem to be associated with an increased risk of dyslipidemia.

Data regarding the effects of FGA on lipid levels are limited, but high-potency drugs (eg, haloperidol) seem to carry a lower risk of hyperlipidemia than low-potency drugs (eg, chlorpromazine and thioridazine).[64] A recent comprehensive review on the effects of SGA on plasma lipid levels suggested that clozapine, olanzapine, and quetiapine are associated with a higher risk of dyslipidemia.[64] In the CATIE study,[51] olanzapine was associated with significantly greater increases in serum levels of cholesterol and triglycerides than the other drugs, even after adjustment for treatment duration. Ziprasidone and risperidone were the only SGA associated with reductions in serum levels of cholesterol and triglycerides. In a recent literature review, Melkersson and Dahl[45] concluded that the relative risk for hyperlipidemia is highest for clozapine and olanzapine, moderate for quetiapine, and low for risperidone and ziprasidone. Aripiprazole has a low risk of causing dyslipidemia. Furthermore, a retrospective chart review of patients who switched to aripiprazole from other SGA showed a decrease in levels of total cholesterol and LDL-cholesterol.[66]

The different AP incidence on lipid profile seems to be primarily related to their effects on BW and adiposity, but the development of glucose intolerance also seems to be involved, as insulin resistance is a key factor in the pathophysiology of serum lipids.[63] A few reports of substantial elevations in triglyceride levels with only modest weight gain raise the possibility of a direct AP effect on lipid levels by some as yet unknown mechanisms.[63]

METABOLIC SYNDROME

Weight gain, glucose dysregulation and dyslipidemia may contribute to the development of the metabolic syndrome in people with schizophrenia. The recent definition by the International Diabetes Federation (IDF) states that a subject to be defined as having the metabolic syndrome must have central obesity plus any 2 of the other 4 factors shown in **Table 2**.[67] In the general population, the presence of metabolic syndrome is a strong predictor of CVD, CVD mortality, and diabetes, although considerable doubt regarding its value as a CVD risk marker has recently been raised.[67–69] Studies in different ethnic patient samples consistently show an enhanced prevalence of metabolic syndrome in individuals with schizophrenia with a two to threefold higher rate of incidence compared with the general population.[70] A large Belgian study found a similar rate of metabolic syndrome, which was two- to threefold higher than in an age-adjusted population sample.[71,72] In the CATIE study, approximately one-third of patients met criteria for metabolic syndrome at baseline.[73,74] A troubling finding was that 88% of patients with dyslipidemia were not receiving treatment, as were 62% of the hypertensive patients and 38% of those with diabetes. Furthermore, as reviewed above, APs are associated with significant adverse effects on weight, lipids, and glucose metabolism,[10,75,76] which may increase the incidence of metabolic syndrome in individuals with schizophrenia. In a recent study of metabolic syndrome in patients diagnosed with schizophrenia in 2000 to 2006 compared with 1984 to 1995, those started on SGA had more than twice the rate of new incident cases of metabolic

Table 2
Clinical definition of metabolic syndrome by the IDF

	Risk Factors	Abnormal Values
Primary defining feature (required)	Visceral obesity	Waist circumference
	Men	≥94 cm
	Women	≥80 cm
Secondary defining features (at least 2 required)	Increased triglycerides	≥150 mg/dL
	Increased FPG	≥110 mg/dL
	Reduced HDL-cholesterol	≤40 mg/dL (men)
		≤50 mg/dL (women)
	Increased blood pressure	≥130/85 mmHg

Abbreviation: FPG, fasting plasma glucose.

syndrome after 3 years, compared with those treated with FGA (27.8% vs 9.8%).[77] In patients without metabolic syndrome at baseline, the risk of developing this combination of metabolic abnormalities was significantly greater in patients started on SGA.

The causes of metabolic syndrome are not fully understood, but a central role of visceral adiposity and insulin resistance has been demonstrated.[63] For the increased risk of metabolic syndrome and other metabolic abnormalities in patients with schizophrenia, 3 complementary and partially overlapping causes are put forward in the literature: lifestyle factors, aspects of the psychotic disorder, and AP medications. People with schizophrenia, on average, conduct a lifestyle which raises their risk for the development of metabolic syndrome: sedentary lifestyle, lack of regular physical activity, nutritionally poor food intake, substance use, and high rates of smoking.[10,47,78] Some of these lifestyle factors are influenced by aspects of the illness, such as negative symptoms and vulnerability to stress. Moreover, drug-naive first-episode patients were shown to have increased visceral adiposity, elevated glycemia, and higher cortisol levels,[10,75,79] which might explain the increased liability of subjects with schizophrenia to develop metabolic abnormalities even in the absence of AP medications.[10,36,47] The increased risk of developing metabolic syndrome under AP medications is in part related to their potential to induce weight gain; however, in up to 25% of cases of metabolic syndrome under AP treatment, no weight gain, or increased abdominal adiposity, was present, suggesting a direct link between the AP agent and the development of metabolic abnormalities.[10]

CLINICAL MANAGEMENT OF WEIGHT GAIN, DIABETES, AND OTHER METABOLIC ABNORMALITIES

It has been documented that a reduction of 10% in cholesterol levels results in a 30% reduction of CVD risk, a lowering of blood pressure of 4% to 6% decreases CVD risk 15%, and smoking cessation would result in a 50% to 70% lowering of CVD prevalence. Maintaining a BMI less than 25 lowers CVD risk 35% to 55%, and having an active lifestyle (20-minute walk a day) results in a similar decrease of risk.[80] There is a general consensus that physical activity has a mild to moderate positive effect on many metabolic and cardiovascular risk factors that constitute, or are related to, the metabolic syndrome.[81] Indeed, it has been shown that regular physical activity is effective in prevention and treatment of hypertension,[82,83] obesity,[84] IGT, diabetes,[85] and dyslipidemia.[86] Therefore, appropriate dieting, lowering blood pressure, increasing physical activity, and cessation of smoking should be important components in multidisciplinary programs for people with schizophrenia to prevent or treat the metabolic syndrome or single metabolic aberrations that frequently occur in these patients.

Weight should be routinely monitored in all patients with schizophrenia, and BMI should be used to monitor weight gain. Patients should be encouraged to monitor their own weight and report changes to the treating clinician. Ethnicity should be considered when determining weight classification, particularly in individuals of South Asian origin, for whom the BMI definition of overweight varies from greater than 23 and obesity from greater than 25. Ethnic group cutoff points should be used for people of the same ethnic group, regardless of their place or country of residence.[87] If the psychiatric team is adequately trained, measurement of waist circumference could be used instead of, or to supplement, BMI, as it gives an indication of visceral adiposity, which seems to determine the greatest health risks and has been shown to be associated with particularly high rates of type 2 diabetes, dyslipidemia, hypertension, and metabolic syndrome regardless of BMI.[88] Ideally, measurement of waist circumference should be taken at the start and during treatment.

All patients receiving an AP that is associated with significant weight gain (**Table 3**) and their care-givers should be informed of the risk of weight gain and the health risks associated with excessive weight. This requirement is especially important for patients who are overweight or obese at the start of therapy, or who have a family history of obesity or diabetes. Advice should be simple and focused on the importance of diet (reducing caloric intake) and exercise (increasing physical activity) in preventing initial weight gain, as subsequent weight loss is more difficult to achieve. Advice should also consider lifestyle and dietary issues commonly occurring in individuals with schizophrenia. Information on local facilities for exercise and physical activity, relevant support groups, and weight management groups should be made available to individuals who are already overweight.[89]

All schizophrenic patients receiving treatment with APs should be evaluated for undiagnosed diabetes or IGT at the start of therapy. Several factors should be screened, including family history of diabetes, ethnicity, age, obesity (especially abdominal obesity), poor diet, lack of exercise, high blood pressure, and dyslipidemia. Initial testing should be conducted regardless of risk factors and the presence of symptoms. Fasting plasma glucose level is considered to be the gold standard, although random glucose levels are acceptable in patients for whom fasting levels are impractical. Following initial evaluation, glucose monitoring is recommended. Monitoring every 6 months seems to be adequate in individuals with no change

Table 3
Metabolic and endocrine risk profile of SGAs

	Weight Gain Risk	Diabetes Risk	Dyslipidemia Risk	Hyperprolactinemia Risk
Clozapine	+++	++	++	±
Olanzapine	+++	++	++	+
Risperidone	++	+	±	++
Quetiapine	++	±	±	+
Aripiprazole	±	Insufficient data	Insufficient data	±
Ziprasidone	±	Insufficient data	Insufficient data	±
Amisulpride	±	Insufficient data	Insufficient data	+++

+, increased effect; –, no effect.

from initial measurement. More frequent monitoring is recommended in individuals with significant risk factors for diabetes and those gaining weight. If high glucose levels are found, referring to the general practitioner or to a specialist is recommended. The psychiatric team should ask patients with schizophrenia about the symptoms of diabetes. These include polyuria, nocturia, polydipsia, tiredness, visual disturbance, and vulvitis (in women). Diabetic ketoacidosis is a life threatening condition and requires emergency treatment. Symptoms include rapid onset of polyuria, polydipsia, weight loss, nausea/vomiting, dehydration, rapid respiration, and visual disturbance. Although it is unlikely to be detected during routine monitoring, the psychiatric team should be aware of and inquire about the symptoms, especially in patients receiving treatment with drugs associated with this condition. In a suspected diabetic ketoacidosis, urine test with Labstick or similar tests can effectively confirm the presence of ketones.

A pretreatment fasting (or random if fasting is difficult) lipid profile is highly advisable and should be obtained for all schizophrenic patients receiving treatment with AP medications. This profile should ideally include measurement of total cholesterol, LDL-cholesterol, HDL-cholesterol, and triglycerides, and should be repeated at least every 6 months after starting AP therapy.[63]

Metabolic risks should be taken into consideration by the psychiatrist when making appropriate treatment choices. There is evidence suggesting differences in the weight gain liability of SGA (see **Table 3**); evidence for differing effects of SGA on glucose and lipid metabolism is less convincing, although clozapine and olanzapine have been more frequently associated with a higher incidence of new-onset diabetes and dyslipidemia. The treating clinician should also consider the dismetabolic potential of other medications the patient is receiving (mood stabilizers, antidepressants, sedatives). If a patient develops metabolic abnormalities or a weight gain corresponding to 1 BMI unit, or greater than 5% increase of baseline BW, following initiation of AP therapy, consideration should be given to switching the patient to another AP with a less dismetabolic potential. When considering switching, the clinician must evaluate the risk of exacerbation of psychosis against the risk of metabolic adverse effects.

In conclusion, baseline screening and follow-up monitoring of metabolic parameters seems to be mandatory in patients with schizophrenia undergoing AP therapy (**Table 4**). Psychiatrists should be responsible for implementation of the necessary screening assessment, and should strictly collaborate with general practitioners and other specialists, when necessary, to pharmacologically treat hypertension, hyperglycemia/diabetes, or dyslipidemia. Education of the mental health team should not be

Table 4
Recommendations for initial and ongoing metabolic monitoring in schizophrenic patients

	Treatment Start	First Month	Second Month	Third Month	Six-Monthly	Annually
Personal/family risk factors	X					X
BMI/waist circumference	X	X	X	X	X	
Blood pressure	X			X	X	
FPG	X	X	X	X	X	
FLP	X			X	X	

Abbreviations: FPG, fasting plasma glucose; FLP, fasting lipid profile.

forgotten. Many psychiatrists, nurses, and other health professionals may be unfamiliar with the notion of metabolic risk and the means of assessing and treating it. These topics should be included in continuing professional development programs. Psychiatric treatment facilities should offer and promote healthy lifestyle interventions.

HYPERPROLACTINEMIA

Prolactin (PRL) is a polypeptide hormone produced by lactotroph cells of the anterior pituitary gland. Although it is best known as the hormone that elicits lactation in mammals, it is involved in a broad spectrum of functions beyond lactation and reproduction, including roles in metabolism, behavior, immunomodulation, and osmoregulation.[90] Generally, patients with schizophrenia have PRL levels within the normal range before receiving treatment for psychosis. It is the antagonist action of APs on D2 dopamine receptors in the tuberoinfundibular dopaminergic system that causes the elevation of PRL.

Although hyperprolactinemia may be clinically silent in most cases, AP-induced PRL elevation is endowed with short-term and long-term health issues. In the short-term, amenorrhea, or irregularities in the menstrual cycle with or without galactorrhea, are the most common clinical consequences of elevated PRL in women, whereas gynecomastia may be observed in men.[91] Hyperprolactinemia may also cause sexual dysfunctions with loss of libido or fertility and the inability to reach orgasm in both sexes.[91] Men may experience prolonged erection, or priapism.[92] Because PRL inversely affects estrogens and testosterone levels, prolonged hyperprolactinemia may induce bone mineral density loss, which may predispose patients to osteoporosis.[93,94] This is a serious issue in persons with schizophrenia, because they tend to have other risk factors for osteoporosis, such as sedentary lifestyle, smoking, poor nutrition, and pathologic water drinking.[95] Hyperprolactinemia has also been linked to an increased risk of developing breast and endometrial cancer in women,[95–97] but more research in this area is needed. Finally, there has been recognition that hyperprolactinemia may be temporally associated with insulin resistance.[98,99]

Hyperprolactinemia has long been recognized to occur in patients receiving FGA, ranging from 33% to 87% of patients treated.[100] The potential impact on PRL levels varies among SGA (see **Table 3**).[91] Amisulpride is probably the SGA with the maximum potential for PRL elevation. Kopecek and colleagues[101] suggested that doses of amisulpiride as low as 50 mg/d can induce hyperprolactinemia in almost all cases, with significantly higher values in women than men. Aripiprazole is associated with a low rate of hyperprolactinemia (<5%), consistent with its pharmacology as a D2 partial agonist.[102] Clozapine has a weak binding affinity for dopamine D2 receptors and is not expected to be associated with elevations in PRL plasma levels, with studies reporting a prevalence of hyperprolactinemia ranging from 0% to 5%.[103–105] The occasional finding of hyperprolactinemia in clozapine-treated patients may be explained by transient drug level elevations in the first hours after medicating,[106] and seems to have no clinical relevance. Risperidone is probably the SGA for which the major clinical data are available. Fourteen clinical trials from 1999 to 2008 reported risperidone as able to induce hyperprolactinemia in 72% to 100% of patients, with plasma levels of the hormone almost double in women than in men.[100] The dose used may be important, as less than 4 mg/d risperidone may have lower PRL-elevating potential.[107] Paliperidone, a recently licensed SGA, is the major active metabolite of risperidone and is probably predominantly responsible for the PRL elevation found with both drugs.[108] Although 2 RCTs have supported the notion that quetiapine is a PRL-sparing AP,[109,110] some studies have reported a prevalence of hyperprolactinemia ranging from 0% to 29%.[100] Olanzapine is associated with mild and transient hyperprolactinemia, with an estimated prevalence of the alteration ranging from 6% to 40%.[100]

MANAGING HYPERPROLACTINEMIA

The PRL-raising potential of AP drugs should be considered when starting treatment, and, ideally, should be discussed with the patient. However, there may be clinical situations in which the discussion may be postponed until the mental state improves. Recent guidance from the American Psychiatric Association suggests that PRL-screening should be done only in those patients with relevant symptoms[111]; however, some investigators suggest that it may be appropriate to assess PRL levels before starting any AP medication with PRL-raising potential.[112] The subsequent monitoring will assess the development of relevant symptoms (gynecomastia, galactorrhea, infertility, menstrual irregularities, and sexual dysfunction including decreased libido, impaired arousal, and impaired orgasm). The decision on how to treat a patient with raised PRL should follow a careful risk/benefit analysis. The management options include: (1) decreasing current AP dose; (2) switching to a PRL-sparing AP; (3) introducing a dopamine agonist or estrogen (for women). The effectiveness of decreasing AP doses has not been systematically studied, and although it is uncertain whether this strategy can decrease PRL levels, it can certainly raise the risk of deteriorating mental state. The evidence is probably best for the strategy of switching to a PRL-sparing AP that leads to a lowered PRL level, but this may still present a significant risk of relapse.[112] If it is not possible, or desirable, to switch or decrease an AP, hyperprolactinemia can be successfully treated with dopamine agonists (bromocriptine, amantadine, cabergoline). Current opinion is that these agents can be effective in reducing PRL levels; however, the potential for exacerbating psychotic symptoms suggests extreme caution in using these drugs in people with schizophrenia. In women for whom switching AP is not the preferable option, combined oral contraceptives can prevent symptoms associated with estrogen deficiency,[91] although PRL-related symptoms will persist, so this strategy should be carefully considered.

SUMMARY

Individuals with schizophrenia are more likely to be overweight/obese, and to have hyperglycemia/diabetes and dyslipidemia, which, together with the higher prevalence of other modifiable risk factors for CVD, such as smoking and hypertension, put them at higher risk of CVD. Indeed, it is widely accepted that the mortality for CVD in patients with schizophrenia is 2 to 3 times higher than in the general population.[3] Although these cardio-metabolic risk factors are attributable to the unhealthy lifestyle of individuals with schizophrenia, such as poor diet and sedentary behavior, recent evidence has shown that the APs have a significant negative impact on the metabolic risk factors.[113] Part of this negative impact can be explained by the liability of some APs, especially SGA, to induce significant weight gain. Data reviewed above show that young patients experiencing FEP are particularly susceptible to rapid and severe weight gain and to experiencing physical adverse effects related to AP drugs, such as metabolic disturbances and increase in abdominal fat mass.[114,115] Moreover, young patients are more sensitive to body image and self-esteem issues, thus transforming weight gain into social discrimination and stigma.[116,117] This may exacerbate the natural pharmacological noncompliance that characterizes younger patients, less disposed to adhering to medication regimens.[118] At present, there is no way to predict which patients will experience AP-induced metabolic abnormalities. Pharmacogenomic studies certainly would be extremely valuable to clinicians to identify individuals at high risk, but, although some interesting findings have been produced by genetic association studies and whole genome and linkage studies, no conclusive data have been provided so far. Therefore, more studies are needed to cope with weight gain and other metabolic abnormalities of people suffering from schizophrenia.

Psychiatrists should be aware of the cardio-metabolic risk carried by schizophrenia itself and of the different potentials of APs to increase such risk.[119,120] They should make every effort to prevent or minimize this risk to improve the quality of life of their patients with schizophrenia.

REFERENCES

1. Harris EC, Barraclough B. Excess mortality of mental disorder. Br J Psychiatry 1998;173:11–53.
2. Colton CW, Manderscheid RW. Congruencies in increased mortality rates, years of potential life lost, and causes of death among public mental health clients in eight states. Prev Chronic Dis 2006;3:A42.
3. Osby U, Correia N, Brandt L, et al. Mortality and causes of death in schizophrenia in Stockholm County, Sweden. Schizophr Res 2000;45(1–2):21–8.
4. World Health Organization. Body mass index (BMI). Available at: www.euro.who.int/nutrition/20030507. Accessed March, 2009.
5. Willet WC, Dietz WH, Colditz GA. Guidelines for healthy weight. N Engl J Med 1999;341:427–34.
6. Colditz GA, Willet WC, Stampfer MJ, et al. Weight as a risk factor for clinical diabetes in women. Am J Epidemiol 1990;132:501–13.
7. Mokdad AH, Ford ES, Bowman BA, et al. Prevalence of obesity, diabetes, and obesity-related health risk factors. J Am Med Assoc 2003;289:76–9.
8. Must A, Spadano J, Coakley EH, et al. The disease burden associated with overweight and obesity. J Am Med Assoc 1998;282:1523–9.
9. Marder SR, Essock SM, Miller AL, et al. Physical health monitoring of patients with schizophrenia. Am J Psychiatry 2004;161:1334–49.
10. Newcomer JW. Second generation (atypical) antipsychotics and metabolic effects. A comprehensive literature review. CNS Drugs 2005;19(1):1–93.
11. Green AI, Patel JK, Goisman RM, et al. Weight gain from novel antipsychotic drugs: need for action. Gen Hosp Psychiatry 2000;22(4):224–35.
12. Sussman N. Review of atypical antipsychotics and weight gain. J Clin Psychiatry 2001;62(23):5–12.
13. Weiden PJ, Mackell JA, McDonnell DD. Obesity as a risk factor for antipsychotic noncompliance. Schizophr Res 2004;66(1):51–7.
14. Allison DB, Mentore JL, Heo M, et al. Antipsychotic-induced weight gain: a comprehensive research synthesis. Am J Psychiatry 1999;156:1686–96.
15. Lieberman JA, Stroup TS, McEvoy JP, et al. Effectiveness of antipsychotic drugs on patients with chronic schizophrenia. N Engl J Med 2005;353:1209–23.
16. Dossenbach M, Arango-Davila C, Silva IH, et al. Response and relapse in patients with schizophrenia treated with olanzapine, risperidone, quetiapine or haloperidol: 12-month follow-up of the Intercontinental Schizophrenia Outpatient Health Outcomes (IC-SOHO) Study. J Clin Psychiatry 2005;66:1021–30.
17. Lieberman J, McEvoy JP, Perkins D, et al. Comparison of atypicals in first-episode psychosis: a randomized, 52-week comparison of olanzapine, quetiapine and risperidone [abstract]. Eur Neuropsychopharmacol 2005;15(3):S525.

18. Brecher M, Leong RW, Stening G, et al. Quetiapine and long-term weight change: a comprehensive data review of patients with schizophrenia. J Clin Psychiatry 2007;68:597–603.
19. McEvoy JP, Lieberman JA, Perkins DO, et al. Efficacy and tolerability of olanzapine, quetiapine and risperidone in the treatment of early psychosis: a randomized, double-blind 52-week comparison. Am J Psychiatry 2007;164:1050–60.
20. Kolotkin RL, Corey-Lisle PK, Crosby RD. Changes in weight and weight-related quality of life in a multicentre, randomized trial of aripiprazole versus standard of care. Eur Psychiatry 2008;23(8):561–6.
21. Pigott TA, Carson WH, Saha AR, et al. Aripiprazole for the prevention of relapse in stabilized patients with chronic schizophrenia: a placebo-controlled 26-week study. J Clin Psychiatry 2003;64:1048–56.
22. Kane JM, Carson WH, Saha AR, et al. Efficacy and safety of aripiprazole and haloperidol versus placebo in patients with schizophrenia and schizoaffective disorder. J Clin Psychiatry 2002;63:763–71.
23. Potkin SG, Saha AR, Kujawa MJ, et al. Aripiprazole, an antipsychotic with a novel mechanism of action, and risperidone vs placebo in patients with schizophrenia and schizoaffective disorder. Arch Gen Psychiatry 2003;60:681–90.
24. McQuade RD, Stock E, Marcus R, et al. A comparison of weight change during treatment with olanzapine or aripiprazole: results from a randomized, double-blind study. J Clin Psychiatry 2004;65(18):47–56.
25. Alvarez-Jimenez M, Gonzalez-Blanch C, Crespo-Facorro B, et al. Antipsychotic-induced weight gain in chronic and first-episode psychotic disorders. A systematic critical reappraisal. CNS Drugs 2008;22(7):547–62.
26. Alvarez E, Ciudad A, Olivares JM, et al. A randomized, 1-year previous atypical antipsychotic follow-up study of olanzapine and risperidone in the treatment of negative symptoms in outpatients with schizophrenia. J Clin Psychopharmacol 2006;26(3):238–49.
27. Whirshing DA, Whirshing WC, Kysar L, et al. Novel antipsychotics: comparison of weight gain liabilities. J Clin Psychiatry 1999;60:358–63.
28. Roth BL, Sheffler DJ, Kroeze WK. Magic shotguns versus magic bullets: selectively nonselective drugs for mood disorders and schizophrenia. Nat Rev Drug Discov 2004;3:353–9.
29. Matsui-Sakata A, Ohtano H, Sawada Y. Receptor occupancy-based analysis of the contributions of various receptors to antipsychotics-induced weight gain and diabetes mellitus. Drug Metab Pharmacokinet 2005;20:368–78.
30. Sussman N. The implication of weight changes with antipsychotic treatment. J Clin Psychopharmacol 2003;23:S21–6.
31. Muller DJ, Kennedy JL. Genetics of antipsychotic treatment emergent weight gain in schizophrenia. Pharmacogenomics 2006;7(6):863–87.
32. Lu ML, Lane HY, Lin SK, et al. Adjunctive fluvoxamine inhibits clozapine-related weight gain and metabolic disturbances. J Clin Psychiatry 2004;65:766–71.
33. Monteleone P, Fabrazzo M, Tortorella A, et al. Pronounced early increase in circulating leptin predicts a lower weight gain during clozapine treatment. J Clin Psychopharmacol 2002;22:424–6.
34. Report of the Expert Committee on the Diagnosis and Classification of Diabetes Mellitus. Diabetes Care 1997;20:1183–97.
35. American Diabetes Association. Diagnosis and classification of diabetes mellitus. Diabetes Care 2004;27(1):S5–10.
36. Kohen D. Diabetes mellitus and schizophrenia: historical perspective. Br J Psychiatry 2004;184(47):S64–6.

37. Haupt DW, Newcomer JW. Abnormalities in glucose regulation associated with mental illness and treatment. J Psychosom Res 2002;53(4):925–33.
38. Tabata H, Kikuoka M, Kikuoka H, et al. Characteristics of diabetes mellitus in schizophrenic patients. J Med Assoc Thai 1987;70(2):90–3.
39. Mukherjee S, Decina P, Bocola V, et al. Diabetes mellitus in schizophrenic patients. Compr Psychiatry 1996;37:68–73.
40. Dixon L, Weiden P, Delahanty J, et al. Prevalence and correlates of diabetes in national schizophrenia samples. Schizophr Bull 2000;26:903–12.
41. Ryan MC, Collins P, Thakore JH. Impaired fasting glucose tolerance in first-episode, drug naive patients with schizophrenia. Am J Psychiatry 2003; 160(2):284–9.
42. Ryan MC, Flanagan S, Kinsella U, et al. The effects of atypical antipsychotics on visceral fat distribution in first episode, drug-naive patients with schizophrenia. Life Sci 2004;74(16):1999–2008.
43. Henderson DC. Schizophrenia and comorbid metabolic disorders. J Clin Psychiatry 2005;66(6):11–20.
44. Hedenmalm K, Hagg S, Stahl M, et al. Glucose intolerance with atypical antipsychotics. Drug Saf 2002;25:1107–16.
45. Melkersson K, Dahl ML. Adverse metabolic effects associated with atypical antipsychotics: literature review and clinical implications. Drugs 2004;64(7):701–23.
46. Newcomer JW, Haupt DW. The metabolic effects of antipsychotic medications. Can J Psychiatry 2006;51:480–91.
47. Scheen AJ, De Hert MA. Abnormal glucose metabolism in patients treated with antipsychotics. Diabete Metab 2007;33:169–75.
48. Haddad PM, Sharma SG. Adverse effect of atypical antipsychotics. Differential risk and clinical implications. CNS Drugs 2007;21(11):911–36.
49. Bushe CJ, Leonard BE. Blood glucose and schizophrenia: a systematic review of prospective randomized clinical trials. J Clin Psychiatry 2007;68:1682–90.
50. Smith M, Hopkins D, Peveler RC, et al. First- v. second-generation antipsychotics and risk for diabetes in schizophrenia: systematic review and meta-analysis. Br J Psychiatry 2008;192:406–11.
51. Lieberman JA, Stroup TS, McEvoy JP, et al. For the Clinical Antipsychotic Trials of Intervention Effectiveness (CATIE) Investigators. Effectiveness of antipsychotic drugs in patients with chronic schizophrenia. N Engl J Med 2005;353: 1209–23.
52. Scheen AJ, De Hert MA, Hanssens L, et al. Anomalies de la tolérance au glucose chez les patients schizophrènes traités par antipsychotiques de seconde génération: étude comparative prospective de trois mois. Diabete Metab 2007;68(1):1S129.
53. De Hert M, Hanssens L, Van Winkel R, et al. Reversibility of antipsychotic treatment-related diabetes in patients with schizophrenia. A case series of switching to aripiprazole. Diabetes Care 2006;29:2329–30.
54. Newcomer JW, Ratner RE, Eriksson JW, et al. A 24-week, multicenter, open-label, randomized study to compare changes in glucose metabolism in patients with schizophrenia receiving treatment with olanzapine, quetiapine, or risperidone. J Clin Psychiatry 2009;70(4):487–99.
55. Lieberman JA, Phillips M, Gu H, et al. Atypical and conventional antipsychotic drugs in treatment-naive first episode schizophrenia: a 52-week randomized trial of clozapine vs. chlorpromazine. Neuropsychopharmacology 2003;28:995–1003.
56. Saddichha S, Manjunatha N, Ameen S, et al. Diabetes and schizophrenia - effect of disease or drug? Results from a randomized, double-blind, controlled

prospective study in first-episode schizophrenia. Acta Psychiatr Scand 2008; 117(5):342–7.
57. Koller EA, Cross JT, Doraiswamy PM, et al. Pancreatitis associated with atypical antipsychotics: from the Food and Drug Administration's MedWatch surveillance system and published reports. Pharmacotherapy 2003;23:1123–30.
58. Bergman RN, Ader M. Atypical antipsychotics and glucose homeostasis. J Clin Psychiatry 2005;66:504–14.
59. Ader M, Kim SP, Catalano KJ, et al. Metabolic dysregulation with atypical antipsychotics occurs in the absence of underlying disease: a placebo-controlled study of olanzapine and risperidone in dogs. Diabetes 2005;54: 862–71.
60. Johnson DE, Yamazaki H, Ward KM, et al. Inhibitory effects of antipsychotics on carbachol-enhanced insulin secretion from perifused rat islets. Role of muscarinic antagonism in antipsychotic-induced diabetes and hyperglycemia. Diabetes 2005;54:1552–8.
61. Holt AIG, Peveler RC. Association between antipsychotic drugs and diabetes. Diabetes Obes Metab 2006;8:125–35.
62. NCEP Expert Panel. Third Report of the National Cholesterol Education Program (NCEP) Expert Panel on detection, evaluation, and treatment of high blood cholesterol in adults (Adult Treatment Panel III) final report. Circulation 2002; 106(25):3143–421.
63. Barnett AH, Mackin P, Chaudry I, et al. Minimising metabolic and cardiovascular risk in schizophrenia: diabetes, obesity and dyslipidemia. J Psychopharmacol 2007;21(4):357–73.
64. Meyer JM, Koro CE. The effects of antipsychotic therapy on serum lipids: a comprehensive review. Schizophr Res 2004;70:1–17.
65. Redelmeier DA, Tan SH, Booth GL. The treatment of unrelated disorders in patients with chronic medical diseases. N Engl J Med 1998;338:1516–20.
66. Spurling RD, Lamberti JS, Olsen D, et al. Changes in metabolic parameters with switching to aripiprazole from another second-generation antipsychotic: a retrospective chart review. J Clin Psychiatry 2007;68(3):406–9.
67. Ford ES, Giles WH, Mokdad AH. Increasing prevalence of the metabolic syndrome among US adults. Diabetes Care 2004;27:2444–9.
68. Hu G, Qiao Q, Tuomilehto J, et al. Prevalence of the metabolic syndrome and its relation to all-cause and cardiovascular mortality in nondiabetic European men and women. Arch Intern Med 2004;164:1066–76.
69. Sacks FM. Metabolic syndrome: epidemiology and consequences. J Clin Psychiatry 2004;65:3–12.
70. De Hert M, Schreurs V, Vancampfort D, et al. Metabolic syndrome in people with schizophrenia: a review. World Psychiatry 2009;8:15–22.
71. De Hert M, van Winkel R, Van Eyck D, et al. Prevalence of the metabolic syndrome in patients with schizophrenia treated with antipsychotic medication. Schizophr Res 2006;83:87–93.
72. De Hert M, van Winkel R, Van Eyck D, et al. Prevalence of diabetes, metabolic syndrome and metabolic abnormalities in schizophrenia over the course of the illness: a cross-sectional study. Clin Pract Epidemol Ment Health 2006; 2:14.
73. McEvoy JP, Meyer JM, Goff DC, et al. Prevalence of the metabolic syndrome in patients with schizophrenia: baseline results from the Clinical Antipsychotic Trials of Intervention Effectiveness (CATIE) schizophrenia trial and comparison with national estimates from NHANES III. Schizophr Res 2005;80:19–32.

74. Meyer JM, Nasrallah HA, McEvoy JP, et al. The Clinical Antipsychotic Trials of Intervention Effectiveness (CATIE) Schizophrenia Trial: clinical comparison of subgroups with and without the metabolic syndrome. Schizophr Res 2005;80: 9–18.
75. Tschoner A, Engl J, Laimer M, et al. Metabolic side effects of antipsychotic medication. Int J Clin Pract 2007;61:1356–70.
76. Meyer JM, Davis VG, Goff DC, et al. Change in metabolic syndrome parameters with antipsychotic treatment in the CATIE Schizophrenia Trial: prospective data from phase 1. Schizophr Res 2008;101:273–86.
77. De Hert M, Hanssens L, Wampers M, et al. Prevalence and incidence rates of metabolic abnormalities and diabetes in a prospective study of patients treated with second-generation antipsychotics. Schizophr Bull 2007;33:560.
78. Scheen AJ, De Hert M. Drug induced diabetes mellitus: the example of atypical antipsychotics. Rev Med Liege 2005;60:455–60.
79. Thakore JH. Metabolic syndrome and schizophrenia. Br J Psychiatry 2005;186: 455–6.
80. Hennekens CH, Hennekens AR, Hollar D, et al. Schizophrenia and increased risks of cardiovascular disease. Am Heart J 2005;150:1115–21.
81. Lakka TA, Laaksonen DE. Physical activity in prevention and treatment of the metabolic syndrome. Appl Physiol Nutr Metab 2007;32:76–88.
82. Fagard R. Exercise characteristics and the blood pressure response to dynamic physical training. Med Sci Sports Exerc 2001;33:484–92.
83. Pescatello LS, Franklin BA, Fagard R, et al. Exercise and hypertension. Med Sci Sports Exerc 2004;36:533–53.
84. Blair SN, Brodney S. Effects of physical inactivity and obesity on morbidity and mortality: current evidence and research issues. Med Sci Sports Exerc 1999;31: S646–62.
85. Lambers S, Van Laethem C, Van Acker K, et al. Influence of combined exercise training on indices of obesity, diabetes and cardiovascular risk in type 2 diabetes patients. Clin Rehabil 2008;22:483–92.
86. Saltin B, Helge JW. Metabolic capacity of skeletal muscles and health. Ugeskr Laeger 2000;162:59–64.
87. Tan CE, Ma S, Wai D, et al. Can we apply the national cholesterol education program adult treatment panel definition of the metabolic syndrome to Asians? Diabetes Care 2004;27:1182–6.
88. Janssen I, Katzmarzyk PT, Ross R. Body mass index, waist circumference, and health risk: evidence in support of current National Institutes of Health guidelines. Arch Intern Med 2002;162:2074–9.
89. National Obesity Forum. Guidelines on management of adult obesity and overweight in primary care. National Obesity Forum; 2004. Available at: www.nationalobesityforum.org.uk. Accessed March, 2009.
90. Fitzgerald P, Dinan TG. Prolactin and dopamine: what is the connection? A review article. J Psychopharmacol 2008;22(2):12–9.
91. Haddad PM, Wieck A. Antipsychotic-induced hyperprolactinaemia: mechanisms, clinical features and management. Drugs 2004;64(20):2291–314.
92. Knegtering H, van der Moolen AEGM, Castelein S, et al. What are the effects of antipsychotics on sexual dysfunctions and endocrine functioning? Psychoneuroendocrinology 2003;28(2):109–23.
93. Becker D, Liver O, Mester M, et al. Risperidone but not olanzapine decreases bone mineral density in female premenopausal schizophrenia patients. J Clin Psychol 2003;64:761–6.

94. O'Keane V. Antipsychotic-induced hyperprolactinaemia, hypogonadism and osteoporosis in the treatment of schizophrenia. J Psychopharmacol 2008; 22(2):70–5.
95. Tworoger SS, Sluss P, Hankinson SE. Association between plasma prolactin concentrations and risk of breast cancer among predominantly premenopausal women. Cancer Res 2006;66:2476–82.
96. Tworoger SS, Eliassen H, Sluss P, et al. A prospective study of plasma prolactin concentrations and the risk of premenopausal and postmenopausal breast cancer. J Clin Oncol 2007;25:1482–8.
97. Yamazawa K, Matsui H, Seki K, et al. A case-control study of endometrial cancer after antipsychotics exposure in premenopausal women. Oncology 2003;64(2): 116–23.
98. Schernthaner C, Prager R, Punzengruber C, et al. Severe hyperprolactinaemia is associated with decreased insulin binding in vitro and insulin resistance in vivo. Diabetologia 1985;28:138–42.
99. Foss MC, Paula F, Paccola G, et al. Peripheral glucose metabolism in human hyperprolactinaemia. Clin Endocrinol 1995;43:721–6.
100. Bushe C, Shaw Michael, Peveler RC. A review of the association between antipsychotic use and hyperprolactinaemia. J Psychopharmacol 2008;22(2):46–55.
101. Kopecek M, Bares M, Svarc J, et al. Hyperprolactinemia after low dose of amisulpride. Neuro Endocrinol Lett 2004;25(6):419–22.
102. Kane JM, Meltzer HY, Carson WH Jr, et al. Aripiprazole for treatment-resistant schizophrenia: results of a multicenter, randomized, double-blind, comparison study versus perphenazine. J Clin Psychiatry 2007;68(2):213–23.
103. Bushe C, Shaw M. Prevalence of hyperprolactinaemia in a naturalistic cohort of schizophrenia and bipolar outpatients during treatment with typical and atypical antipsychotics. J Psychopharmacol 2007;21(7):768–73.
104. Wong J, Seeman MV. Prolactin, menstrual irregularities, quality of life. Schizophr Res 2007;91(13):270–1.
105. Bushe C, Yeomans D, Floyd T, et al. Categorical prevalence and severity of hyperprolactinaemia in two UK cohorts of patients with severe mental illness during treatment with antipsychotics. J Psychopharmacol 2008;22(2):56–62.
106. Turrone P, Kapur S, Seeman MV, et al. Elevation of prolactin levels by atypical antipsychotics. Am J Psychiatry 2002;159(1):133–5.
107. Kleinberg DL, Davis JM, De Coster R. Prolactin levels and adverse effects in patients treated with risperidone. J Clin Psychopharmacol 1999;19:57–61.
108. Knegtering R, Baselmans P, Castelein S. Predominant role of the 9-hydroxy metabolite of risperidone in elevating blood prolactin levels. Am J Psychiatry 2005;162(5):1010–2.
109. Arvanitis LA, Miller BG. Multiple fixed doses of "Seroquel" (quetiapine) in patients with acute exacerbation of schizophrenia: a comparison with haloperidol and placebo. The Seroquel Trial 13 Study Group. Biol Psychiatry 1997; 42(4):233–46.
110. Potkin SG, Gharabawi GM, Greenspan AJ, et al. A double-blind comparison of risperidone, quetiapine and placebo in patients with schizophrenia experiencing an acute exacerbation requiring hospitalization. Schizophr Res 2006; 85(1–3):254–65.
111. Lehman AF, Lieberman JA, Dixon LB, et al. Practice guideline for the treatment of patients with schizophrenia, second edition. Am J Psychiatry 2004;161(2):1–56.
112. Walters J, Jones I. Clinical questions and uncertainty – prolactin measurement in patients with schizophrenia. J Psychopharmacol 2008;22(2):82–9.

113. Ucok A, Gaebel W. Side effect of atypical antipsychotics: a brief overview. World Psychiatry 2008;7:58–62.
114. Graham KA, Perkins DO, Edwards LJ, et al. Effect of olanzapine on body composition and energy expenditure in adults with first-episode psychosis. Am J Psychiatry 2005;162(1):118–23.
115. Perez-Iglesias R, Crespo-Facorro B, Amado JA, et al. A 12-week randomized controlled trial to evaluate metabolic changes in drug-naive first-episode patients treated with haloperidol, olanzapine or risperidone. J Clin Psychiatry 2007;68(11):1733–40.
116. Van Bruggen J, Tijssen J, Dingemans P, et al. Symptom response and side-effects of olanzapine and risperidone in young adults with recent onset schizophrenia. Int Clin Psychopharmacol 2003;18(6):341–6.
117. Gortmaker SL, Must A, Perrin JM, et al. Social and economic consequences of overweight in adolescence and young adulthood. N Engl J Med 1993;329(14):1008–12.
118. Coldham EL, Addington J, Addington D. Medication adherence of individuals with a first episode of psychosis. Acta Psychiatr Scand 2002;106(4):286–90.
119. Maj M. Physical health care in persons with severe mental illness: a public health and ethical priority. World Psychiatry 2009;8:1–2.
120. Sartorius N. Physical illness in people with mental disorders. World Psychiatry 2007;6:3–4.

Clinical Perspectives on Autoimmune Processes in Schizophrenia

Sun Young Yum, MD[a], Sun Kyoung Yum, MD[b], Tak Kim, MD, PhD[b], Michael Y. Hwang, MD[a,c,d,*]

KEYWORDS

• Schizophrenia • Autoimmune • Glia • Immune system

It is not uncommon to see a diagnosis of schizophrenia on the medical charts of patients with systemic autoimmune conditions being treated in psychiatric settings. These patients are often resistant to antipsychotic treatment and have volatile clinical courses. More frequently, we may encounter patients diagnosed with schizophrenia with multiorgan diseases. Sometimes, we wonder only in retrospect whether the patient's condition may have been autoimmune in origin. Chronic autoimmune illnesses (eg, systemic lupus erythematosus [SLE]) as well as acute autoimmune illnesses (eg, Sydenham chorea or chorea insaniens[1]) can mimic symptoms of schizophrenia, such as psychosis, obsessionality, and abnormal involuntary movements. Such symptoms wax and wane with changes in systemic antibody titers. It has long been speculated that autoimmune processes may be involved in the etiopathogenesis of schizophrenia. Rothermundt[2] summarized three main hypotheses for the involvement of immunopathological mechanisms in the pathogenesis of schizophrenia: infectious, autoimmune, and Th1/Th2 imbalance.

This article reviews the epidemiology of autoimmune conditions in schizophrenia, symptom manifestations of autoimmune conditions resembling schizophrenia, and the immunological changes observed in schizophrenia; and reflects on their associations with neurodevelopment, neurodegeneration, clinical course, and management of schizophrenia.

[a] Department of Psychiatry, The Commonwealth Medical College of Pennsylvania, Scranton, PA, USA

[b] Department of Obstetrics and Gynecology, Korea University Anam Hospital, Seoul, Korea

[c] Department of Psychiatry, Robert Wood Johnson Medical School, UMDNJ, Piscataway, NJ, USA

[d] Mental Health Service, Franklin Delano Roosevelt Hospital, Veterans Affairs Hudson Valley Healthcare System, PO Box 100, Montrose, NY 10548, USA

* Corresponding author. Mental Health Service, Franklin Delano Roosevelt Hospital, Veterans Affairs Hudson Valley Healthcare System, PO Box 100, Montrose, NY 10548, USA

E-mail address: michael.hwang@va.gov (M.Y. Hwang).

Psychiatr Clin N Am 32 (2009) 795–808

doi:10.1016/j.psc.2009.09.003 psych.theclinics.com

EPIDEMIOLOGICAL EVIDENCE

Patients with schizophrenia in general have been reported to have an increased risk of suffering from autoimmune conditions.[3] Patients with a first-degree relative with schizophrenia were reported to be significantly more likely to also have a parent or sibling with an autoimmune disease.[4] On the other hand, specific autoimmune conditions, especially organ-specific ones, have been reported to have negative associations with schizophrenia (eg, insulin-dependent diabetes mellitus[5] and rheumatoid arthritis[6]).

The largest epidemiological study on this topic, which used data from the Danish national registry,[7] showed that the prevalence of several autoimmune diseases was significantly higher among people with schizophrenia and their parents than in an unaffected control sample population. The study involved 7704 patients treated for schizophrenia, their parents, and 92,509 age-sex matched nonaffected subjects and their parents. Patients with schizophrenia and their parents had nearly 50% higher incidence of autoimmune diseases compared with control. Of 29 autoimmune diseases identified in the population, 9 were significantly more prevalent among schizophrenia patients compared with those identified in the control group, and 12 had higher rates among parents of schizophrenia patients than among parents of the unaffected group. Five diseases (thyrotoxicosis, celiac disease, acquired hemolytic anemia, interstitial cystitis, and Sjogren syndrome) showed higher prevalence among both patients and parents versus control subjects. Because the study design required the onset of autoimmune diseases to precede the diagnosis of schizophrenia, late-onset autoimmune conditions may have been missed.

According to criteria assessing the stringency of evidence determining whether a condition is autoimmune in origin,[8] these epidemiological studies linking schizophrenia with autoimmune diseases in the patients and their families offer only circumstantial evidence.

The criteria propose three levels of evidence: direct evidence (ie, transmissibility by lymphoid cells or antibody of the characteristic lesions of the disease from human to human or from human to animal, or reproduction of the functional defects characteristic of the disease in vitro), indirect evidence (ie, reproduction of the autoimmune disease in experimental animals or isolation of autoantibodies or autoreactive T cells from the target organ), and circumstantial evidence (ie, the presence of markers that are descriptive of autoimmune disease).

AUTOIMMUNE CONDITIONS IN PATIENTS WITH SCHIZOPHRENIA

Neuropsychiatric Lupus

The most studied indirect evidence of autoimmune etiology of schizophrenia is from neuropsychiatric disease in SLE (NPSLE). Prevalence of neuropsychiatric syndromes in SLE is estimated to be up to 90%.[9] Neuropsychiatric lupus can present with various neurological and psychiatric symptoms and signs, including psychosis.[10] The lack of vasculitis or cellular infiltrate in patients with NPSLE suggests that the pathogenesis may be different from the immune complex deposition of lupus involvement in other organs, such as the kidney.[11]

While there is no immune complex vasculitis and no reliable test for NPSLE, cerebrospinal fluid (CSF) immunoglobulin indices have been shown to reflect disease state in SLE. In 1998, Hirohata and colleagues[12] reported a case of SLE in which steroid-induced psychosis was associated with more manic features, normal CSF immunoglobulin indices, and unresponsiveness to antipsychotic treatment, whereas central nervous system SLE was associated with grimacing, catalepsy, negativism, elevated CSF immunoglobulin indices, and response to antipsychotic and steroid combination treatment.

More specific antibodies were identified subsequently, including ribosomal anti-P antibodies (anti-P), anti–endothelial-cell antibodies, antiphospholipid antibodies, or anti–N-methyl-D-aspartate receptor antibodies (NMDAR), which are often associated in an antibody-mediated injury to the nervous system.[13–17]

Anti-P had been proposed to help distinguish lupus psychosis from primary psychosis in childhood.[18] In a study of 20 patients with psychosis secondary to SLE, 18 patients had anti-P. Longitudinal studies of anti-P activity in 2 patients with psychosis revealed that anti-P levels increased before and during the active phase of psychosis but not during other exacerbations of SLE.[19] The elevations were selective for anti-P. Since this study, many subsequent studies have provided conflicting results.[20–22] These studies have used various immunoassay methods with varied reliability in detecting anti-P. One study reported that anti-P was associated with malar rash in Berlin and Shanghai, with lupus nephritis in Berlin, and with NPSLE in Japan and Berlin.[23] SLE patients with anti-P were found to have a greater frequency of anticardiolipin antibody.[24] Anticardiolipin antibody has also been associated with NPSLE.[25] Another study found no patient with NPSLE with anticardiolipin antibody to have anti-P.[20]

Lupus anticoagulant and anticardiolipin antibody are autoantibodies associated with thromboembolism. Antipsychotic medications have been associated with such antibodies,[26–31] and in a dose-dependent manner.[32]

A subset of lupus autoantibodies, anti-DNA, binds a peptide sequence in the NR2A and NR2B subunits of the NMDAR.[33,34] Serum with reactivity to DNA and NMDAR extracted from lupus patients elicited cognitive impairment in mice.[35] This study provides solid direct evidence that lupus autoantibody causes deficits in brain function. However, because the distributions of NMDAR subtypes vary with species, it is uncertain what kind of deficit this will translate to in humans.

Neurosarcoidosis, Neuro-Behçet

Other systemic autoimmune diseases can also present with symptoms resembling schizophrenia, a topic that has not been well studied. Bona[36] described a patient with several years of refractory psychosis and multiple psychiatric hospitalizations until the diagnosis of neurosarcoidosis. In a Rorschach study of 40 patients with neuro-Behçet disease, 30% of patients had rigid and extremely concrete thoughts while disturbances in perception or reality distortion were observed in 40%.[37] Psychotic symptoms were detected in varied rates (0.6%–2%) in those with neuro-Behçet disease.[38,39]

Celiac Disease

The large epidemiological study cited above[7] reported higher occurrence of celiac disease in patients with schizophrenia and their parents. A 1976 study suggested that wheat gluten had primary schizophrenia-promoting effects. Patients with schizophrenia were placed on a gluten-free diet with improvement of symptoms, but their symptoms worsened with reintroduction of gluten.[40] Higher levels of anti–gliadin IgA was observed in a subgroup of schizophrenia patients.[41] This is related to the theory that schizophrenia may not have existed before agriculture, which introduced neuroactive peptides from gluten. After observing a decrease in hospital admissions for schizophrenia in countries that had limited bread consumption during World War II, Dohan[42] suggested a possible relationship between bread and schizophrenia. He then observed that overt schizophrenia was rare in remote tribal areas of several South

Pacific islands where grains were rare, as compared with similar populations that had a higher prevalence of overt schizophrenia and grain consumption.[43]

NEUROTROPIC VIRUSES AND SCHIZOPHRENIA

It was suggested as early as 1857 that psychosis can be contagious.[44] Since then, various attempts to find proof of infectious etiology of schizophrenia ensued, ranging from epidemiological studies showing that first episode of psychosis occurs more frequently in people who live in apartment blocks with schizophrenia patients, to animal transmission experiments.

Many infections resulted in psychotic manifestations resembling schizophrenia, including encephalitis lethargica, prion diseases, toxoplasmosis, and retroviruses. An influenza epidemic was followed by observation of increased risk of later developing schizophrenia.[45] A prospective birth cohort showed maternal viral respiratory infection to be associated with an increased chance of schizophrenia in the offspring.[46] Rabbits inoculated with influenza A virus produced antibodies that cross-reacted with a brain-specific protein in the human hippocampus, cortex, and cerebellum.[47] It was thought that maternal antibodies may cross the placenta and cross-react with fetal brain tissues, interfering with normal neurodevelopment. Pregnant mice with respiratory infection produced a syndrome similar to schizophrenia in the offspring, including defects in prepulse inhibition, thinning of the neocortex and hippocampus, and pyramidal cell atrophy.[48]

Herpes simplex virus has been linked to cognitive impairment in schizophrenia.[49] Cytomegalovirus,[50] Epstein-Barr virus,[51] and Borna disease virus[52] are among the many viruses reported to be associated with schizophrenia.

HIV has been associated with various neuropsychiatric manifestations, including psychotic illness.[53] Valproate[54] and lithium[55] may provide neuroprotective effects against HIV encephalitis. Moreover, antipsychotics may have antiviral activity against HIV.[56]

Human Endogenous Retroviruses

The most innovative thought on the infectious etiology of schizophrenia probably came from Crow[44] 25 years ago. He hypothesized that schizophrenia may be due to infection with a virus that becomes integrated in the genome and is sometimes passed from one generation to the next. Exogenously acquired viral genes can be integrated in the germ line. Retrovirus in particular carries genes for enzyme reverse transcriptase, which permits viral RNA to be transcribed into DNA, which can then be integrated into the host genome. Because the retroviral integration sites within the genome are random, the clinical consequences vary. Support for Crow's theory came only recently with studies reporting increased activity of human endogenous retroviruses (HERVs) in plasma, CSF, and brain tissues in patients with schizophrenia.[57–59] HERVs comprise about 8% of our genome. These fossil viruses were thought to be remnants of ancestral infections and constitute silent areas of the genome with no function.

How HERV is involved in schizophrenia is still unknown. Two hypotheses have been proposed. According to one hypothesis, the long-term terminal repeat regions of retroviruses contain binding sites for a variety of transcription factors, including those for hormonal and inflammatory mediators that can activate human genes. According to the other hypothesis, expression of viral proteins may directly affect cellular function, particularly immune/autoimmune responses.[57]

Dickerson[60] reported a strong association between the risk of type 2 diabetes in individuals with schizophrenia and the presence of genetic polymorphisms within the envelope region of the Herv K-18 endogenous retrovirus. Herv K-18 is located within the CD48 gene in the q22 region of chromosome 1, one of the more frequently proposed locations for schizophrenia-susceptibility genes. He concluded that polymorphisms in endogenous retroviruses, which are located near immunomodulatory genes, may constitute risk factors for diabetes in individuals with schizophrenia.

The genetic studies in schizophrenia have largely excluded repetitive regions of the genome, such as those that contain HERVs. Given the exciting latest developments, these are targets for further examination.

Another potential source of future exploration may be the prion protein gene. In a retrospective review of 100 cases of variant Creutzfeldt-Jakob disease (vCJD), some patients manifested with psychotic features, including auditory and visual hallucinations, paranoid behaviors, and delusions.[61] In sporadic Creutzfeldt-Jakob disease (sCJD), 53 of 126 patients had psychotic symptoms, including hallucinations, delusions, disorganized thoughts, and behavior.[62]

A suggestion for prevention of schizophrenia has been to design vaccines that eliminate infectious pathogens. Perhaps this should be done in consideration with Vaughan's findings that patients with schizophrenia may have decreased ability to produce antibodies in response to vaccines.[63] On the other hand, based on results showing an antipsychotic-induced increase in antibody production, perhaps antipsychotic medications may aid appropriate B cell activation and antibody production to vaccine antigens.

BACTERIAL INFECTION AND PSYCHOSES

Post–streptococcal neuropsychiatric syndromes have also been implicated in psychoses. People with a history of Sydenham chorea and/or rheumatic fever were at high risk for developing psychopathology later in life with a relative risk for schizophrenia as high as 8.9 in a 10-year follow-up of 29 Sydenham patients.[64]

IMMUNE SYSTEM ALTERATIONS

Leukocytes

Numerous studies in the 1990s have examined absolute and relative numbers of cells involved in immunological processes in schizophrenia, including $CD8^+$ and $CD4^+$ T-cells, monocytes, and natural killer cells, with varied results. These will not be discussed here as they do not provide specific information about the immunological processes in schizophrenia.

Autoantibodies Against Brain Structures

Heath[65,66] provided one of the earliest direct pieces of evidence of immunological etiology of schizophrenia. Abnormal electroencephalogram recordings in the caudate nucleus and septal area of schizophrenic patients were reproduced in monkeys after injection of IgG isolated from acutely ill schizophrenic patients.

In addition to antibodies associated with NPSLE, numerous other autoantibodies have been studied in association with schizophrenia. Antibodies to specific brain regions, neurotransmitter receptors, and organ nonspecific autoantibodies have been studied and reviewed.[67]

Microglia

Microglia are the macrophages of the brain and are thought to be involved in neurodevelopment, neurodegeneration, and neuroregeneration. It seems that activated microglia function as a "double-edged sword," with neuroprotective features predominating in the healthy nervous system and neurodestructive properties observed in various disease states.[68] Activated microglia have been suggested to be the culprits for inflammatory and degenerative diseases, such as multiple sclerosis, Alzheimer disease, Parkinson disease, amyotrophic lateral sclerosis, Huntington disease, and traumatic brain injury. Microglia are also demonstrated to have pathological effects on neural stem cells.

Activated microglia cells were observed in a subset of patients with schizophrenia from postmortem studies.[69,70] More recently, such cells were observed in a similar subset of patients in vivo via nuclear imaging.[71] Microglia quantification has also been suggested to be useful as a clinical predictor of suicide in schizophrenia. Significant microgliosis was observed in the dorsolateral prefrontal cortex, anterior cingulate cortex, mediodorsal thalamus, and hippocampus of patients with schizophrenia and depression who committed suicide.[72]

Reduction of activated microglia in schizophrenia may be a potential future treatment consideration. Sustained treatment with nonsteroidal anti-inflammatory drugs (NSAIDs) has shown to lower the risk of Alzheimer dementia by 55%, delay disease onset, attenuate symptom severity, and slow cognitive decline. The main cellular target for NSAIDs is thought to be microglia. In patients taking NSAIDs, the number of activated microglia is decreased by 65%.[73] Some antipsychotics have been shown to inhibit release of inflammatory cytokines and free radicals from activated microglia.[74–77]

Microglial activity in association with female sex steroids in schizophrenia is an unexplored area of research that may hold promise. Autoimmune conditions in general occur more frequently in women. Numerous animal and human studies support effects of sex steroids in immune modulation. Female sex steroids have been studied in autoimmune conditions whose symptoms are altered during pregnancy and the menstrual cycle. This effect may be regulated in part by hormonal alteration of microglial activation.[78] Since clinical symptoms of schizophrenia fluctuate with the menstrual cycle[79–81] in some women patients, examination of the gender differences in the immunological activity of schizophrenia may render better treatment strategies for volatile women patients.

Astroglia

Astrocytes serve as immunocompetent cells within the brain. They express major histocompatibility complex (MHC) class II antigens and costimulatory molecules (B7 and CD40) critical for antigen presentation and T-cell activation. As immune effector cells, astrocytes influence aspects of inflammation and immune reactivity within the brain by, for example, promoting Th2 responses. In addition, astrocytes produce a wide array of chemokines and cytokines.[82]

The most studied marker of astrocytic function is the S100B. Liu[83] in 2005 reported an association between a certain haplotype of the S100B-gene (four single nucleotide polymorphisms examined) and schizophrenia. S100B protein concentration has been associated with symptom severity, quality, and treatment response time.[84]

Cytokines

Cytokines represent one of the most widely studied areas in psychoneuroimmunology during the past decade. They have been studied in their absolute and relative quantities in schizophrenia during different illness states, and the results of these studies have often conflicted.

Various cytokines seem to influence the release of neurotransmitters studied in schizophrenia. Interleukin-1beta (IL-1beta) caused a profound decrease of glutamate transmission in the rat brain, but not γ-aminobuteric acid–ergic (GABAergic) inhibition, in hippocampal CA1 pyramidal neurons. This decrease by IL-1beta was prevented by pharmacological blockade of adenosine A1 receptors.[85] Some have suggested that IL-1alpha plays an important role in MPTP (1-methyl-4-phenyl-1,2,3,6-tetrahydropyridine)–induced plasticity of dopaminergic neurons.[86] IL-2 potentiates dopamine release. Interferon-alpha decreased dopamine activity in mouse brain[87,88] and chronic interferon-alpha potentiated latent inhibition.[89] IL-2 was found to reduce dopamine turnover in the caudate and substantia nigra in mice when administered repeatedly.[90]

Cytokines have been implicated as potential markers of illness states. Psychotic episodes have been shown to be preceded by raised levels of certain cytokines in the cerebrospinal fluid,[91] and treatment with cytokines can provoke psychiatric symptoms.[92] Cytokines are known to affect brain development and adult synaptic transmission and plasticity.

Numerous studies have reported antipsychotic-induced changes in cytokine concentrations, especially reduction of serum IL-2 concentrations in schizophrenia.[93] However, these finding have been conflicting. In fact, Muller's Th1-Th2 imbalance theory in schizophrenia is based on evidence of decreased IL-2 production in schizophrenia, with subsequent increase with antipsychotic treatment.[94] Patients presenting with low concentrations of serum IL-2 and IL-8 concentrations at baseline showed less improvement after treatment.[93] Increased IL-6 has been associated with treatment resistance.[95] Clozapine-induced agranulocytosis has been associated with the inhibitory effects of cytokines.[96]

One important consideration in reading research measuring cytokines is that, according to Haack and colleagues,[97] cytokine levels are affected by age, body mass index, gender, smoking, infections, and medication history. These investigators found that, after controlling for these confounders, plasma levels of cytokines yielded little information about the immunopathology in schizophrenia. The gender effects may be more difficult to control. Sex steroids, with cyclical fluctuations in reproductive women, play complex roles to enhance or inhibit cytokine productions.

A clinical question pertaining to obstetrics is what the benefit/risk ratio is for anti-inflammatory or antiviral agents during pregnancy versus that of untreated maternal infection leading to changes in cytokine levels in the fetus, potentially leading to neurodevelopmental changes.

Major Histocompatibility Complex

The MHC is highly polymorphic and each individual inherits a unique combination of alleles. It was previously believed that the brain is immunologically privileged because normal, uninfected neurons were not thought to express MHC class I molecules. It is now established that neurons normally express MHC molecules,[98] which function not only in immune capacity, but also play critical roles in normal brain development, neuronal differentiation, synaptic plasticity, and behavior. Numerous studies have noted a genetic correlation between schizophrenia and MHC.[99]

In a mouse model of MHC class I deficiency, the main phenotypic presentation is the anatomical defect in normal developmental pruning of synaptic connection.[100] An enlarged lateral ventricle is also occasionally observed. These two features have also been reported in schizophrenia.

Human leukocyte antigen (HLA) genotyping of German schizophrenic patients showed that clozapine-induced agranulocytosis was significantly associated with both MHC I and II antigens, namely, HLA-Cw*7, DQB*0502, DRB1*0101, and DRB3*0202.[101] However, as the investigators point out, it is uncertain whether this association is due to causal involvement or linkage disequilibrium. Associations between increased HLA-DR7 and chlorpromazine-induced lupus anticoagulant have also been reported.[102]

MHC may be an important factor in determining the individual responses to infectious agents in the brain. Why some people manifest with psychosis and others don't in the presence of infectious microorganisms may depend on the different ability of HLA alleles to express peptide products to elicit immune response.

Semaphorin

A topic worth exploring in association with autoimmune processes in schizophrenia is the role of semaphorin. Semaphorins are best known for their roles in nervous system development. Semaphorins are also widely expressed in many organ systems and their derivatives, including the cardiovascular, endocrine, gastrointestinal, hepatic, immune, musculoskeletal, renal, reproductive, and respiratory systems. In the immune system, semaphorins are critical for various phases of the immune response.[103] Altered semaphorin function has been linked to schizophrenia,[104] and a semaphorin receptor, PLXNA2, has been identified as a potential candidate for schizophrenia susceptibility locus.[105]

SUMMARY

Similar to schizophrenia, many autoimmune diseases have complex etiopathologies, according to various theories, with numerous potential markers and varied clinical manifestations. There is so much published about each autoimmune condition and each immune component, often with conflicting results, that a clinical model to conceptualize autoimmune processes in schizophrenia is needed for effective patient care.

However, whether autoimmune conditions and schizophrenia are etiologically linked or merely coincidental, recognition of the immunological factors in individual patients with schizophrenia can have treatment implications. It is important to consider autoimmune or inflammatory processes even if the patients present with classic symptoms and signs of schizophrenia.

Immunotherapy may be considered as one augmentation option for refractory schizophrenia with possible autoimmune or inflammatory pathology. Immunotherapy may involve manipulations of genetic vulnerabilities, restoration of immune system homeostasis, or prevention through protection from infectious agents. In the future, stem cell transplants may be used to reset homeostasis of regulatory cells.

Although common understanding of antipsychotic mechanism has been largely reduced to a handful of neurotransmitters, a better understanding of the immunological mechanisms of antipsychotic and other psychotropic medications will be important, given the evidence of immune-modulatory and antiviral functions of antipsychotics.

Exploration of gender differences in immunological activities in schizophrenia may be helpful in developing individualized treatment strategies for women patients.

REFERENCES

1. Swedo SE, Leonard HL, Schapiro MB, et al. Sydenham's chorea: physical and psychological symptoms of St Vitus dance. Pediatrics 1993;91(4):706–13.
2. Rothermundt M, Arolt V, Leadbeater J, et al. Cytokine production in unmedicated and treated schizophrenic patients. Neuroreport 2000;11(15):3385–8.
3. Ganguli R, Rabin BS, Kelly RH, et al. Clinical and laboratory evidence of autoimmunity in acute schizophrenia. Ann NY Acad Sci 1987;496:676–85.
4. Wright P, Sham PC, Gilvarry CM, et al. Autoimmune diseases in the pedigrees of schizophrenic and control subjects. Schizophr Res 1996;20(3):261–7.
5. Finney GO. Juvenile onset diabetes and schizophrenia? Lancet 1989;2(8673): 1214–5.
6. Eaton WW, Hayward C, Ram R. Schizophrenia and rheumatoid arthritis: a review [review]. Schizophr Res 1992;6(3):181–92.
7. Eaton WW, Byrne M, Ewald H, et al. Association of schizophrenia and autoimmune diseases: linkage of Danish national registers. Am J Psychiatry 2006; 163(3):521–8.
8. Rose NR, Bona C. Defining criteria for autoimmune diseases (Witebsky's postulates revisited). Immunol Today 1993;14(9):426–30.
9. Brey RL, Holliday SL, Saklad AR, et al. Neuropsychiatric syndromes in lupus: prevalence using standardized definitions. Neurology 2002;58(8):1214–20.
10. West SG. Neuropsychiatric lupus. Rheum Dis Clin North Am 1994;20(1):129–58.
11. Hanly JG. Neuropsychiatric lupus. Rheum Dis Clin North Am 2005;31(2):273–98.
12. Hirohata S, Iwamoto S, Miyamoto T, et al. A patient with systemic lupus erythematosus presenting both central nervous system lupus and steroid induced psychosis. J Rheumatol 1988;15(4):706–10.
13. Conti F, Alessandri C, Bompane D, et al. Autoantibody profile in systemic lupus erythematosus with psychiatric manifestations: a role for anti-endothelial-cell antibodies. Arthritis Res Ther 2004;6(4):R366–72.
14. Karassa FB, Ioannidis JP, Touloumi G, et al. Risk factors for central nervous system involvement in systemic lupus erythematosus. QJM 2000;93(3):169–74.
15. Toubi E, Khamashta MA, Panarra A, et al. Association of antiphospholipid antibodies with central nervous system disease in systemic lupus erythematosus. Am J Med 1995;99(4):397–401.
16. Isshi K, Hirohata S. Association of anti-ribosomal P protein antibodies with neuropsychiatric systemic lupus erythematosus. Arthritis Rheum 1996;39(9): 1483–90 [Erratum in: Arthritis Rheum 1997;40(5):977].
17. Zandman-Goddard G, Chapman J, Shoenfeld Y. Autoantibodies involved in neuropsychiatric SLE and antiphospholipid syndrome. Semin Arthritis Rheum 2007;36(5):297–315.
18. Press J, Palayew K, Laxer RM, et al. Antiribosomal P antibodies in pediatric patients with systemic lupus erythematosus and psychosis. Arthritis Rheum 1996;39(4):671–6.
19. Bonfa E, Golombek SJ, Kaufman LD, et al. Association between lupus psychosis and anti-ribosomal P protein antibodies. N Engl J Med 1987;317(5):265–71.
20. Gerli R, Caponi L, Tincani A, et al. Clinical and serological associations of ribosomal P autoantibodies in systemic lupus erythematosus. prospective evaluation in a large cohort of Italian patients. Rheumatology (Oxford) 2002;41(12):1357–66.
21. Isshi K, Hirohata S. Differential roles of the anti-ribosomal P antibody and antineuronal antibody in the pathogenesis of central nervous system involvement in systemic lupus erythematosus. Arthritis Rheum 1998;41(10):1819–27.

22. Nojima Y, Minota S, Yamada A, et al. Correlation of antibodies to ribosomal P protein with psychosis in patients with systemic lupus erythematosus. Ann Rheum Dis 1992;51(9):1053–5.
23. Mahler M, Kessenbrock K, Szmyrka M, et al. International multicenter evaluation of autoantibodies to ribosomal P proteins. Clin Vaccine Immunol 2006;13(1):77–83.
24. Schneebaum AB, Singleton JD, West SG, et al. Association of psychiatric manifestations with antibodies to ribosomal P proteins in systemic lupus erythematosus. Am J Med 1991;90(1):54–62.
25. Yoshio T, Masuyama J, Ikeda M, et al. Quantification of antiribosomal P0 protein antibodies by ELISA with recombinant P0 fusion protein and their association with central nervous system disease in systemic lupus erythematosus. J Rheumatol 1995;22(9):1681–7.
26. Schwartz M, Kormilachev M, Kushnir M, et al. Lupus anticoagulant and anticardiolipin antibodies in serum of patients treated with risperidone. J Clin Psychiatry 2009;70(5):769–71.
27. Iyer HV, Moudgil H, Newman P, et al. Chlorpromazine-associated antiphospholipid antibody syndrome. Ann Pharmacother 2007;41(3):528.
28. Schwartz M, Rochas M, Toubi E, et al. The presence of lupus anticoagulant and anticardiolipin antibodies in patients undergoing long-term neuroleptic treatment. J Psychiatry Neurosci 1999;24(4):351–2.
29. Ducloux D, Florea A, Fournier V, et al. Inferior vena cava thrombosis in a patient with chlorpromazin-induced anticardiolipin antibodies. Nephrol Dial Transplant 1999;14(5):1335–6.
30. Kanjolia A, Valigorsky JM, Joson-Pasion ML. Clozaril-induced lupus anticoagulant. Am J Hematol 1997;54(4):345–6.
31. Matsukawa Y, Satoh M, Itoh T, et al. Plasmapheresis for a schizophrenic patient with drug-induced lupus anti-coagulant. J Int Med Res 1996;24(1):147–50.
32. Shen H, Li R, Xiao H, et al. Higher serum clozapine level is associated with increased antiphospholipid antibodies in schizophrenia patients. J Psychiatr Res 2009;43(6):615–9.
33. Gaynor B, Putterman C, Valadon P, et al. Peptide inhibition of glomerular deposition of an anti-DNA antibody. Proc Natl Acad Sci U S A 1997;94(5):1955–60.
34. Katz JB, Limpanasithikul W, Diamond B. Mutational analysis of an autoantibody: differential binding and pathogenicity. J Exp Med 1994;180(3):925–32.
35. Kowal C, Degiorgio LA, Lee JY, et al. Human lupus autoantibodies against NMDA receptors mediate cognitive impairment. Proc Natl Acad Sci U S A 2006;103(52):19854–9.
36. Bona JR, Fackler SM, Fendley MJ, et al. Neurosarcoidosis as a cause of refractory psychosis: a complicated case report. Am J Psychiatry 1998;155(8):1106–8.
37. Koptagel-Ilal G, Tunçer O, Enbiyaoğlu G, et al. A psychosomatic investigation of Behçet's disease. Psychother Psychosom 1983;40(1–4):263–71.
38. Siva A, Kantarci OH, Saip S, et al. Behçet's disease: diagnostic and prognostic aspects of neurological involvement. J Neurol 2001;248(2):95–103.
39. Akman-Demir G, Serdaroglu P, Tasçi B. Clinical patterns of neurological involvement in Behçet's disease: evaluation of 200 patients. The Neuro-Behçet Study Group. Brain 1999;122(Pt 11):2171–82.
40. Singh MM, Kay SR. Wheat gluten as a pathogenic factor in schizophrenia. Science 1976;191(4225):401–2.
41. Cascella NG, Kryszak D, Bhatti B, et al. Prevalence of celiac disease and gluten sensitivity in the United States clinical antipsychotic trials of intervention effectiveness study population. Schizophr Bull 2009 [Epub ahead of print].

42. Dohan FC. Cereals and schizophrenia data and hypothesis. Acta Psychiatr Scand 1966;42(2):125–52.
43. Dohan FC, Harper EH, Clark MH, et al. Is schizophrenia rare if grain is rare? Biol Psychiatry 1984;19(3):385–99.
44. Crow TJ. A re-evaluation of the viral hypothesis: is psychosis the result of retroviral integration at a site close to the cerebral dominance gene? Br J Psychiatry 1984;145:243–53.
45. Cooper SJ. Schizophrenia after prenatal exposure to 1957 A2 influenza epidemic. Br J Psychiatry 1992;161:394–6.
46. Brown AS, Schaefer CA, Wyatt RJ, et al. Maternal exposure to respiratory infections and adult schizophrenia spectrum disorders: a prospective birth cohort study. Schizophr Bull 2000;26(2):287–95.
47. Laing P, Knight JG, Hill JM, et al. Influenza viruses induce autoantibodies to a brain-specific 37-kDa protein in rabbit. Proc Natl Acad Sci U S A 1989; 86(6):1998–2002.
48. Fatemi SH, Earle J, Kanodia R, et al. Prenatal viral infection leads to pyramidal cell atrophy and macrocephaly in adulthood: implications for genesis of autism and schizophrenia. Cell Mol Neurobiol 2002;22(1):25–33.
49. Dickerson FB, Boronow JJ, Stallings C, et al. Infection with herpes simplex virus type 1 is associated with cognitive deficits in bipolar disorder. Biol Psychiatry 2004;55(6):588–93.
50. Dickerson F, Kirkpatrick B, Boronow J, et al. Deficit schizophrenia: association with serum antibodies to cytomegalovirus. Schizophr Bull 2006;32(2):396–400.
51. Delisi LE, Smith SB, Hamovit JR, et al. Herpes simplex virus, cytomegalovirus and Epstein-Barr virus antibody titres in sera from schizophrenic patients. Psychol Med 1986;16(4):757–63.
52. Waltrip RW 2nd, Buchanan RW, Summerfelt A, et al. Borna disease virus and schizophrenia. Psychiatry Res 1995;56(1):33–44.
53. De Ronchi D, Bellini F, Cremante G, et al. Psychopathology of first-episode psychosis in HIV-positive persons in comparison to first-episode schizophrenia: a neglected issue. AIDS Care 2006;18(8):872–8.
54. Dou H, Birusingh K, Faraci J, et al. Neuroprotective activities of sodium valproate in a murine model of human immunodeficiency virus-1 encephalitis. J Neurosci 2003;23(27):9162–70.
55. Dou H, Ellison B, Bradley J, et al. Neuroprotective mechanisms of lithium in murine human immunodeficiency virus-1 encephalitis. J Neurosci 2005;25(37):8375–85.
56. Jones-Brando LV, Buthod JL, Holland LE, et al. Metabolites of the antipsychotic agent clozapine inhibit the replication of human immunodeficiency virus type 1. Schizophr Res 1997;25(1):63–70.
57. Huang WJ, Liu ZC, Wei W, et al. Human endogenous retroviral pol RNA and protein detected and identified in the blood of individuals with schizophrenia. Schizophr Res 2006;83(2–3):193–9.
58. Yao Y, Schröder J, Nellåker C, et al. Elevated levels of human endogenous retrovirus-W transcripts in blood cells from patients with first episode schizophrenia. Genes Brain Behav 2008;7(1):103–12.
59. Karlsson H, Bachmann S, Schröder J, et al. Retroviral RNA identified in the cerebrospinal fluids and brains of individuals with schizophrenia. Proc Natl Acad Sci U S A 2001;98(8):4634–9.
60. Dickerson F, Rubalcaba E, Viscidi R, et al. Polymorphisms in human endogenous retrovirus K-18 and risk of type 2 diabetes in individuals with schizophrenia. Schizophr Res 2008;104(1–3):121–6.

61. Spencer MD, Knight RS, Will RG. First hundred cases of variant Creutzfeldt-Jakob disease: retrospective case note review of early psychiatric and neurological features [review]. BMJ 2002;324(7352):1479–82.
62. Wall CA, Rummans TA, Aksamit AJ, et al. Psychiatric manifestations of Creutzfeldt-Jakob disease: a 25-year analysis. J Neuropsychiatry Clin Neurosci 2005;17(4):489–95.
63. Vaughn WT Jr, Sullivan JC, Elmadjian F. Immunity and schizophrenia; a survey of the ability of schizophrenic patients to develop an active immunity following the injection of pertussis vaccine. Psychosom Med 1949;11(6):327–33.
64. Wilcox JA, Nasrallah H. Sydenham's chorea and psychopathology. Neuropsychobiology 1988;19(1):6–8.
65. Heath RG, Krupp IM, Byers LW, et al. Schizophrenia as an immunologic disorder. 3. Effects of antimonkey and antihuman brain antibody on brain function. Arch Gen Psychiatry 1967;16(1):24–33.
66. Heath RG, Krupp IM, Byers LW, et al. Schizophrenia as an immunologic disorder. II. Effects of serum protein fractions on brain function. Arch Gen Psychiatry 1967;16(1):10–23.
67. Jones AL, Mowry BJ, Pender MP, et al. Immune dysregulation and self-reactivity in schizophrenia: do some cases of schizophrenia have an autoimmune basis? Immunol Cell Biol 2005;83(1):9–17.
68. Rock RB, Gekker G, Hu S, et al. Role of microglia in central nervous system infections. Clin Microbiol Rev 2004;17(4):942–64.
69. Bayer TA, Buslei R, Havas L, et al. Evidence for activation of microglia in patients with psychiatric illnesses. Neurosci Lett 1999;271(2):126–8.
70. Radewicz K, Garey LJ, Gentleman SM, et al. Increase in HLA-DR immunoreactive microglia in frontal and temporal cortex of chronic schizophrenics. J Neuropathol Exp Neurol 2000;59(2):137–50.
71. van Berckel BN, Bossong MG, Boellaard R, et al. Microglia activation in recent-onset schizophrenia: a quantitative (R)-[11C]PK11195 positron emission tomography study. Biol Psychiatry 2008;64(9):820–2.
72. Steiner J, Bielau H, Brisch R, et al. Immunological aspects in the neurobiology of suicide: elevated microglial density in schizophrenia and depression is associated with suicide. J Psychiatr Res 2008;42(2):151–7.
73. Landreth GE, Sundararajan S, Heneka MT. Peroxisome proliferator-activated receptor gamma agonists: potential therapeutic agents for neuroinflammation. In: Wood PL, editor. Neuroinflammation mechanisms and management. 2nd edition. Totowa (NJ): Humana Press; 2003. Chapter 7. p. 152.
74. Zheng LT, Hwang J, Ock J, et al. The antipsychotic spiperone attenuates inflammatory response in cultured microglia via the reduction of proinflammatory cytokine expression and nitric oxide production. J Neurochem 2008; 107(5):1225–35.
75. Kato T, Mizoguchi Y, Monji A, et al. Inhibitory effects of aripiprazole on interferon-gamma-induced microglial activation via intracellular Ca2+ regulation in vitro. J Neurochem 2008;106(2):815–25.
76. Bian Q, Kato T, Monji A, et al. The effect of atypical antipsychotics, perospirone, ziprasidone and quetiapine on microglial activation induced by interferon-gamma. Prog Neuropsychopharmacol Biol Psychiatry 2008;32(1):42–8.
77. Kato T, Monji A, Hashioka S, et al. Risperidone significantly inhibits interferon-gamma-induced microglial activation in vitro. Schizophr Res 2007;92(1–3):108–15.
78. Drew PD, Chavis JA. Female sex steroids: effects upon microglial cell activation. J Neuroimmunol 2000;111(1-2):77–85.

79. Dalton K. Menstruation and acute psychiatric illnesses. Br Med J 1959;1(5115): 148–9.
80. Endo M, Daiguji M, Asano Y, et al. Periodic psychosis recurring in association with menstrual cycle. J Clin Psychiatry 1978;39(5):456–66.
81. Riecher-Rössler A, Häfner H, Dütsch-Strobel A, et al. Further evidence for a specific role of estradiol in schizophrenia? Biol Psychiatry 1994;36(7):492–4.
82. Dong Y, Benveniste EN. Immune function of astrocytes [review]. Glia 2001;36(2): 180–90.
83. Liu J, Shi Y, Tang J, et al. SNPs and haplotypes in the S100B gene reveal association with schizophrenia. Biochem Biophys Res Commun 2005;328(1):335–41.
84. Rothermundt M, Ponath G, Arolt V. S100B in schizophrenic psychosis [review]. Int Rev Neurobiol 2004;59:445–70.
85. Luk WP, Zhang Y, White TD, et al. Adenosine: a mediator of interleukin-1beta-induced hippocampal synaptic inhibition. J Neurosci 1999;19(11):4238–44.
86. Ho A, Blum M. Induction of interleukin-1 associated with compensatory dopaminergic sprouting in the denervated striatum of young mice: model of aging and neurodegenerative disease. J Neurosci 1998;18(15):5614–29.
87. Kamata M, Higuchi H, Yoshimoto M, et al. Effect of single intracerebroventricular injection of alpha-interferon on monoamine concentrations in the rat brain. Eur Neuropsychopharmacol 2000;10(2):129–32.
88. Shuto H, Kataoka Y, Horikawa T, et al. Repeated interferon-alpha administration inhibits dopaminergic neural activity in the mouse brain. Brain Res 1997;747(2): 348–51.
89. Bethus I, Stinus L, Goodall G. Chronic interferon-alpha potentiates latent inhibition in rats. Behav Brain Res 2003;144(1–2):167–74.
90. Lacosta S, Merali Z, Anisman H. Central monoamine activity following acute and repeated systemic interleukin-2 administration. Neuroimmunomodulation 2000; 8(2):83–90.
91. McAllister CG, van Kammen DP, Rehn TJ, et al. Increases in CSF levels of interleukin-2 in schizophrenia: effects of recurrence of psychosis and medication status. Am J Psychiatry 1995;152(9):1291–7.
92. Nawa H, Takahashi M, Patterson PH. Cytokine and growth factor involvement in schizophrenia–support for the developmental model. Mol Psychiatry 2000;5(6): 594–603.
93. Zhang XY, Zhou DF, Cao LY, et al. Changes in seruminterleukin-2, -6, and -8 levels before and during treatment with risperidone and haloperidol: relationship to outcome in schizophrenia. J Clin Psychiatry 2004;65(7):940–7.
94. Müller N, Riedel M, Ackenheil M, et al. The role of immune function in schizophrenia: an overview. Eur Arch Psychiatry Clin Neurosci 1999;249(Suppl 4):62–8.
95. Lin A, Kenis G, Bignotti S, et al. The inflammatory response system in treatment-resistant schizophrenia: increased serum interleukin-6. Schizophr Res. 1998; 32(1):9–15.
96. Sperner-Unterweger B, Gaggl S, Fleischhacker WW, et al. Effects of clozapine on hematopoiesis and the cytokine system. Biol Psychiatry 1993;34(8):536–43.
97. Haack M, Hinze-Selch D, Fenzel T, et al. Plasma levels of cytokines and soluble cytokine receptors in psychiatric patients upon hospital admission: effects of confounding factors and diagnosis. J Psychiatr Res 1999;33(5):407–18.
98. Boulanger LM, Shatz CJ. Immune signalling in neural development, synaptic plasticity and disease. Nat Rev Neurosci 2004;5(7):521–31.
99. Wright P, Nimgaonkar VL, Donaldson PT, et al. Schizophrenia and HLA: a review [review]. Schizophr Res 2001;47(1):1–12.

100. Huh GS, Boulanger LM, Du H, et al. Functional requirement for class I MHC in CNS development and plasticity. Science 2000;290(5499):2155–9.
101. Dettling M, Schaub RT, Mueller-Oerlinghausen B, et al. Further evidence of human leukocyte antigen-encoded susceptibility to clozapine-induced agranulocytosis independent of ancestry. Pharmacogenetics 2001;11(2):135–41.
102. Vargas-Alarcón G, Yamamoto-Furusho JK, Zuñiga J, et al. HLA-DR7 in association with chlorpromazine-induced lupus anticoagulant (LA). J Autoimmun 1997;10(6):579–83.
103. Yazdani U, Terman JR. The semaphorins. Genome Biol 2006;7(3):211.
104. Eastwood SL, Law AJ, Everall IP, et al. The axonal chemorepellant semaphorin 3A is increased in the cerebellum in schizophrenia and may contribute to its synaptic pathology. Mol Psychiatry 2003;8(2):148–55.
105. Mah S, Nelson MR, Delisi LE, et al. Identification of the semaphorin receptor PLXNA2 as a candidate for susceptibility to schizophrenia. Mol Psychiatry 2006;11(5):471–8.

Schizophrenia and Eating Disorders

Sun Young Yum, MD[a], Giovanni Caracci, MD[b], Michael Y. Hwang, MD[a,c,d,*]

KEYWORDS

- Schizophrenia • Eating disorder • Comorbidity
- Appetitive behavior • Body image

The heterogeneity of schizophrenia requires diverse and individualized treatment approaches. Accurate identification and subsequent management of comorbid psychiatric syndromes are determinants of outcome. Work has been done examining comorbid anxiety disorders, affective disorders, and medical disorders in patients with schizophrenia, but eating disorders has not been an area of much exploration.

Disturbances in eating behaviors in patients with schizophrenia have been described as pica, gorging, anhedonic displeasure from food, and starvation associated with paranoid delusions. Disturbances in eating and the distorted perception of body image are difficult to separate from the rest of the psychotic phenomena. Recognition of psychiatric symptoms as dynamic points of a continuum is advantageous in long-term clinical care. Schizophrenia and eating disorder symptoms exist on a spectrum and have subsyndromal disturbances.

Eating is a complicated integration of psychoneuroendocrinology. Despite the difficulties in defining the point of distinction between behaviors and cognitive perceptions that are and are not of categorically diagnosable severity, there are patients with clearer coexistence of eating disorders and schizophrenia that carry on independent courses. In this article, the authors present a series of clinical cases that portray a wide spectrum of eating pathology in patients with schizophrenia.

Symptoms have complex and varied sources and manifestations. Psychoanalysts have suggested that they are symbolic consequences of the mind's efforts to cope. Therefore, symptoms substitute one another in the context of remaining underlying conflicts. In this context, it is conceivable that the sources of the manifest symptoms

[a] Department of Psychiatry, The Commonwealth Medical College of Pennsylvania, Scranton, PA, USA
[b] Department of Psychiatry, New Jersey Medical School, UMDNJ, Newark, NJ, USA
[c] Department of Psychiatry, Robert Wood Johnson Medical School, UMDNJ, Piscataway, NJ, USA
[d] Mental Health Service, Franklin Delano Roosevelt Hospital, Veterans Affairs Hudson Valley Healthcare System, PO Box 100, Montrose, NY 10548, USA
* Corresponding author. Mental Health Service, Franklin Delano Roosevelt Hospital, Veterans Affairs Hudson Valley Healthcare System, PO Box 100, Montrose, NY 10548.
E-mail address: michael.hwang@va.gov (M.Y. Hwang).

Psychiatr Clin N Am 32 (2009) 809–819
doi:10.1016/j.psc.2009.09.004 psych.theclinics.com

are the roots of psychiatric comorbidities. This concept might be better understood if we draw an analogy from medicine. Hyperglycemia can result from pancreatic failure to produce insulin, peripheral insulin receptor insensitivities, absence of insulin cofactors, dysfunction of the signaling cascade after insulin-receptor binding, sudden intake of large amount of glucose, increased adrenal production of cortisol, and so on. At first glance, we merely observe a sign—increased blood glucose.

The concept of comorbidity in psychiatry has varied definitions. Comorbidity in this article does not refer to mere coexistence of distinct clinical entities. The concept of comorbidity used here is closer to the medical-genetic concept, referring to two illnesses that coexist at rates greater than that expected by chance. For example, diabetes, hypertension, dyslipidemia, renal failure, stroke, and ischemic heart disease may be comorbidities; whereas a patient with discoid meniscus who develops cataracts is more likely to have unrelated coexisting conditions.

There is lack of systematized examination of eating disorders and schizophrenia. The two diagnostic categories were traditionally thought to be mutually exclusive. Most of the evidence to date is from review of medical databases for coexistence of two diagnoses in the same patient's chart or assessment of eating behaviors in patients with documented history of schizophrenia without adequate assessment of the schizophrenic phenomena. Disturbance in food intake is not an eating disorder in itself, which at the core is a disorder of the self accompanied by the key diagnostic feature of body dissatisfaction or fear of gaining weight. The motives or drives are important considerations in eating disorders, rather than just in the manifest behaviors.[1]

The following cases discuss eating disorders symptoms in relation to schizophrenic psychopathology.

CASE1: UNCONTROLLED EATING WITHOUT COMPENSATION

Mr A was 58 years old with chronic schizophrenia and numerous involuntary admissions due to poor medication compliance and aggressive behaviors at his boarding home. He showed moderate conceptual disorganization, a few unstructured and unstable delusions, affective instability with sudden shifts to extremes, and absorption with autistic experiences, mostly hunger, with little awareness of others or the milieu. He had marked difficulties in delaying gratification, episodically leading to explosive behaviors when his demands, mostly related to food, are not met immediately. He asked for bananas, oranges, and sandwiches multiple times a day everyday then threw tantrums on the floor with complaints of hunger. He once frightened another patient's family by stepping into the visiting room and gulping down a dozen donuts and their coffee.

Discussion

Schizophrenic eating behaviors have often been viewed as lack of control. Kraepelin[2] described it as voracious gorging and Bleuler[3] thought there was "a tendency to swallow all kinds of things, even their own excrement, which is sometimes accompanied by gustatory enjoyment and sometimes not."

Bruch,[4] on the other hand, explored overeating as an adaptive defense against stress, for the maintenance of control. She thought that excess weight functions as an equivalent for or protection against the schizophrenic illness and that overeating and obesity may have positive values in the maintenance of clinical stability. She had described three cases that illustrated such defensive obesity and the dangers in weight reduction. The following case illustrates the adaptive function and simultaneously the maladaptive features of overeating.

CASE 2: EMOTIONAL OR REACTIVE EATING WITH PERIODS OF COMPENSATION

Ms B was 45 years old with diagnosis of undifferentiated schizophrenia and morbid obesity at body mass index 53.6, hypercholesterolemia, hypertension, and prediabetic range impaired fasting glucose. She had been stable and compliant with her regular depot antipsychotic injections and she had not been hospitalized for more than 4 years. She was college educated, intelligent, and pleasant. Her positive psychotic symptoms were not overt on examination, but she reported "constant noises" which she was able to ignore and cope with. She had more prominent negative symptoms, including blunted affect, some rigidity in beliefs, and apathy. Although she preferred to be alone, and tended to withdraw, she was very considerate and often displayed altruistic behaviors without expecting return of favor. Owing to her large size, she received unfiltered comments from other patients at her day treatment program about her size and how she should exercise and control what she eats. Although distressed, she would take on such abuse without any form of protest. She had gained more than 200 pounds since illness onset. She reported she could not resist the temptation to eat. What starts out as motivationally salient often resulted in a binge with subjective sense of loss of control, where she quickly ate large amounts of food beyond comfort, followed by feelings of depression and guilt about what she has eaten and over her body weight. Feeling embarrassed, she opted to eat by herself and subsequently tried to buy smaller packages of chips, cookies, then decided to keep food out of her house altogether as a means of controlling her eating. She has undergone numerous periods of fasting, commercial fad diets as compensatory efforts, but her successful reduction was invariably followed by return of binges. Initially she denied ever having experienced a sense of loss of control, but after some consideration, stated that she "used food as a crutch" to assist her through emotional distress.

Discussion

The experience of hunger is not innate, but something that contains important elements of learning. The ability to differentiate "hunger" from other signals of discomfort may have been incorrectly learned throughout development. As a result, emotional tension states aroused by the greatest variety of conflicts and problems can be mistakenly interpreted as physiological hunger.[5] The restraint theory contends that dieting leads to overeating and there may be no binges without prior restrained food intake.[6] We have reported that macronutrient preferences may predict disinhibited eating following highly restrained eating in patients with schizophrenia.[7] Ms B's binges are quite common binge eating observed in non-schizophrenic dieters. Binge is not so much a disturbance in appetitive behavior, but more a disturbance in the termination of eating. It is not the initiation of appetitive behavior that distresses patients, but the inability to stop eating once they start.

CASE 3: RITUALISTIC NIGHT EATING WITH PURGING

Mr C was 54 years old, had long history of schizophrenia with mild residual symptoms. He had vague paranoid ideas and ideas of reference, but has not had overt psychotic symptoms or hallucinatory experiences for many years while on various antipsychotic medications. However, he had moderate-to-marked negative symptoms of schizophrenia, with generally flat affect, emotional distance, apathy, and minimal spontaneous social contacts. He engaged in regular overeating 2 to 4 times a week, only at night after spending the day at his treatment clinic. What he ate during these large meals were not typical binge foods seen in eating disorders—he had 5 lbs of turkey, ham, or chicken. He denied intentional purging but reported involuntarily vomiting due to inability to tolerate such large intakes. He preferred to eat alone, although denied being embarrassed about eating in front of others. He felt compelled to chew his food a certain number of times before swallowing, and to wipe his mouth with a napkin a fixed number of times after each bite, and had numerous other rituals commonly seen in eating disorders. Although he denied being fearful of becoming fat, he had a defined weight range that he must stay within. He compensated for the food intakes with ritualistic exercise routines.

Discussion

The behaviors observed in Mr C, including eating alone, eating large quantities of food followed by vomiting, and eating and exercise rituals, bear many similarities to bulimia nervosa. However, despite objectively large quantities of food, there is lack of subjective sense of loss of control over food intake, which is inconsistent with categorical diagnosis of eating disorders per *Diagnostic and Statistical Manual of Mental Disorders-Fourth Edition* (*DSM-IV*). Additionally, the ritualistic chewing and diligent napkin wiping are not typical of binge eating that occurs rapidly. The question of insight is a puzzling one in both schizophrenia and eating disorders. Insight too, runs on a continuum. Mr C recognizes his meals as being excessive compared with his regular meals, and purposefully compensates for it.

One of the most distinctive characteristics in anorexia nervosa is lack of appropriate concern or denial of the seriousness of their low body weight.[8] Similarly, in bulimia nervosa the *International Statistical Classification of Diseases, 10th Revision*, criterion of "intrusive dread of fatness" or the *DSM-IV* criterion of "self-evaluation unduly influenced by body shape and weight" are not reflective of good insight.

According to a World Health Organization attempt to arrive at a consensus definition of schizophrenia, there was 97% consensus that schizophrenics showed lack of insight. However, 47% of depressed patients were also characterized as lacking insight.[9] Unbending cognitive schemas in eating disorders share many features with schizophrenic thought: fixity in the idealization of thinness and the disparagement of bigness; body image distortion; perseveration over hips, thighs, and cheeks; and the bizarreness of beliefs or rituals related to eating. Do they have overvalued obsessive ideas or are these ideas perceptual distortions severe enough to be somatic delusions?[10] The question is explored further with the next case.

CASE 4: PREOCCUPATIONS AND RITUALS RELATED TO EATING AND BODY IMAGE

Mr D was 53 years old with diagnosis of obsessive-compulsive schizophrenia, associated with preoccupations revolving around two main themes of recycling and cleansing. For example, he drank his own urine to recycle it, hoarded neighborhood garbage in his apartment in attempts to own a thrifty shop, ate popcorn from the garbage cans at theaters so as not to waste them, and engaged in superficial cutting to recycle color with the generous intent of donating red color to the world so little kids won't be disappointed when they want Kool-Aid. The ritualistic cutting also signified purification, which he religiously performed by drinking bleach. Although he denied preoccupations and rituals related to eating and body shape, he had a fixed numeric range in which his weight had to remain (155–160 pounds). He expressed not wanting to look like his friends who are getting rounder, wider, and "shorter in proportion." He felt compelled to put vinegar on all his foods, including sweet potato pie, lemon pie, apple pie, coconut pie, and pumpkin pie. The vinegar sour taste, he believed, helped him maintain his weight. He was not aware that this was at one time an actual fad diet.

He reported that he usually chewed his food to a certain consistency, checked before swallowing and regurgitated if he was not sure that it was right before going down. However, there were occasions when he gulped down large amounts of food with the sense of loss of control. He could not associate these events with any particular stressors including drinking or hunger. He said he did not need to compensate purposely for this uncontrolled eating because his body made more stool.

Discussion

Schizophrenia[11] and eating disorders[12] both have overlapping areas with obsessive-compulsive (OC) phenomena. Eating disorders, in turn, overlap with schizophrenic pathology. Those with anorexia nervosa were shown to have trait obsessionality with inflexible thinking, social introversion, overly compliant behavior, and limited social spontaneity.[13] These traits resemble schizophrenic negative symptoms. Patients with eating disorders present with a wide range of eating-related preoccupations or rituals as reflected in the Yale-Brown-Cornell Eating Disorder Scale.[14] These thoughts and rituals were shown to be largely ego-syntonic in both anorexics and bulimics,[15] similar to psychotic obsessive-compulsive disorder, which is somewhat nearer to a delusion than an obsession according to classic dichotomy along the spectrum.[16]

Disturbed eating behaviors are more overt in patients in their acute psychotic states. Disturbed body image and excessive weight preoccupations are also more readily disclosed in acute psychotic states. However, once schizophrenic patients are more stabilized to the point of being able to live independently, patient's own perception of body weight, body image as well as eating behaviors become more discrete. In order to obtain information about secretive and ritualistic eating behaviors, it is helpful to first inquire about the importance of body image and body weight in determining the patient's self-esteem. Once this is established, the patient may offer very rich details of his/her eating disorders.

A remaining question is whether OC phenomena are stable features in patients with eating disorders, or a consequence of malnutrition. In the Minnesota starvation study,[16] physically and psychologically healthy subjects were carefully selected out of a large group of volunteers. However, as starvation continued, subjects became increasingly preoccupied with food. Some even pursued new food-related vocations after refeeding and study termination.

It is not uncommon to meet a patient whose first psychotic episode was immediately preceded by preoccupations with body weight/image and periods of fasting. These patients recollect this period to be intensely distressing, and in some patients, it seems that obsessive compulsive reactions offered them a certain level of comfort.

Whereas patients with eating disorders generally have, albeit a smokescreen, reasons for their behaviors, only some patients with schizophrenia have explanations. For those patients without even fantastical explanations (such as Mr D), it seems that what started out as purposeful behaviors lose their purpose as psychotic states progress and only repetitive behaviors remain.

Another interesting feature of schizophrenic patients' restrictive diets is that some of them appear to be able to maintain monotonous diets for an extended period, eg, one man reported having eaten nothing but cottage cheese during the past year, while another patient reported eating only Cheerios for a month.

There are other patients that are stuck on idiosyncratic features of food, eg, only eating purple foods, only eating foods having perfect square sides, eating only in even numbers. Anecdotally, when different authors rated the same patients' positive and negative syndrome scale (PANSS) scores on the same day, one during a regular clinical follow-up interview, and another during a research interview focused on eating disorders symptoms, the latter interviewer picked up much richer symptoms and rated higher scores.

CASE 5: RESTRICTIVE EATING ASSOCIATED WITH POSITIVE PSYCHOTIC SYMPTOMS

Ms E was 43 years old, with numerous psychiatric admissions for medication noncompliant schizophrenia. She was brought in by family for refusing to eat because she "[did] not wish to be immortal." She was initially admitted to the psychiatric inpatient unit, continued to refuse solid food, drank little amounts of fluid, and was transferred to medicine 9 days later because of dehydration (blood urea nitrogen/creatinine [BUN/Cr] 18/0.7 = 25.7). Upon transfer, she was malodorous, unkempt, and made no eye contact. Her speech was barely audible, yet she had excessive verbal output and was tangential and derailing with little content. She had bizarre persecutory delusions and delusions of reference. As starvation progressed, she became increasingly preoccupied with food, yet refusing to eat owing to appetites for bizarre concoctions, for example shellfish with little infants' heads on them. She was force-fed via nasogastric tube. Despite paranoid ideas and furious resistance against the nasogastric tube, she never attempted to pull it out. She appeared to have no volition or motivation of any kind. After one day of aggressive hydration, her hydration status improved to BUN/Cr 7/0.6 = 11.7. She was gradually advanced to full-strength tube feeding which she tolerated well with transient refeeding thermogenesis. Meanwhile, her antipsychotic had not been given to her because of a transcription error. She became more alert, awake, and still bizarrely delusional, but her thought process was more goal-directed by day 3 (brief psychiatric rating scale score improvement from 64 to 38), after which she started to receive olanzapine. At day 6, Ms E stated she was hungry, asked for ice cream, fresh fish, fresh vegetables, and she was transferred back to psychiatry.

Discussion

It is unclear whether Ms E's malnutrition is entirely or partly attributable to psychotic decompensation or vice versa. Common clinical intuition is likely to suggest that the presence of disorganized thinking and poor insight led to an illogical self-induced starvation. Nevertheless, refeeding alone resulted in significant symptom improvement. Accounts of famine[17] and systematized psychological study of starvation[18] have established that starvation alone can precipitate psychotic symptoms. Aside from Ms E's underlying diagnosis of chronic schizophrenia, her initial presentation bears striking resemblance to subject number 234 in the Minnesota starvation study, who was a 24-year-old man with normal baseline Minnesota Multiphasic Personality Inventory and stellar physical health that volunteered to undergo 24-week semistarvation. In the first week, he was troubled by dreams of "eating senile and insane people" and by week 9 began voluminous writings that consisted of "ramble" and was noted to be "talkative, emotionally unstable, and somewhat elated." Whether he went on to develop schizophrenia is unknown, but the case illustrated that malnutrition, or perhaps subjective distress related to deprivation, can lead to psychotic breakdown in normal individuals.

Patients with anorexia nervosa often reach a point of complete refusal to eat accompanied by an unrealistic fear of gaining weight or delusional belief that they are fat despite being severely emaciated. Starvation leads to further distortion of body image and subsequent food refusal, which becomes a self-perpetuating cycle. Starvation itself is a psychosomatic phenomenon that comprises the behavioral, emotional, and social manifestations. In the broad sense, starvation is a state resulting from complex interactions between anatomical, physiological, individual-psychological, and social-psychological factors.[18]

CASE 6. RESTRICTIVE EATING RELATED TO NEGATIVE PSYCHOTIC SYMPTOMS AND DEPRESSION

Mr F was 50 yeas old, with residual negative symptoms of schizophrenia, heightened general anxiety, and associated depression, who punished himself by not eating. He had weight fluctuations of about 50 pounds because, when he started to eat in response to improvements in mood, it often led to binge eating with a subjective sense of loss of control, which he described as being "automatic." Because of shame and guilt related to delusional interpretations of his illness, he led a life of asceticism. Although he provided for his daughter throughout college and beyond, he feels too ashamed and inadequate to see her.

Discussion

Lack of self-esteem is frequently seen in schizophrenia and comorbid depression. Such self-esteem issues also appear to lie at the core of eating pathology and disturbed experience of self and body image in eating disorders.

CASE 7. RESTRICTIVE EATING NOT ASSOCIATED WITH PSYCHOSIS

Ms G was 29 years old, had a brief modeling career before being diagnosed with schizophrenia. She was most recently committed to psychiatric treatment because of poor food intake. Her thoughts were loose; she played with clang associations, verbigerations, neologism, and was often incoherent. She was frequently engaged in hallucinatory behaviors and displayed multiple systematized delusions of grandeur and persecution, which included bizarre somatic complaints including pseudocyesis. In addition, she was highly conscious of her petite figure and was very difficult to please in her dietary demands. She could not eat most of what was given to her and listed different food allergies with each tray. Occasionally, she would take a piece of chicken into her room, eat in bed by herself while carefully scrutinizing the food, tearing it in small pieces; it would take her half an hour to eat one chicken leg. Then she would be seen doing jumping jacks, throwing jabs while doing the boxing steps, and other calisthenics. She refused her medications because she was "the prettiest person on the ward" and had to stay that way. With forced medications, her thoughts became organized and her behaviors became socially inhibited and appropriate. However, even with improvements in positive psychotic symptoms, body image preoccupations and food restriction persisted.

Discussion

Ms E from case 5 appears to have had concurrent psychosis and starvation that had related clinical course. However, Ms G's positive psychotic symptoms, including conceptual disorganization, hallucinatory behaviors, and hostility, appeared to have independent clinical courses from those associated with anorectic cognition and behavior.

Bleuler[19] stated that, "In psychoses, food intake as well as general intestinal activity is dependent to the highest degree upon psychic factors … in no other mental disease does complete refusal of food occur so frequently and so persistently as in schizophrenia."

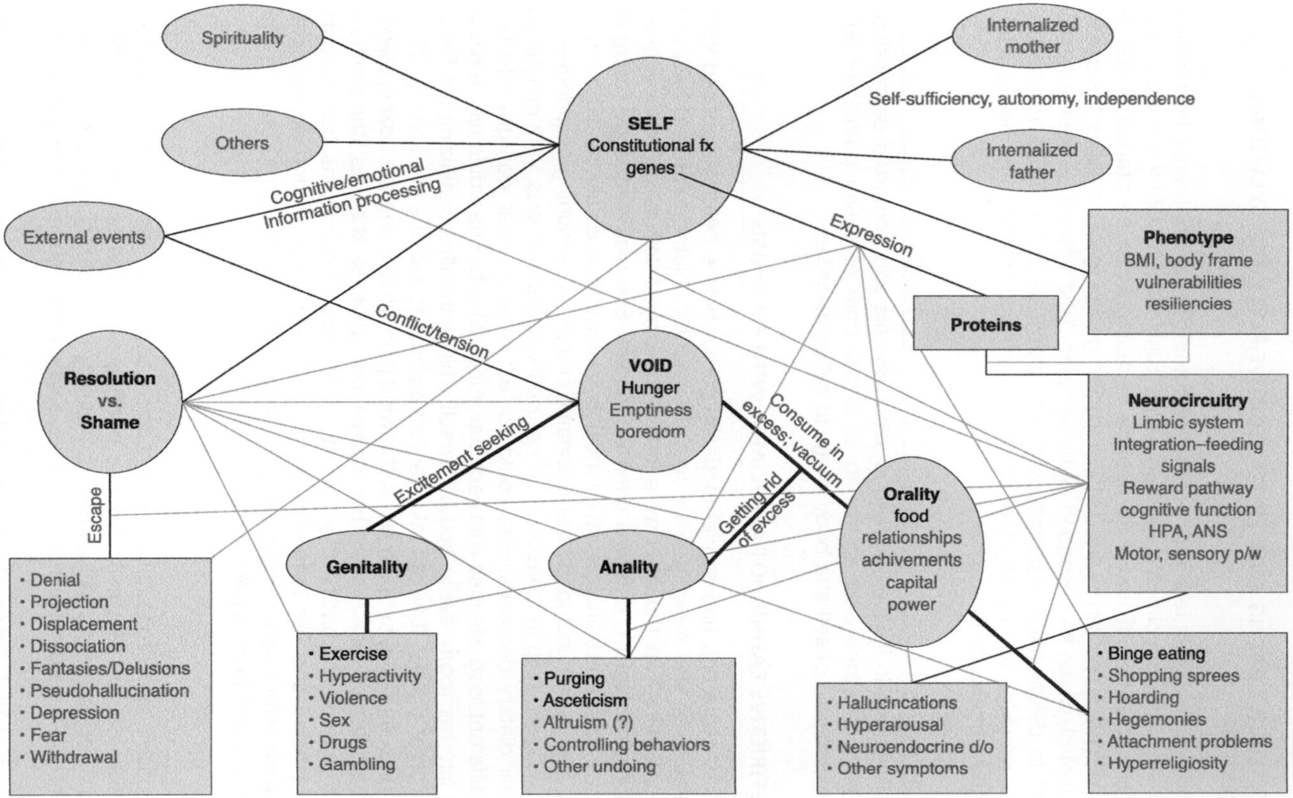

Fig. 1. Simplified model of symptom manifestation in patients with schizophrenia and eating disorders. BMI, body-mass index; HPA, hypothalamic-pituitary adrenal axis; ANS, autonomic nervous system.

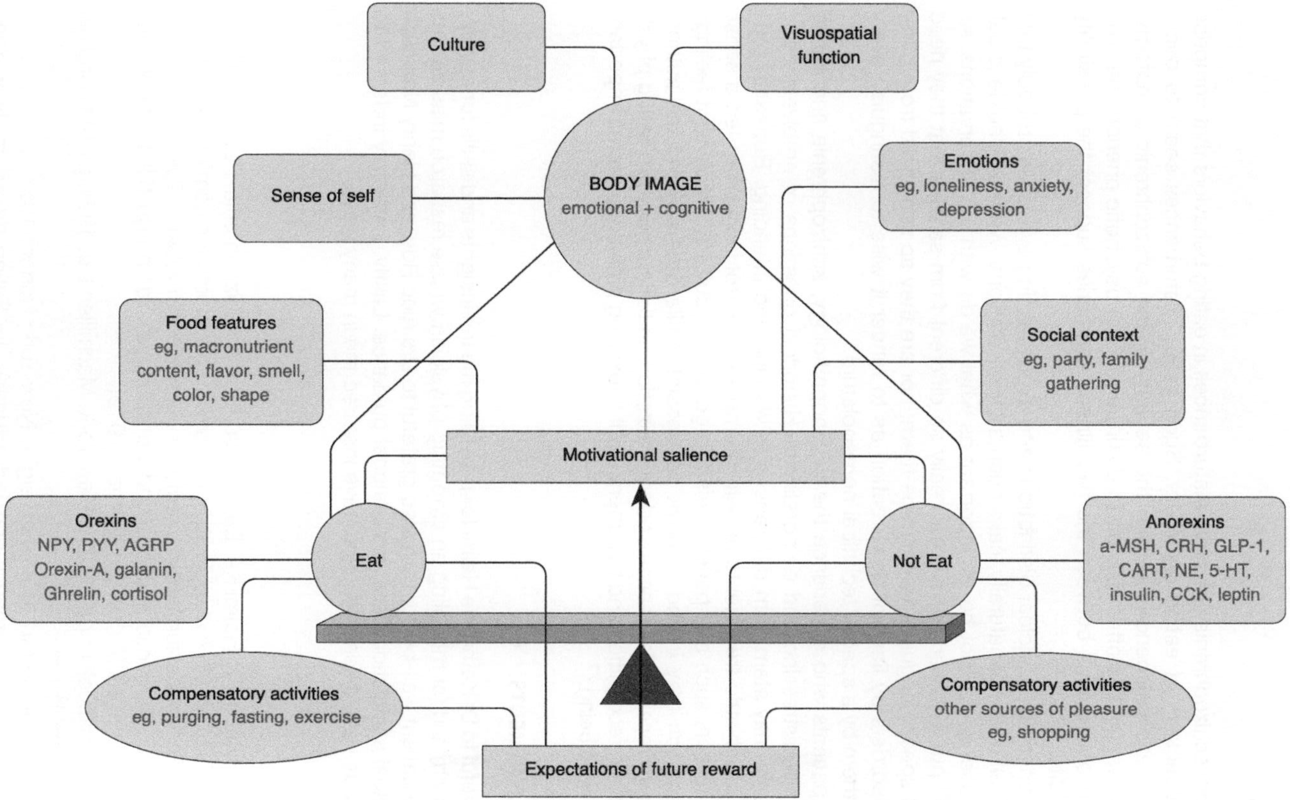

Fig. 2. Processes leading to the act of eating. NPY, neuropeptide Y; PYY, peptide YY; AGRP, agouti-related peptide; MSH, melanocyte-stimulating hormone; CRH, corticotropin-releasing hormone; GLP, glucagon-like peptide; CART, cocaine-amphetamine regulated transcript; NE, norepinephrine; 5-HT, serotonin; CCK, cholecystokinin.

The psychic factors potentially involved in eating disturbances based on clinical experience is shown in **Fig. 1**. The processes leading to the act of eating are shown in **Fig. 2**.

SUMMARY

Patients with schizophrenia can have disturbances in eating behaviors that comprise an entire spectrum of eating disorders. Such eating disturbances seem to occur concurrently and independently from the severity of the schizophrenic symptoms. Eating disorder itself is often difficult to distinguish from psychotic phenomena. The overlapping phenomena between the two illness categories suggest the possibility of comorbidity.

The reason for such unclear distinctions and overwhelming overlap is probably that the brain itself does not naturally make such artificial divisions. What we decide to call what we observe may not be as important as what we do with our observations. As Maudsley[20] put it, "Insanities are not really so different from sanities that they need a new and special language to describe them; nor are they so separated from other nervous disorders by lines of demarcation as to render it wise to distinguish every feature of them by a special technical nomenclature."

For the patients who experience the psychopathology, schizophrenia and eating disorders are distressing and demoralizing. Historical questions of ambivalence in schizophrenia may stem from differences in wanting and intending. Repeated past failures in psychiatric treatments or self-attempts of control have often left a sense of demoralization, such that patients wish to get better, but with ambivalent feelings about how much they intend to work on possibly futile efforts. What the authors observe more recently, is a sense of demoralization on the part of the treating physician. However, recognition and treatment of all coexisting pathology seems important for patient well being.[21]

ACKNOWLEDGMENTS

I am grateful to Dr Katherine Halmi for providing me the insights and skills for psychiatric research, and for modeling an empathic physician whose research mission was to improve patient well-being. I am also grateful to Drs Alec Roy, and Henry Nasrallah for intellectual stimulations and professional guidance. Lastly, I am truly indebted to the numerous patient-teachers who have inspired me in many ways.

REFERENCES

1. Yum SY, Hwang MY, Halmi KA. Eating disorders in schizophrenia. Psychiatr Times Vol XXIII, No 7, 2006. Available at: http://www.psychiatrictimes.com/display/article/10168/51311?pageNumber=2&verify=0. Accessed October 8, 2006.
2. Kraepelin E. Dementia praecox and paraphrenia. Edinburgh (UK): Thoemmes Press; 2002. p. 87 [Original published 1919].
3. Bleuler E. Textbook of psychiatry. New York: Macmillan Co. 1924. p. 149 [Original published 1911].
4. Bruch H. The importance of overweight. New York: Norton; 1957.
5. Bruch H. Hunger awareness and individuation. In: Eating disorders. New York: Basic Books Inc; 1976. p. 44–5.
6. Stunkard AJ, Messick S. The three-factor Eating questionnaire to measure dietary restraint, disinhibition and hunger. J Psychosom Res 1985;29(1):71–83.

7. Yum SY, Hwang MY, Yum SK. Predictors of disinhibited eating in restrained eaters in patients with schizophrenia. NAASO Annual Meeting. Vancouver, Canada, October, 2005.
8. Casper RC, Heller W. 'La douce indifference' and mood in anorexia nervosa: neuropsychological correlates. Prog NeuroPsychopharmacol Biol Psychiatry 1990; 15:15–23.
9. World Health Organization. The international pilot study of schizophrenia. vol. 1. Geneva (Switzerland): World Health Organization; 1973.
10. Yum SY. The starved brain: eating behaviors in schizophrenia. Psychiatr Ann 2005;35(1):82–9.
11. Hwang MY, Opler LA. Schizophrenia with obsessive-compulsive features: assessment and treatment. Psychiatr Ann 1994;24:468–72.
12. Halmi KA, Sunday SR, Strober M, et al. Perfectionism in anorexia nervosa: variation by clinical subtype, obsessionality, and pathological eating behavior. Am J Psychiatry 2000;157(11):1799–805.
13. Strober M. Personality and symptomatological features in young, nonchronic anorexia nervosa patients. J Psychosom Res 1980;24(6):353–9.
14. Mazure CM, Halmi KA, Sunday SR, et al. The Yale-Brown-Cornell Eating Disorder Scale: development, use, reliability, and validity. J Psychiatr Res 1994;28:425–45.
15. Sunday SR, Halmi KA, Einhorn A. The Yale-Brown-Cornell Eating Disorder Scale: a new scale to assess eating disorder symptomatology. Int J Eat Disord 1995; 18(3):237–45.
16. Hwang MY, Yum SY, Kwon JS, et al. Management of schizophrenia with obsessive-compulsive disorder. Psychiatr Ann 2005;35(1):36–43.
17. Dols M, van Arcken D. Food supply and nutrition in the Netherlands during and immediately after World War II. Milbank Mem Fund Q 1946;24:319–55.
18. Keys A. Psychology. In: The biology of human starvation. Minneapolis (MN): Univ Minnesota Press; 1950. p. 767–920.
19. Bleuler E. Dementia praecox or the group of schizophrenias. New York: International Universities Press; 1950.
20. Maudsley H. Preface. In: The pathology of mind. London: Macmillan; 1879.
21. Yum SY, Hwang MY, Lee YH, et al. Non-dieting approaches to the management of obesity in schizophrenia. Washington: Paradigm; Fall, 2006. p. 12, 13, 22.

Management of Schizophrenia with Substance Use Disorders

Janice Lybrand, MD[a,*], Stanley Caroff, MD[a,b]

KEYWORDS

- Schizophrenia • Substance use disorders
- Alcohol • Cannabis • Nicotine • Cocaine

Around 50% of patients with schizophrenia develop a co-occurring substance use disorder involving alcohol or illicit substances at some time during their lives. The comorbid substance abuse will markedly affect the course of illness of schizophrenia. In this article, we review the epidemiology, theories of causation, effect on the course of illness, and treatment of co-occurring schizophrenia and substance use disorder.

EPIDEMIOLOGY

Three decades of epidemiologic studies have examined the prevalence of substance use disorder in schizophrenia. The landmark Epidemiologic Catchment Area study, published in 1990, reported that 47% of individuals in the United States who had a diagnosis of schizophrenia or schizophreniform disorder also had a substance abuse or dependence diagnosis.[1] The Epidemiologic Catchment Area study found that the odds ratio for the presence of a substance abuse diagnosis were 4.6 times higher for persons with schizophrenia than for the general population. The odds ratio for alcohol disorders were 3.3 times higher and the odds of other drug use disorders were 6.2 times higher than those for the general population. The most prevalent substance used (other than nicotine) was alcohol, followed by cannabis and cocaine. Subsequent studies have confirmed a lifetime prevalence of substance use disorder in patients with schizophrenia of 40% to 60%.[2] Chambers and colleagues[3] reported the range of alcohol abuse from 20% to 60%, with cannabis abuse from 12% to 42% and cocaine abuse from 15% to 50%. Data from different geographic areas show that

[a] Department of Psychiatry, Philadelphia VA Medical Center, 3900 Woodland Avenue, Philadelphia, PA 19104, USA
[b] Department of Psychiatry, University of Pennsylvania School of Medicine, 3900 Woodland Avenue, Philadelphia, PA 19104, USA
* Corresponding author.
E-mail address: janice.lybrand@va.gov (J. Lybrand).

Psychiatr Clin N Am 32 (2009) 821–833
doi:10.1016/j.psc.2009.09.002
0193-953X/09/$ – see front matter. Published by Elsevier Inc.

cocaine is less often abused in rural regions but is more common in urban areas.[1,4] Abuse of amphetamines among patients with schizophrenia is less frequent in studies published thus far. However, as the prevalence of amphetamine use has recently risen in the general population, future studies among the population of patients with schizophrenia may reveal a similar rise. Abuse of opiates and sedative hypnotics remains relatively uncommon.

Although many studies of comorbidity of schizophrenia and substance abuse omit nicotine, it is an important substance to consider because of its very high prevalence and the extent of medical harm caused by smoking. Among the general population in the United States, the prevalence of smoking among adults is about 20%.[5] In various studies, the prevalence of smoking among persons with schizophrenia in the United States ranges from about 50% to greater than 90%, or 2.5 to 4.5 times the prevalence of smoking in the general population.[6,7] In addition, persons with schizophrenia are disproportionately heavy smokers. In one population-based study of a discrete geographic area (Nithsdale, Scotland), Kelly and McCreadie[8] found that, among schizophrenic smokers, 68% used more than 25 cigarettes per day, whereas among the general population, only 11% of smokers used more than 25 cigarettes per day.

Certain demographic characteristics affect the probability that a schizophrenic patient will have a substance use disorder. Younger age and male gender increase the likelihood of abuse of drugs and alcohol among those with schizophrenia.[9] Earlier age of onset of schizophrenia is also associated with increased substance abuse.[10] An often-cited study by Salyers and Mueser[11] of recently hospitalized patients with schizophrenia showed a lower level of negative symptoms among those patients who use drugs and alcohol. Those who use substances had greater social motivation and more social contacts than those with no substance abuse. The Epidemiologic Catchment Area study found that the prevalence of lifetime substance use diagnoses was about doubled in persons with mental illness who are institutionalized as compared with those with mental illness who are not treated. The rate of substance use disorder in prisoners with schizophrenia was found to be over 90%.[1] The rate of substance abuse among homeless persons with schizophrenia (including male and female) is around 70%.[12]

THEORIES OF CAUSATION

Efforts to account for the very high comorbidity of schizophrenia and substance use have led to several hypotheses:

- That schizophrenia leads to substance use
- That substance use leads to schizophrenia
- That substance use and schizophrenia have a common origin
- That the increased rate of substance use results from multiple risk factors, including affect dysregulation and poor coping skills
- That the substance use is a response to reward circuitry dysfunction

Schizophrenia Leads to Substance Use

The most common form of the hypothesis that schizophrenia leads to substance use is one proposed by Khantzian[13,14] and referred to as the self-medication hypothesis. He proposes that substance abuse is an attempt to treat the symptoms of schizophrenia. If true, this hypothesis implies that the pharmacologic properties of the substances selected would match the symptoms experienced by schizophrenic patients. For example, it implies that stimulant abuse should be preferred by patients with prominent negative symptoms, and also that the extent of substance abuse should correlate with the extent of the symptoms experienced. However, studies have not borne out this hypothesis, but instead have revealed that schizophrenic patients tend to use the substances most available and affordable to them.[3,15] Also, the order of substances most commonly chosen (alcohol, cannabis, then stimulants) is the same for both schizophrenic patients and the general population. Self-report by patients with schizophrenia on the reasons that they abuse substances are similar to the self-report data by persons without schizophrenia. In the study by Dixon and colleagues[16] in 1991, the reasons for substance abuse cited by the schizophrenic patients were to get high (72%), to decrease depression (72%), to relax (64%), to increase pleasure (62%), to increase energy (56%), and to go along with the group (55%). These are similar to the reasons cited by substance abusers without schizophrenia. A smaller number of patients (8%) reported using substances to decrease medication side effects. Duke and colleagues[17] found that akathesia may correlate with increased alcohol use, but Salyers and Mueser[11] found no correlation between substance abuse and akathesia.

In contrast to other substances of abuse, nicotine, it is thought, may be used to self-medicate the symptoms of schizophrenia. In the central nervous system, nicotine modulates the activity of the dopaminergic and glutamatergic systems implicated in the pathophysiology of schizophrenia.[18] During smoking, nicotine binds nicotine acetylcholine receptors in the midbrain. These neurons project from the ventral tegmental area to the prefrontal cortex, where they activate dopamine release. It is thought that hypofunction of dopamine in the prefrontal cortex mediates both negative symptoms and cognitive deficits of schizophrenia. By activating dopamine release to the prefrontal cortex, smoking may reduce some negative symptoms and cognitive deficits of schizophrenia and this may be a contributing factor to the high prevalence of addiction to nicotine in schizophrenia.

One example of this is in the abnormalities seen in schizophrenia in auditory processing. One of these abnormalities is in the prepulse inhibition of the acoustic startle reflex. In schizophrenia, this function is improved by smoking and it is worsened in acute smoking abstinence.[19]

Another cognitive function impaired in schizophrenia is visual-spatial working memory. Performance accuracy in this task is associated with cortical dopamine level. The hypofunction of cortical dopamine in schizophrenia leads to impaired performance of this task, and smoking leads to temporary improvement in task performance.[20]

Substance Use Leads to Schizophrenia

If substance abuse leads to schizophrenia, then we should expect to find that the age of onset of substance abuse precedes the age of onset of schizophrenia. Studies examining this have revealed that, in general, the age of onset of substance abuse is earlier than that of schizophrenia. However, these data have proven difficult to interpret, both because the age of onset of substance abuse in the general population is younger than the typical age of onset of schizophrenia, and also because the prodromal symptoms of schizophrenia may already be present at the time of onset of substance abuse and may be increasing the risk to develop substance abuse.[16,21]

Mueser and colleagues[22] point out that if substance abuse is a causative factor in the onset of schizophrenia, then we should expect to find the greatest evidence of that correlation with the substance that has the highest prevalence of abuse, which is alcohol. Instead, alcohol is rarely proposed as a cause of schizophrenia. It appears that alcohol worsens the course of illness in schizophrenia but does not cause the illness.[23] The drugs most commonly proposed as causative factors in schizophrenia are hallucinogens, stimulants, and cannabis, rather than alcohol. One often-cited study by Andreasson and colleagues[24] was a prospective cohort study of Swedish conscripts. The cohort was followed through the Swedish health registry for 14 years. Those who reported cannabis use at the time of entry into the military were 2.4 times more likely to develop schizophrenia during the follow-up period. Persons who reported heavy cannabis use (defined as more than 50 times) were six times more likely to develop schizophrenia during the follow-up period. The investigators noted that these data cannot determine whether cannabis was the cause or effect. The drug abuse may have been associated with other psychiatric diagnoses at the time of onset of use, or, as noted above, with the prodromal symptoms of schizophrenia. Hambrecht and Haffner[25] examined 232 first-episode patients with comorbid cannabis abuse and found that 27.5% had cannabis abuse more than a year before their prodromal symptoms began, 34.6% had the onset of cannabis abuse and prodromal symptoms in the same month, and 37.9% had symptoms of schizophrenia before onset of cannabis abuse.

Substance Use and Schizophrenia Have a Common Origin

If substance abuse and schizophrenia have a common origin, we would expect to find that persons with schizophrenia have more relatives with substance abuse than people in the general population have, or that persons with substance abuse have more relatives with schizophrenia than the general population has. The studies examining this hypothesis have yielded inconsistent results, providing little support for this as a major factor in the extent of comorbidity seen between schizophrenia and substance use disorders.[26,27]

Multiple Risk Factors: the Affect Regulation Model

Blanchard, Brown, and colleagues[28] have proposed an affect regulation model that focuses on stable personality traits that affect long-term risk for substance abuse. They note that if longstanding traits of individuals are implicated in the onset of substance abuse, then onset of substance abuse can occur independent of the onset of symptoms of schizophrenia. This is consistent with the mixed data on this question, as noted above in the study by Hambrecht and Haffner.[25]

The model by Blanchard, Brown, and colleagues[28] integrates data showing that, in the general population, the trait-cluster of negative affect/neuroticism is associated with increased risk of substance abuse. This stable trait reflects a general lowering of mood, lower threshold for frustration, and magnification of problems. They hypothesize that the link between the trait and substance abuse is a dispositional tendency to negative affective states, which the individual then attempts to reduce by substance abuse. These persons often report that they use substances to help them cope with stress. Blanchard and colleagues[28] note that negative affect is elevated among persons with schizophrenia and that this tendency to negative emotional states is a "critical feature" of the disorder. This finding is consistent with the self-report data asking patients with schizophrenia and substance abuse their reasons for substance abuse. The psychiatric symptom most reported as a reason is depression.

The affect regulation model also builds on the stress-vulnerability model of Cooper.[29] Blanchard and colleagues[28] cite data indicating that maladaptive coping strategies used to respond to stress, such as denial, emotional outbursts, and avoidance, increase vulnerability to substance use disorders. They note that substance abuse is associated with deficits in interpersonal skills and problem-solving abilities in the general population. Deficiency in social behavior is one of the defining features of schizophrenia and deficits in problem-solving skills are also well documented.

In sum, they hypothesize that, in schizophrenia, many individuals have an increase in negative affect/neuroticism, which leads to an increased exposure to stress and interpersonal conflicts. These individuals approach the stressors with poor coping and problem-solving skills, which further weaken their ability to navigate the stressors, worsening their negative affect. They then attempt to reduce the negative affect with substance abuse.

A second cluster of traits associated with substance abuse is disinhibition/impulsiveness, which is characterized by increased risk taking and sensation seeking and reduced concern for the future. These traits are associated with both increased risk of substance abuse and with increased frequency of antisocial personality disorder. In samples of persons with comorbid schizophrenia and antisocial personality disorder, substance use disorders are found to be exceptionally high.

Reward Circuitry Dysfunction

This neurobiological model by Chambers and colleagues[3] hypothesizes that the neuropathology of schizophrenia affects the neural circuitry that mediates drug reward, which then leads to increased vulnerability to addiction. They propose that dysregulated dopamine-mediated mesocorticolimbic pathways underlie both the symptoms of schizophrenia and abnormalities of the brain reward circuitry. Substance abuse may relieve the deficit temporarily, although ultimately worsening the course of illness.

EFFECTS OF SUBSTANCE USE ON COURSE OF ILLNESS

Comorbid substance use disorder and schizophrenia is associated with greater morbidity than schizophrenia alone. In one 18-month longitudinal study of 100 patients with schizophrenia, the patients with comorbid substance use disorder showed a deterioration of function over time that was missing from those who had schizophrenia alone.[30] Tracy and colleagues[31] have noted reduced memory and attention in persons with comorbid schizophrenia and substance abuse, as compared with schizophrenics without substance abuse. Dual-diagnosis patients also have decreased adherence to medications and increased frequency of hospitalization.[32–35] Unsurprisingly, the cost of care for individuals with dual diagnosis is significantly higher than for patients with schizophrenia alone.[36,37]

Those with comorbid substance use disorders and schizophrenia also have higher rates of relapse, decreased employment, and increased homelessness.[12,33,38] Dual diagnosis is associated with increases in suicidal ideation, risk of victimization, violence, and risk of incarceration.[39–43]

In addition, comorbidity of schizophrenia and substance use disorder is associated with increased risk of numerous medical problems, including hepatitis B, hepatitis C, HIV, purified protein derivative (PPD) reactivity, and traumatic injury.[44–47] Chronic use of cocaine or cannabis may also lead to a higher risk of tardive dyskinesia.[48,49] The increased prevalence and intensity of smoking among schizophrenic patients can be expected to lead to increased morbidity from conditions for which smoking is a known risk factor. Studies examining the mortality of cardiovascular illness in schizophrenia have shown an increased relative risk of 1.87 to 2.3. The increased relative risk of respiratory disease ranges from a factor of 2.1 to 3.17.[50,51] A comparison by Himmelhoch, Lehman, and colleagues[52] found the prevalence of chronic obstructive pulmonary disease among persons with schizophrenia to be 22.6%, as compared with the prevalence in the general population of 7.6%.

GENERAL TREATMENT STRATEGIES

Detection

Given the large effect that substance abuse has on the course of illness in schizophrenia, it is important to explore carefully the possibility of a substance use diagnosis with each patient. The interviewer should also bear in mind that relatively small amounts of substances may lead to larger than expected effects in persons with schizophrenia.[53] It is therefore important to consider not just amounts of substances used, but the amount of time spent recovering from the consequences of use. Multiple sources of information can be used to aid in identifying substance abuse, including patient interviews, chart reviews, and information from family members and from other clinicians involved in the patient's care. Clinicians should also be alert to behaviors that are consistent with substance abuse, such as financial problems beyond those expected for the patient's income level and frequent missed appointments. A nonjudgmental therapeutic alliance facilitates more honest reporting about substance abuse.

Urine and blood toxicology tests provide objective screens for substance abuse. In interpreting the results of these tests, it is important to be aware of the maximum detection times for the various substances. Alcohol use will be detected for only about 24 hours. For occasional marijuana users, detection may be positive for 3 days, but for those with frequent, heavy use, it can be detected for up to 12 weeks. Cocaine is detectable for 7 days; amphetamines for 4 days; and benzodiazepines for 6 weeks.[54] Standardized screening tools that clinicians find helpful include the Alcohol Use Disorder Identification Test (AUDIT), the Drug Abuse Screening Test (DAST), the Michigan Alcohol Screening Test (MAST), and the Dartmouth Assessment of Lifestyle Inventory (DALI), an instrument developed specifically for persons with mental illness.[55,56]

Psychosocial Treatments

Integrated treatment is treatment of both the substance abuse and schizophrenia simultaneously by one clinician or team of clinicians. The treatment includes both psychosocial treatments and pharmacotherapy for schizophrenia. Integrated treatment has been well established as the most successful approach to treatment for this patient population.[57] The cognitive and social-skill deficits associated with schizophrenia lead to impaired ability to solve problems and to form and maintain social support. The psychosocial aspect of integrated treatment emphasizes daily functioning, social support, and problem solving.

Because the patients needing treatment are often minimally engaged and little motivated to reduce substance use, the early stage of integrated treatment emphasizes development of a strong therapeutic alliance. This is fostered by empathy and respect. The initial goal is to assist the patient with primary needs, such as housing, and to establish regular contact. As the patient moves forward in treatment, the use of motivational techniques gradually increases the patient's awareness of the problems and risks associated with substance use until a desire to change develops. Throughout treatment, it remains important to continue efforts to increase motivation and promote hope that change is possible, as clinician and patient work together to identify specific steps to achieve the desired change.

After initial engagement and a period of time to help the patient develop increased motivation for change, the patient enters active treatment. Some approaches to this phase of treatment have been adapted from evidence-based treatments for schizophrenia. These approaches include assertive community treatment and social skills training. Other approaches have been adapted from the traditional approaches to addiction. These approaches include cognitive-behavioral strategies and 12-step programs. There is little evidence demonstrating the superiority of any one particular program. In general, effective treatment programs emphasize a long-term perspective and collaboration with the patient, the patient's case managers, and the people or institutions that provide the patient with social, housing, and vocational support.[58]

A study by Bellack and colleagues[59] found that the most effective approaches were those that included group counseling with both a motivational and cognitive-behavioral aspect.

Contingency management techniques, in which reinforcement is given for negative urine drug tests or attendance at clinic, have proven helpful in some studies.[60] In addition, patients with comorbid schizophrenia and substance use disorders benefit from the conventional evidence-based treatments for schizophrenia, such as family psychoeducation and supported employment. Patients unable to respond to outpatient treatment may respond to long-term residential programs.[61]

PHARMACOTHERAPY

General Considerations

Due to the problems that dual-diagnosis patients have with medication adherence,[32] it is important to choose strategies that simplify the medication schedule. This includes use of longer-acting oral medications so that the frequency of dosing can be minimized, and possible use of depot neuroleptics. It may also be helpful to use instrumental and environmental supports, such as use of medication organizers and engagement of family members or case managers to assist in reminding patients to take medications. Prescribers also must consider the interaction of prescribed drugs with substances of abuse. For example, it is necessary to weigh the relative risk of seizures for a patient whose substance use creates an increased risk of seizure activity. Likewise, prescribers must be attentive to the effects of hepatically metabolized drugs in patients with substance-induced or hepatitis-associated liver damage. Another frequent problem is additive sedation or confusion from prescription drugs combined with drugs of abuse. This can be a particular problem with drugs that have strong anticholinergic effects. Because these patients already suffer from addiction, it is important to avoid prescribing medications with addiction potential, such as benzodiazepines.

Smoking has a marked effect on the cytochrome P450 system, inducing CYP1A2 isoenzymes, which metabolize some medications more efficiently, increasing the metabolic rate of some antipsychotic medications by 50%. Some of the medications metabolized through the CYP1A2 system include haloperidol, fluphenazine, thioridazine, chlorpromazine, olanzapine, and clozapine. Smokers, especially heavy smokers, who take these antipsychotic medications may require doses up to twice as high as nonsmokers. Finally, caffeine is metabolized through the same system and very heavy caffeine consumption also reduces the serum level of these drugs.

Choice of Antipsychotic Medication

The conventional antipsychotic agents appear to be less effective for dual diagnosis patients than for patients with schizophrenia alone. These agents do not reduce use of substances, and may increase it in some cases. In particular, some studies have shown an association between haloperidol and increased smoking.[62] One study compared atypical antipsychotics to conventional antipsychotics in 45 smokers with schizophrenia who were using a nicotine transdermal patch. Among the patients taking atypical antipsychotics, more than twice as many stopped smoking as among those taking conventional antipsychotics.[63]

Of the atypical agents, the one most thoroughly studied for use in dual-diagnosis patients is clozapine. Numerous studies of clozapine have shown it to be associated with reduction not only of psychotic symptoms but also of substance abuse. McEvoy[64] studied 70 schizophrenic patients—55 smokers and 15 nonsmokers—over 12 weeks. He found that the smokers smoked less on clozapine. In a 3-year retrospective study by Zimmet and colleagues[65] of 58 patients with schizophrenia and schizoaffective disorder with comorbid alcohol use disorder, the patients taking clozapine showed decreased substance use. Drake and colleagues,[66] in a naturalistic study of patients with schizophrenia and schizoaffective disorder, compared 36 patients on clozapine and 115 patients on conventional antipsychotics, all of whom had a comorbid alcohol use disorder. Among the patients on clozapine, 79% had remission of alcohol use, whereas, among the patients on conventional antipsychotics, the remission rate was only 33.7%.

Studies of the other atypical agents have yielded inconsistent results. An open-label crossover study by Smelson and colleagues[67] of patients with comorbid schizophrenia and cocaine dependence showed that patients using risperidone had less cue-elicited craving and fewer substance abuse relapses than patients taking conventional antipsychotic agents. A retrospective study by Green[68] of patients with schizophrenia or schizoaffective disorder and alcohol and/or cannabis dependence, some taking risperidone and some taking clozapine, found that patients were more likely to abstain from alcohol and cocaine if taking clozapine. Green and colleagues[69] have proposed that the strong dopamine-2 (D-2) blockade of conventional antipsychotic agents does not improve the function of the mesocorticolimbic reward system, and that clozapine, with its reduced D-2 blockade, decreases the dysfunction of this reward system in schizophrenic patients, leading to reduction in substance abuse.

Several studies and case reports have suggested that olanzapine may decrease cravings in cocaine addicts with schizophrenia, but the findings are inconsistent. In 2005, a double-blind, randomized, 26-week trial comparing olanzapine to haloperidol for 24 patients with co-occurring schizophrenia and cocaine-dependence by Sayers and colleagues[70] found no decrease in cravings with olanzapine as compared with haloperidol. In 2006, a similar but shorter (6-week) double-blind, randomized trial compared the same two drugs among patients with the same pair of diagnoses. This trial showed significant reduction in cocaine cravings in the olanzapine group.[71] There are fewer studies thus far of quetiapine, aripiprazole, and ziprasidone.

PHARMACOTHERAPY FOR SPECIFIC SUBSTANCES

The medications reducing use of alcohol and other substances in the general population include naltrexone, disulfiram, acamprosate, and desipramine. Few studies have examined the use of these medications for patients with comorbid schizophrenia. One randomized study of naltrexone versus placebo by Petrakis and colleagues[72] provides evidence of reduction in the number of days of heavy drinking. Mueser and colleagues[73] reported a comprehensive chart review of 33 patients with schizophrenia or schizoaffective disorder and alcoholism who had been treated with disulfiram. Sixty-four percent had at least a 1-year remission of alcoholism over a 3-year period of monitoring. Seventy-six percent reported having used alcohol while taking disulfiram, and 28% reported having had a negative reaction to the alcohol. There were no psychiatric complications reported. One open-label study by Ziedonis and colleagues[74] of patients with schizophrenia or schizoaffective disorder and comorbid cocaine dependence who were treated with adjunctive desipramine or placebo showed that the patients receiving desipramine had a higher rate of retention in treatment and fewer cocaine-positive urines.

Agents to promote smoking cessation include nicotine replacement systems, bupropion, and varenicline. Both nicotine replacement therapy and sustained-release bupropion have been tested in patients with schizophrenia. Nicotine replacement appears to be effective in reducing smoking cessation rates, although less effective than in patients without schizophrenia. George and colleagues[63] found that for patients with schizophrenia using the nicotine patch while taking typical neuroleptics, the rate of cessation was 22.2%, while for those taking atypical neuroleptics the rate was 55.6%. Evins and colleagues[75] reported a 12-week, double-blind, placebo-controlled study of sustained-release bupropion along with high-dose nicotine replacement therapy and cognitive behavioral therapy. Subjects on bupropion had a greater smoking cessation rate at week 8 (52% vs 19% with placebo) but relapse rates were very high when the nicotine taper began. There is little information on use of varenicline in patients with schizophrenia.

SUMMARY

Around half of patients with schizophrenia develop a substance-abuse diagnosis. The most commonly abused drugs are alcohol, cannabis, and cocaine. The use of these substances markedly worsens the course of illness. In addition, 50% to 90% of schizophrenic patients smoke cigarettes, contributing to increased mortality from medical illness. Treatment is most effective when offered in an integrated program that combines the treatment of substance abuse and schizophrenia. Treatment includes both psychosocial treatments and medications. Effective psychosocial treatments include tailoring of interventions to the patient's stage of treatment, providing intensive case management, and ensuring social, housing, and employment support. Atypical antipsychotic medications, especially clozapine, appear to offer significant advantages in reducing rates of substance abuse.

REFERENCES

1. Regier DA, Farmer ME, Rae DS, et al. Comorbidity of mental disorders with alcohol and other drug abuse: results from the Epidemiologic Catchment Area (ECA) Study. JAMA 1990;264:2511–8.
2. Cantor-Graee E, Nordstrom LG, McNeil TF. Substance abuse in schizophrenia: a review of the literature and a study of correlates in Sweden. Schizophr Res 2001;48:69–82.
3. Chamber RA, Krystal JH, Self DW. A neurobiological basis for substance abuse co-morbidity in schizophrenia. Biol Psychiatry 2001;50:71–83.
4. Mueser KT, Essock SM, Drake RE, et al. Rural and urban differences in patients with a dual diagnosis. Schizophr Res 2001;48:93–107.
5. Thorne SL, Malarcher A, Maurice E, et al. Cigarette smoking among adults—United States 2007. Morb Mortal Wkly Rep 2008;57:1221.
6. Lasser K, Boyd JW, Woolhandler S, et al. Smoking and mental illness: a population-based prevalence study. JAMA 2000;284(20):2606–10.

7. deLeon J, Diaz FJ. A meta-analysis of world-wide studies demonstrating an association between schizophrenia and tobacco smoking behaviors. Schizophr Res 2005;76:135–57.
8. Kelly C, McCreadie RM. Smoking habits, current symptoms, and premorbid characteristics of schizophrenic patients in Nithsdale, Scotland. Am J Psychiatry 1999;156(11):1751–7.
9. Gregg L, Barrowclough C, Haddock G. Reasons for increased substance abuse in psychosis. Clin Psychol Rev 2007;27:494–510.
10. Mauri M, Volonteri L, DeGaspari I, et al. Substance abuse in first-episode schizophrenic patients; a retrospective study. Clin Pract Epidemiol Ment Health 2006; 23:2–4.
11. Salyers MP, Mueser KT. Social functioning, psychopathology, and medication side effects in relation to substance use and abuse in schizophrenia. Schizophr Res 2001;48:109–23.
12. Caton CL, Shrout PE, Eagle PF, et al. Risk factors for homelessness among schizophrenic men: a case-control study. Am J Public Health 1994;84:265–70.
13. Khantzian EJ. The self-medication hypothesis of addictive disorders: focus on heroin and cocaine dependence. Am J Psychiatry 1985;142:1259–64.
14. Khantzian EJ. The self-medication hypothesis of substance use disorder: a reconsideration and recent applications. Harv Rev Psychiatry 1997;4:231–44.
15. Mueser KT, Bellack AS, Blanchard JJ. Comorbidity of schizophrenia and substance abuse: implications for treatment. J Consult Clin Psychol 1992;60: 845–56.
16. Dixon L, Haas G, Weiden PJ, et al. Drug abuse in schizophrenic patients: clinical correlates and reasons for use. Am J Psychiatry 1991;148:224–30.
17. Duke PJ, Pantelis C, Barnes TRE. South Westminster schizophrenia survey: alcohol use and its relationship to symptoms, tardive dyskinesia and illness onset. Br J Psychiatry 1994;164:630–6.
18. Dalack GW, Healy DJ, Meador-Woodruff JH. Nicotine dependence in schizophrenia: clinical phenomena and laboratory findings. Am J Psychiatry 1998; 155:1490–501.
19. Kumari V, Soni W, Sharma T. Influence of cigarette smoking on prepulse inhibition of the acoustic startle response in schizophrenia. Hum Psychopharmacol 2001; 16:321–6.
20. George TP, Vessicchio JC, Termine A, et al. Effects of smoking abstinence on visuospatial working memory function in schizophrenia. Neuropsychopharmacology 2002;26:75–85.
21. Grant BF. Prevalence and correlates of alcohol use and DSM-IV alcohol dependence in the United States: results of the national longitudinal alcohol epidemiologic survey. J Stud Alcohol 1997;58:464–73.
22. Mueser KT, Drake RE, Wallach MA. Dual diagnosis: a review of etiological theories. Addict Behav 1998;23:717–34.
23. Hambrecht M, Hafner H. Substance abuse and the onset of schizophrenia. Biol Psychiatry 1996;40:1155–63.
24. Andreasson S, Allebeck P, Engstrom A, et al. Cannabis and schizophrenia: a longitudinal study of Swedish conscripts. Lancet 1987;2(8574):1483–6.
25. Hambrecht M, Hafner H. Cannabis, vulnerability, and the onset of schizophrenia: an epidemiologic perspective. Aust N Z J Psychiatry 2000;34:468–75.
26. Kendlar KS, Gardner CO. The risk for psychiatric disorders in relative of schizophrenia and control probands: a comparison of three independent studies. Psychol Med 1997;27:411–9.

27. Kendlar KS. A twin study of individuals with both schizophrenia and alcoholism. Br J Psychiatry 1985;147:48–53.
28. Blanchard JB, Brown SA, Horan WP, et al. Substance use disorders in schizophrenia: review, integration, and a proposed model. Clin Psychol Rev 2000; 20(2):207–34.
29. Cooper ML, Russell M, Skinner JB, et al. Stress and alcohol use: moderating effects of gender, coping, and alcohol expectancies. J Abnorm Psychol 1992; 101:139–52.
30. Choulijan TL, Shumway M, Balanzio E, et al. Substance use among schizophrenia outpatients: prevalence, course and relation to financial status. Ann Clin Psychiatry 1995;7:19–24.
31. Tracy H, Josiassen RC, Bellak AS. Neuropsychology of dual diagnosis: understanding the combined effects of schizophrenia and substance use disorders. Clin Psychol Rev 1995;15:67–97.
32. Owens RR, Fisher EP, Booth BM, et al. Medication non-compliance and substance abuse among patients with schizophrenia. Psychiatr Serv 1998;47:853–8.
33. Mason P, Harrison G, Glazebrook C, et al. The course of schizophrenia over 13 years: a report from the International Study on Schizophrenia (ISoS) coordinated by the World Health Organization. Br J Psychiatry 1996;169:580–6.
34. Swofford CD, Kasackow JW, Schellen-Gilkey C, et al. Substance use: a powerful predictor of relapse in schizophrenia. Schizophr Res 1996;20:145–51.
35. Gupta S, Hendricks S, Kendel A, et al. Relapse in schizophrenia: is there a relationship to substance abuse? Schizophr Res 1998;20:153–6.
36. Bartels SJ, Teague GB, Drake RE, et al. Service utilization and costs associated with substance abuse among rural schizophrenic patients. J Nerv Ment Dis 1993; 181:227–32.
37. Dickey B, Azeni H, Drake RE, et al. Persons with dual diagnosis of substance abuse and major mental illness: their excess costs of psychiatric care. Am J Public Health 1996;86:973–7.
38. Cuffel BJ. Prevalence of estimates of substance abuse in schizophrenia and their correlates. J Nerv Ment Dis 1992;180:589–92.
39. Cuffel BJ, Sumway M, Choulijan T. A longitudinal study of substance use and community violence in schizophrenia. J Nerv Ment Dis 1994;182:704–8.
40. Seibyl JP, Satel SL, Anthony D, et al. Effects of cocaine on hospital course in schizophrenia. J Nerv Ment Dis 1993;181(1):31–7.
41. Goodman LA, Slayers MP, Mueser KT, et al. Recent victimization in women and men with severe mental illness: prevalence and correlates. J Trauma Stress 2001;14:615–32.
42. Cuffel BJ. Violent and destructive behavior among the severely mentally ill in rural areas; evidence from Arkansas' community mental health system. Community Ment Health J 1994;30:495–504.
43. Abram KM, Teplin LA. Co-occurring disorders among mentally ill jail detainees: implications for public policy. Am J Psychol 1991;46:1036–45.
44. Cividini A, Pistorio A, Regazetti A, et al. Hepatitis C virus infection among institutionalized psychiatric patients: a regression analysis of indicators of risk. J Hepatol 1997;27:455–63.
45. Rosenberg SD, Goodman LA, Osher FC, et al. Prevalence if HIV, hepatitis B and hepatitis C in people with severe mental illness. Am J Public Health 2001;91: 31–7.
46. Taubes T, Galanter A, Dermatis H, et al. Crack cocaine and schizophrenia as risk factors for PPD reactivity in the dually diagnosed. J Addict Dis 1998;17(3):63–74.

47. Dickey B, Azeni H, Weiss R, et al. Schizophrenia, substance use disorders and medical co-morbidity. J Ment Health Policy Econ 2000;3:27–33.
48. Brady K, Anton R, Ballenger JC. Cocaine abuse among schizophrenic patients. Am J Psychiatry 1990;147:1164–7.
49. Zaretsky A, Rector NA, Seeman MV, et al. Current cannabis use and tardive dyskinesia. Schizophr Res 1993;11:3–8.
50. Harris EC, Barraclough B. Excess mortality of mental disorders. Br J Psychiatry 1998;173:11–53.
51. Brown S, Inskip H, Barraclough B. Causes of excess mortality of schizophrenia. Br J Psychiatry 2000;177:212–7.
52. Himmelhoch S, Lehman A, Kreyenbuhl J, et al. Prevalence of chronic obstructive pulmonary disease among those with serious mental illness. Am J Psychiatry 2004;161(12):2317–9.
53. Drake RE, Mueser KT. Substance abuse comorbidity. In: Lieberman JA, Murray RM, editors. Comprehensive care of schizophrenia. London: Martin Dunitz; 2001. p. 243.
54. Ziedonis DM, Smelson D, Rosenthal RN, et al. Improving the care of individuals with schizophrenia and substance use disorder: consensus recommendations. J Psychiatr Pract 2005;11(5):315–37.
55. Maisto SA, Carey MP, Carey KB, et al. Use of AUDIT and the DAST-10 to identify alcohol and drug use disorders among adults with severe and persistent mental illness. Psychol Assess 2000;12:186–92.
56. Rosenberg SD, Drake RE, Wolford GL, et al. The Dartmouth Assessment of Lifestyle Instrument (DALI): a substance use disorder screen for people with severe mental illness. Am J Psychiatry 1998;155:232–8.
57. Drake RE, Essock SM, Shaner A, et al. Implementing dual diagnosis services for clients with severe mental illness. Psychiatr Serv 2001;52:469–76.
58. Drake RE, O'Neal EL, Wallach MA. A systematic review of psychosocial research on psychosocial interventions for people with co-occurring severe mental illness and substance use disorders. J Subst Abuse Treat 2008;34(1):123–38.
59. Bellack AS, Bennett ME, Gearon JS, et al. A randomized clinical trial of a new behavioral treatment for drug abuse in people with severe and persistent mental illness. Arch Gen Psychiatry 2006;63:426–32.
60. Haddock G, Barrowclough C, Tarrier N, et al. Cognitive-behavioural therapy and motivational intervention for schizophrenia and substance misuse: 18-month outcomes for a randomized controlled trial. Br J Psychiatry 2003;183:418–26.
61. Brunette MF, Mueser KT, Drake RE. A review of research on residential programs for people with severe mental illness and co-occurring substance use disorders. Drug Alcohol Rev 2004;23:471–81.
62. McEvoy JP, Freundenreich O, Levin ED, et al. Haloperidol increases smoking in patients with schizophrenia. Psychopharmacology 1995;119:124–6.
63. George TP, Ziedonis DM, Feingold A, et al. Nicotine transdermal patch and atypical antipsychotic medication for smoking cessation in schizophrenia. Am J Psychiatry 2000;157:1835–42.
64. McEvoy JP, Freudenreich O, Wilson WH. Smoking and therapeutic response to clozapine in patients with schizophrenia. Biol Psychiatry 1999;46:125–9.
65. Zimmet SV, Strous RD, Burgess ES, et al. Effects of clozapine on substance use in patients with schizophrenia and schizoaffective disorder: a retrospective survey. J Clin Psychiatry 2000;20:94–8.
66. Drake RE, Xie H, McHugo GI, et al. The effects of clozapine on alcohol and drug use disorder among patients with schizophrenia. Schizophr Bull 2000;26:441–9.

67. Smelson DA, Losonczy MF, Davis CW, et al. Risperidone decreases craving and relapses in individuals with schizophrenia and cocaine dependence. Can J Psychiatry 2002;47:671–5.
68. Green AI, Burgess ES, Dawson R, et al. Alcohol and cannabis use in schizophrenia: effects of clozapine vs. risperidone. Schizophr Res 2003;60:81–5.
69. Green AI, Zimmet SV, Strous RD, et al. Clozapine for comorbid substance use disorder and schizophrenia: do patients with schizophrenia have a reward-deficiency syndrome that can be ameliorated by clozapine? Harv Rev Psychiatry 1999;6:287–96.
70. Sayers S, Campbell EC, Kondrich J, et al. Cocaine abuse in schizophrenic patients treated with olanzapine versus haloperidol. J Nerv Ment Dis 2005;193: 379–86.
71. Smelson DA, Ziedonis D, Williams J, et al. The efficacy of olanzapine for decreasing cue-elicited cravings in individuals with schizophrenia and cocaine dependence. J Clin Psychopharmacol 2006;26:9–12.
72. Petrakis IL, O'Malley S, Rounsaville B, et al. Naltrexone augmentation of neuroleptic treatment in alcohol abusing patients with schizophrenia. Psychopharmacology 2004;172(3):291–7.
73. Meuser KT, Noordsy DL, Wolfe R. Disulfiram treatment for alcoholism in severe mental illness. Am J Addict 2003;12(3):242–52.
74. Ziedonis D, Richardson T, Lee E, et al. Adjunctive desipramine in the treatment of cocaine abusing schizophrenics. Psychopharmacol Bull 1992;28(3):309–14.
75. Evins AE, Cather C, Culhane MA, et al. A 12-week double-blind placebo-controlled study of bupropion SR added to high-dose dual nicotine replacement therapy for smoking cessation or reduction in schizophrenia. J Clin Psychopharmacol 2007; 27(4):380–6.

Management of Schizophrenia with Obsessive-Compulsive Features

Michael Y. Hwang, MD[a,b,c,*], Sung-Wan Kim, MD, PhD[a,d], Sun Young Yum, MD[a,c,e], Lewis A. Opler, MD, PhD[a,f]

KEYWORDS

- Schizophrenia • Obsessive-compulsive • Comorbidity
- Atypical antipsychotics • Amisulpride • SSRI

The obsessive-compulsive (OC) phenomenon in psychotic disorders has been extensively described and debated over the years. Early clinicians believed that these affective and anxiety symptoms are a reactive manifestation to the perceived external or internal stressors in the psychotic patient. Hierarchical diagnostic methodologies hindered systematic examination of this complex and challenging clinical condition, and contributed to the lack of effective treatment interventions.

The *Diagnostic and Statistical Manual of Mental Disorders* (DSM)-III, -III-R, and -IV diagnostic modifications, by allowing diagnosis of coexisting disorders, have promoted clinical and research interest in schizophrenia with coexisting psychiatric conditions.[1] The current emphasis on identifying specific symptom dimensions in preliminary discussions that will help shape DSM-V[2] underscores the need to address multiple dimensions of pathology and to treat comorbid conditions.

The OC phenomena observed in patients with psychotic disorder are similar to those of the traditional neurotic obsessive-compulsive disorder (OCD). These phenomena include contamination, sexual, somatic, religious, aggressive, and somatic themes with or without accompanying compulsions and intrusiveness.

[a] Mental Health Service, Franklin Delano Roosevelt Hospital, Veterans Affairs Hudson Valley Healthcare System, PO Box 100, Montrose, NY 10548, USA
[b] Robert Wood Johnson Medical School – UMDNJ, Piscataway, New Jersey, USA
[c] The Commonwealth Medical College of Pennsylvania, Scranton, Pennsylvania, USA
[d] Department of Psychiatry, Chonnam National University Medical School, Gwangju, Korea
[e] Lilly Pharmaceutical, Seoul, Korea
[f] Department of Psychiatry, Columbia University College of Physicians & Surgeons, New York, NY, USA
* Corresponding author. Mental Health Service, Franklin Delano Roosevelt Hospital, Veterans Affairs Hudson Valley Healthcare System, PO Box 100, Montrose, NY 10548, USA.
E-mail address: michael.hwang@va.gov (M.Y. Hwang).

Psychiatr Clin N Am 32 (2009) 835–851
doi:10.1016/j.psc.2009.08.002
0193-953X/09/$ – see front matter. Published by Elsevier Inc.

Many early clinicians including Westphal,[3] Kraepelin,[4] Stengel,[5] and Bleuler[6] considered such OC phenomena as a prodrome or an integral part of psychotic illness, and some considered the presence of OCS in schizophrenia a predictor of better clinical outcome. However, such diagnostic practice remained controversial until the 1980s as the presence of OCS in schizophrenia contradicted the diagnostic convention based on distinguishing 3 unique, nonoverlapping diagnostic categories in mental illness: neurotic versus psychotic disorders, with borderline personality organization emerging to capture those individuals who fell between this dichotomy. In the 1980s a more descriptive and less psychoanalytically driven nosology emerged, coining various terms such as "malignant OCD," "psychotic OCD," and "schizo-obsessive compulsive disorder" to describe coexisting OCS in schizophrenia. In clinical practice, however, the presence of OCS was frequently overlooked and therefore not treated.

During the past decade epidemiological and clinical studies, as well as advances in understanding of the neurobiological basis of mental illness, have led to psychiatrists in general, and the American Psychiatric Association in particular, endorsing the concept of comorbidity in schizophrenia.

The classic subtyping strategy based on phenomenology (eg, simple, paranoid, disorganized or hebephrenic, and undifferentiated) and more recently the positive and negative symptom subtyping[7] are based on the assumption that a specific psychopathological symptom dimension in schizophrenia is driven by specific underlying neurobiological pathogenesis. However, clinical and research evidence indicate that current subtyping is inadequate. Further understanding of the neurobiological basis in the specific psychopathological dimension and coexisting disorders may be necessary to construct clinically meaningful and biologically relevant diagnostic classification and subtyping strategies for psychotic disorders in general and schizophrenia in particular.[8]

In the hope of advancing this effort regarding OC phenomena in schizophrenia, this article reviews clinical profiles, current neurobiological evidence, and treatment studies and strategies.

EPIDEMIOLOGY AND PATHOGENESIS

Epidemiology

The epidemiological and clinical evidence for interface and overlap between OC phenomena and some neuropsychiatric disorders has been well established over the years.[9] Neuropsychiatric disorders often associated with OCD include Tourette syndrome, autism, Sydenham chorea, trichotillomania, body dysmorphic disorder, hypochondriasis, and dissociative and eating disorders. During the course of the illness, these patients often show an overlap of overvalued ideations and delusional manifestations. Epidemiological studies have indicated that the risk of psychosis is greater in patients with OCD than in the general population.[10,11]

Many clinicians debated this seeming co-occurrence of what they considered neurotic OC phenomena and psychotic illnesses. Westphal[3] noted that OC manifestation was a variant or a prodrome of psychotic illness, whereas Bleuler[6] suggested that some of these psychotic patients with unremitting obsession were schizophrenic. Stengel[5] proposed a possible interaction between neurotic OC manifestations and psychotic reactions during psychotic illness as a part of an adaptive defense mechanism. Early epidemiological studies by Jaherresis[12] and Rosen[13] found a low prevalence rate of OCS in schizophrenia, 1.1% and 3.5% respectively, and argued that OCS in schizophrenia predict a more benign clinical course and better outcome.

Insel and Akiskal[14] proposed that the OCD constitutes a psychopathological spectrum disorder, varying along a continuum of insight; thus, a patient at the severe end of the spectrum may have an obsessive-compulsive psychosis in contrast to one with neurotic OCD possessing intact insight. These investigators note that a shift from neurotic obsession (neurosis) to a psychotic obsessive state may occur when loss of resistance to intrusive thoughts occurs and insight is diminished. Furthermore, in contrast to the earlier belief that presence of OCS may serve as a defense mechanism against psychotic decompensation by maintaining psychological integrity,[5,6] recent studies[15] suggest greater neurobiological dysfunction and worse clinical course and long-term outcome in patients with OC schizophrenia. Based on this concept of resistance and insight allowing schizophrenia and OCD to coexist, along with the appreciation that Axis I disorders (eg, schizophrenia, OCD) and Axis II disorders (eg, borderline personality disorder) can also exist, recent studies have examined the comorbidity issues and overlapping of the psychopathological symptoms between schizophrenia and OCD, as well as between other disorders, without earlier arbitrary constraints.

The National Institute of Mental Health Epidemiological Catchment Area (ECA) study that used the diagnostic interview schedule (DIS) to examine comorbidity in mental disorders reported a prevalence rate of co-occurring OCD and schizophrenia of 12.2%.[15] The ECA study also found that the OC schizophrenic subgroup generally suffer from worse clinical course and outcome than non-OC schizophrenic patients. Other investigators have reported greater symptom severity, suicide risk, and functional impairment, as well as worse long-term outcome, in OC schizophrenia compared with non-OC schizophrenia.[16–18]

Subsequent systematic studies, many using the Structured Clinical Interview of the DSM-III-R or -IV (SCID), found a high prevalence in recent years of comorbid OCD and schizophrenia ranging from 4% to 50%, with an average prevalence of 23%.[19] This high variability in prevalence rate is due to differing methodologies, including sample size, sampling method, study design (cross-sectional vs prospective), method of evaluation (structured interview vs chart review), definition of comorbidity (OCD vs OCS), diversity in psychotic disorders of subjects (schizophrenia vs affective psychosis), chronicity of the illness (first episode vs multiple episodes), type of antipsychotic treatment (typical vs atypical), and other demographic and clinical characteristics (eg, acute vs stable status; inpatients, outpatients, or community residents).[20] For example, studies conducted in patients with first-episode psychosis showed a relatively lower OCD prevalence rate (4%–14%) than did those with chronic schizophrenia,[21,22] suggesting an increase in comorbidity with age and chronicity of the illness. Also, the prevalence of OCS in patients with schizophrenia is generally higher (10%–64%) than those with OCD.[19]

In a recent prospective study, Craig and colleagues[22] investigated first-admission psychotic patients diagnosed with schizophrenia, schizoaffective disorder, and affective disorders for coexisting Axis I disorders. The 2-year, prospective, longitudinal study design allowed ascertainment of the diagnostic validity of psychotic and comorbid anxiety disorders at more than one point in time, thus verifying the diagnostic validity, a weakness in most earlier studies. This methodological approach significantly improved the diagnostic reliability and established a new onset and resolution of the anxiety symptoms during the 2-year study period. In addition, a longitudinal examination of 2 coexisting sets of anxiety symptoms across 3 diagnostic groups of psychotic disorders enabled the investigators to address the specificity of comorbid associations between disorders and their impact on clinical course.

The study verified the following findings: (1) a high prevalence rate for comorbid anxiety disorders in newly diagnosed schizophrenia and schizoaffective disorders

(10.5%); (2) diagnostic validity and reliability of coexisting anxiety disorders in patients with psychotic disorders; and (3) a significant new onset and resolution of the anxiety symptoms/disorders during the first 24 months of psychotic illness. The study also found that primary clinicians diagnosed only about 10% of the patients with comorbid OCD; however, more than 20% of OC schizophrenic patients received pharmacological treatment appropriate for the coexisting anxiety symptoms.

Neurobiological Basis of Obsessive-Compulsive Symptoms

The neurobiological basis of OCD and schizophrenia has been extensively studied in recent years; however, there is a paucity of controlled studies in OC schizophrenia. The current evidence suggests dorsolateral prefrontal cortical dysfunction in schizophrenia, and a corticostriatal-thalamic-cortical circuitry abnormality in OCD. Neuroimaging studies of patients with schizophrenia have shown significant degenerative changes in the orbitofrontal cortex, cingulate, and caudate nucleus; however, although these areas are also implicated in OCD, no gross anatomical changes have been found in patients with OCD.[23] A recent neuroimaging study in patients with OCD and with schizophrenia found that volume reduction of the hippocampus is common in both diseases, but with a greater reduction of insular volume in patients with schizophrenia and enlargement of the amygdala in OCD.[24,25] Functional neuroimaging studies also revealed differences between OCD and schizophrenia; hyperactivity in the orbitofrontal cortex, caudate nucleus, and thalamus has been often observed in OCD patients, whereas dorsolateral prefrontal cortex dysfunction is a dominant finding in schizophrenic patients.[26,27] This diversity in neurobiological abnormalities in 2 disorders suggests that schizophrenia and OCD constitute 2 distinct disorders with significant unique pathogenesis, but with some overlap in pathogenesis that might explain common clinical features.

Neuropsychological studies in recent years have demonstrated greater prefrontal cortex functional impairment in the OC subgroup compared with non-OC schizophrenia patients.[17,28–30] In an earlier study, Hwang and colleagues[17] investigated demographically matched OC and non-OC schizophrenic patients in an urban, long-term hospital setting. The study applied rigorous and objective OCS criteria in well-established chronic schizophrenia to evaluate and characterize neuropsychological and clinical profiles of OC schizophrenic patients. The study found significant differences between the 2 groups, with the OC subgroup demonstrating greater prefrontal executive function impairments, as well as worse clinical course with poor treatment response and longer hospitalizations. The study also found significantly higher negative symptom scores in the OC subgroup; in contrast, there was no correlation between the positive symptoms scores and presence of the OCS as some investigators have suggested.[29] The greater prefrontal lobe dysfunction and functional impairment in the OC schizophrenic subgroup has been replicated by some investigators while others have disputed the finding.[31,32]

Genetic evidence from the epidemiological and family studies suggests a significant overlap in candidate genes between schizophrenia and affective disorder. A national epidemiological study of Swedish families[33] found evidence for common genetic risk factors for schizophrenia and bipolar illness. Although OCD and schizophrenia constitute distinct diagnostic entities, OCD and schizophrenia share some epidemiological and clinical similarities: both disorders develop in early adulthood, have an equal gender ratio with earlier onset in males, have high prevalence rates of comorbid disorders, and have a chronic course. However, no clear familial relationship or shared genetic etiology between OCD and schizophrenia has been found.[34] Instead, an association between OCD and “schizo-obsessive disorder” (schizophrenia with OCS) has been reported in a recent family study, which found that relatives of schizophrenia probands with OCD had a significantly higher morbid risk for OCD, OC personality disorder, and "schizo-obsessive disorder" than the schizophrenia probands without OCD, whose risk for OCD was similar to the general population.[35] Another recent genetic study revealed that the polymorphisms associated with glutaminergic transmission, also known to be associated with OCD, are involved in developing OCS in schizophrenic patients taking atypical antipsychotics (AAPs).[36] These emerging epidemiological and genetic findings are consistent with the hypothesis that schizophrenia with OCS constitutes a distinct schizophrenic subgroup with a unique neurobiological pathogenesis.

Pathogenesis of Obsessive-Compulsive Symptoms in Schizophrenia

Emerging evidence suggests more than one pathogenesis in OC schizophrenia.[1,8,37] The OCS in patients with schizophrenia may clinically manifest as (1) prodrome in schizophrenic illness, (2) a coexisting independent disorder presenting before the onset of psychotic symptoms, (3) part of active psychotic illness, (4) obsessive ruminations during recovery or the remission phase, or (5) de novo OCS associated with atypical antipsychotic treatment (**Fig. 1**).

The OCS in schizophrenia may manifest as a transient phenomena, or it may persist or even worsen during the course of psychotic illness. OCS may also occur as a prodrome preceding the onset of schizophrenia[38] that may resolve or attenuate after the onset of psychosis. In contrast, OCS that predates onset of schizophrenia may persist or worsen regardless of progress in schizophrenic illness as an independent, coexisting disorder. Patients in this category may have previously met the criteria for OCD, and subsequently develop psychosis in the course of chronic and often treatment-refractory illness that currently meets the criteria for schizophrenia. Patients in this category exhibit variable degrees of insight and resistance regarding their OCS during the course of illness. Patients in this group often have a worse clinical course and outcome than patients with non-OC schizophrenia.[1,17,39] In some patients, OCS develops as a part of an active psychotic process that emerges along with acute psychosis and usually resolves with the overall improvement in psychosis. Patients in this group have an unequivocal diagnosis of schizophrenia, with little or no insight into their OCS. As the psychotic symptoms improve, the OCS may become attenuated and present as obsessive rumination or obsessive doubt, which may resolve with

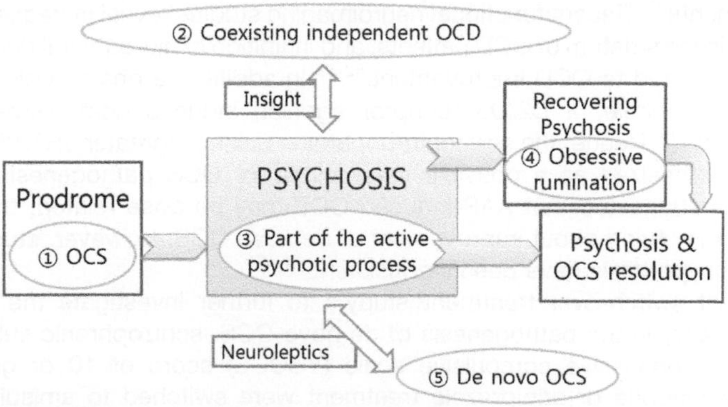

Fig. 1. Pathogenesis of obsessive-compulsive symptoms (OCS) in schizophrenia. OCD, obsessive-compulsive disorder.

further improvement. Patients in this group show varying degrees of insight and resistance regarding their obsessions, and show little difference in clinical course and prognosis compared with non-OC schizophrenia patients. Finally, emergence (de novo) or exacerbation of OCS following treatment with AAPs that possess a potent antiserotonergic receptor profile has challenged clinicians in recent years.[40–46] These AAPs include clozapine, olanzapine, risperidone, quetiapine, aripiprazole, and ziprasidone. In particular, clozapine therapy has been most commonly associated with the emergence of de novo OCS.[44] Due to its diverse nature of clinical presentation and presence of multiple pathogeneses, it is important to be acquainted with the varying presentations of OCS in schizophrenia, as each pathogenesis may require a specific treatment intervention. Ascertaining pathogenesis during a single cross-sectional evaluation is often difficult. OC schizophrenia therefore, may require multiple and longitudinal assessments to ascertain its pathogenesis and formulate treatment strategy.

TREATMENT

Although the therapeutic efficacy of anti-OCD medication and the AAPs in OC schizophrenia has been well investigated in recent years, the findings have been variable. This variation may be attributable to the presence of multiple pathogeneses as previously described, as well as differing pharmacologic profiles of antipsychotics. For example, whereas some AAPs such as clozapine are known to induce de novo OCS in schizophrenia, OCS that is part of a psychotic process may be successfully treated with clozapine monotherapy.[47] On the other hand, amisulpride an antipsychotic medication with negligible 5-HT2a receptor affinity[48] has shown clinical efficacy in the management of medication-induced de novo OCS in schizophrenia.[45,49] Therefore, treatment of OCS in patients with schizophrenia must be individualized based on the possible pathogenesis and clinical status (**Fig. 2**).

Management of De Novo Obsessive-Compulsive Symptoms in Schizophrenia

As previously mentioned, some AAPs cause de novo OCS or exacerbation of preexisting OCS.[40–45] De novo emergence or exacerbation of OCS with AAPs is thought to be related to their antagonist effect on 5-HT2a receptors, whereas D2 receptor blocking activity of antipsychotics is thought to be related to their antiobsessional effect.[45,50] Clomipramine and fluoxetine, both selective serotonin reuptake inhibitors (SSRIs) with mild indirect dopamine blocking properties, are highly effective antiobsessional agents.[51] Recent functional neuroimaging studies reveal increased dopaminergic tone in the striatum of OCD patients, and inhibition of nigrostriatal dopaminergic activity was related to OCD improvement.[52,53] In addition, a pharmacological study found that quinpirole, a D2/D3 receptor agonist, induces compulsive checking behavior in rats.[54] Hence, the serotonin-dopamine balance (greater 5HT2/D2 antagonism) is hypothesized as a possible mechanism for OCS pathogenesis. Previous studies have suggested that AAP-induced OCS may be dose related, thus a dose adjustment may bring about improvement of de novo OCS. However, study findings to verify the hypothesis have been inconsistent.[41,42]

In a recent switch-over treatment study[49] to further investigate the serotonin-dopamine theory in the pathogenesis of de novo OCS, schizophrenic subjects with a Yale-Brown obsessive compulsive scale (YBOCS) score of 10 or greater and receiving risperidone or aripiprazole treatment were switched to amisulpride after baseline assessment. Amisulpride is a novel antipsychotic drug, with selective dopamine D2/D3 receptor antagonism and a negligible affinity for the 5-HT2a receptor. In

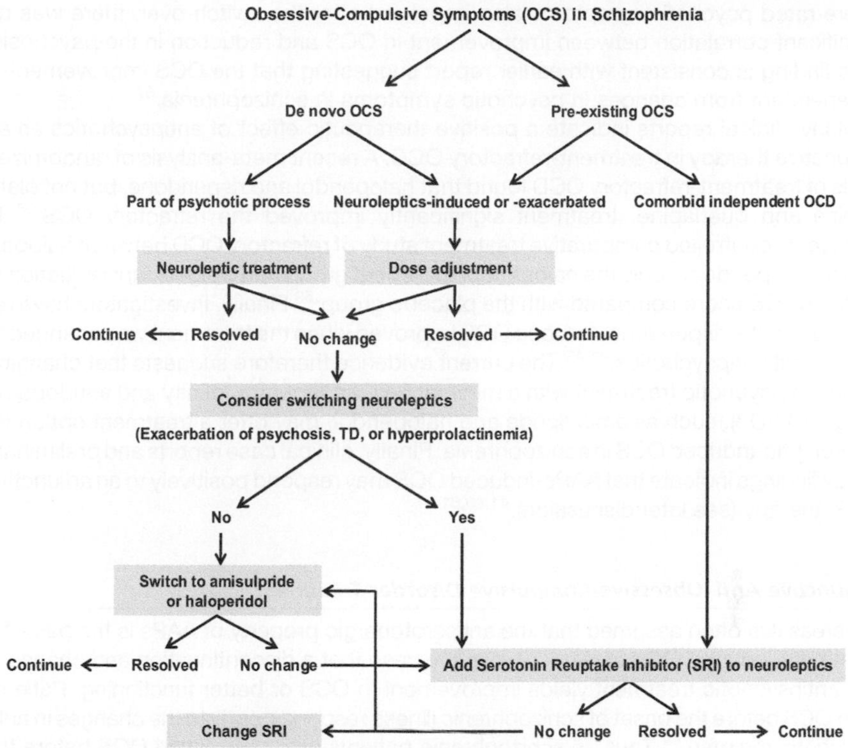

Fig. 2. Treatment guidelines of OCS in schizophrenia.

this study amisulpride was highly effective in improving the AAP-induced OCS in schizophrenic patients, with a YBOCS total score improvement from 16.5 to 5.3. A possible explanation for the OCS relief following switch-over includes withdrawal of the previous AAP, with a potent 5-HT2a antagonist known to activate the OCS in conjunction with D2 receptor blocking effect hypothesized to alleviate the OCS.

In a recent small prospective study,[55] Glick and colleagues reported that a switch from AAPs to aripiprazole treatment improved the de novo OCS in schizophrenia. However, this finding remains controversial as some others noted worsening of OCS with the aripiprazole treatment.[43,45,49] Aripiprazole's unique neuroreceptor profile, primarily dopamine partial agonist unlike the other AAPs, was suggested as a therapeutically useful pharmacological property in the treatment of OC schizophrenia. However, its potent 5-HT2a antagonism with the weak D2 blockade effect may also be related to potential to induce or exacerbate OCS in schizophrenic patients. In a recent 26-week prospective switch-over study, Kim and colleagues[56] found that 4 of 61 patients (7%) developed a new OCS on aripiprazole treatment, and 2 discontinued from the study due to the adverse event. This finding contrasts with Glick's report that 4 of 11 subjects (36%) improved 50% or more on the YBOCS score after the switch to aripiprazole treatment. In addition, the Glick study failed to specify whether the OCS improvement was an independent OC symptom change or was secondary to the overall improvement of psychosis. On the contrary, in another prospective switch-over study with either a risperidone or aripiprazole group swithching to amisulpride,[49] 12 of 16 subjects (75%) demonstrated a robust reduction in OCS rated using the YBOCS (50% or greater). Although positive and negative syndrome score rated psychotic symptoms also improved after the switch-over, there was no significant correlation between improvement in OCS and reduction in the psychosis. This finding is consistent with earlier report suggesting that the OCS improvement is independent from changes in psychotic symptoms in schizophrenia.[57]

Many clinical reports indicate a positive therapeutic effect of antipsychotics as an adjunctive therapy in treatment-refractory OCD. A recent meta-analysis of randomized trials of treatment-refractory OCD found that haloperidol and risperidone, but not olanzapine and quetiapine, treatment significantly improved the refractory OCS.[58] In a placebo-controlled comparative treatment study of refractory OCD between haloperidol and risperidone, only the haloperidol treatment group had a significant reduction in total YBOCS score compared with the placebo group.[59] Finally, investigators have reported that the risperidone-induced OCS improved when the treatment was changed to the typical antipsychotics.[41,42] The current evidence therefore suggests that changing to an antipsychotic treatment with a minimal 5-HT2a receptor affinity and antidopaminergic (D2/D3), such as amisulpride and haloperidol, may offer a treatment option for neuroleptic-induced OCS in schizophrenia. Finally, clinical case reports and preliminary study findings indicate that AAPs-induced OCS may respond positively to an adjunctive SSRI therapy (see later discussion).[41,60,61]

Adjunctive Anti–Obsessive-Compulsive Disorder Treatment

Whereas it is often assumed that the antiserotonergic property of AAPs is the basis for treatment-induced OCS, it is not always the case that a discontinuation and change in the antipsychotic treatment yields improvement in OCS or better functioning. Patients with OCS before the onset of schizophrenic illness respond poorly to the changes in antipsychotic regimen.[49] Thus, in schizophrenic patients with preexisting OCS before the onset of psychosis, adjunctive SSRI treatment should be considered (see **Fig. 2**). Use of the antidopaminergic drugs such as haloperidol or amisulpride in the management of de novo OCS may be constrained in some patients prone to adverse effects such as hyperprolactinemia or tardive dyskinesia (TD).[62] Furthermore, change from clozapine to other antipsychotics due to treatment-induced OCS is often impractical in clinical practice, as they are often refractory to the other treatment. Therefore, in OC schizophrenic patients who fail to respond or are unable to tolerate switching to antidopaminergic medications, the use of adjunctive SSRI may be a first-line treatment option for OCS.

Although there is a scarcity of double-blind controlled studies with an adjunctive anti-OCD medication in OC schizophrenia, several recent studies supported specific efficacy of serotonergic antidepressants in OC schizophrenia.[57,63–67] Some investigators found a marked OCS reduction with clinical and neuropsychological function improvement with an adjunctive anti-OCD regimen,[57,63–67] whereas others have found no significant beneficial effects,[68] and few even reported worsening of the symptoms.[69] To investigate the therapeutic efficacy of adjunctive SSRI in treatment of OC schizophrenia the authors conducted a prospective crossover treatment study in a chronic, treatment-refractory OC schizophrenia.[70] This study assessed the patients' clinical, psychopathological, and neuropsychological profiles over a 6-month period. The authors found a specific OCS reduction accompanied by the prefrontal executive function improvement with the adjunctive treatment. Furthermore, the OCS relief was also accompanied by the negative psychotic symptom reduction and global clinical assessment. This clinical and neuropsychopathological improvement correlated positively with addition of anti-OCD medication and worsened with its removal during the study period. Although this case study finding is limited, the specific anti-OC effect and neurocognitive functional improvement in OC schizophrenia suggests a possible pathogenesis that is unique and distinct in this subgroup of schizophrenic patients.[17]

Pharmacokinetic and pharmacodynamic effects of the SRIs must be carefully considered when used as an adjunctive therapy with the antipsychotic regimen. SRIs competitively inhibit microsomal P450 isoenzymes that can significantly increase the antipsychotic blood level.[71] In fact, fluoxetine and paroxetine may increase the plasma concentrations of clozapine and risperidone by between 20% and 75% via competitive inhibition of the CYP 2D6 or CYP 3A4 isoenzymes.[72–74] Clomipramine, a potent inhibitor of CYP 2D6, can increase risperidone and aripiprazole serum levels[75] and fluvoxamine, which has been effective in OC schizophrenia in several studies,[66,67] may increase plasma concentration of olanzapine up to 100% and clozapine by up to 5 to 10 times by blocking CYP 1A2 enzyme.[76–79] Therefore, augmentation of fluvoxamine to treat OCS should be avoided in patients taking clozapine, while olanzapine dosage should be adjusted with fluvoxamine treatment. These pharmacokinetic interactions of the SSRIs can significantly exacerbate the number of antipsychotic adverse effects such as akathisia and extrapyramidal symptoms. Whereas sertraline, citalopram, and escitalopram may minimally influence metabolism via a CYP enzyme[71,75,79] there are only few reports that indicate their efficacy in OC schizophrenia.[60,61] The pharmacodynamic interactions, which take place at receptor sites and occur between drugs with similar adverse effects, should also be considered.[71] Combining drugs with those having similar pharmacologic action could exaggerate potential adverse effects.[80] For example, combining clomipramine with clozapine exacerbates sedation, orthostatic hypotension, and anticholinergic side effects, which are caused by both drugs. Therefore, clinicians must carefully monitor for potential adverse effects due to adverse pharmacodynamic, as well as, pharmacokinetic effects of the adjunctive drug therapy.[81]

CLINICAL CASES

Patient A

A 45-year-old white man with an extensive psychiatric history presented with treatment-refractory, undifferentiated schizophrenia. He was agitated, psychotic, and revealed several bizarre, stereotyped behaviors. These ritualistic behaviors reportedly persisted over the years and were unresponsive to various antipsychotic treatments, including clozapine. Adjunctive medication trials, including lithium, valproic acid, carbamazepine, propranolol, and benzodiazepines, were ineffective. Electroencephalography and brain computed tomography (CT) scan were unremarkable. Treatment with high-dose chlorpromazine (CPZ) reduced agitation, with a partial reduction in psychosis. His bizarre rituals persisted, and a treatment trial with fluoxetine as an adjunctive therapy with gradual dose titration was initiated. After 2 weeks of fluoxetine, 40 mg/d and CPZ, his rituals lessened and self-care skills improved. He became more engaged in ward routines and treatment milieu. After a year of treatment with marked symptom reduction, fluoxetine was reduced to 20 mg/d, which brought about exacerbation of the rituals. Subsequent increase of fluoxetine to 60 mg/d for 6 weeks once again reduced impulsivity and ritualistic behaviors. The patient remained stable for the next 2 years on a combined CPZ and fluoxetine regimen.[8]

Patient B

A 35-year-old single white man diagnosed at age 12 years with undifferentiated schizophrenia presented with hallucinations and paranoid delusion. He had several psychotic relapses over the years that responded well to a routine antipsychotic medication treatment. During the previous hospitalization precipitated by an acute onset of paranoid delusion and auditory/visual hallucinations, accompanied by catatonic behavior, he failed to respond to multiple antipsychotic treatments. The patient also began to exhibit bizarre rituals such as repetitive touching of objects, opening and closing doors, excessive ritualistic water drinking, and forcefully rubbing and injuring his eyes. The medical workup and brain CT scan were normal. Clomipramine (CMI), 25 mg/d was subsequently added to ongoing fluphenazine decanoate (50 mg/2 wk) and lithium carbonate (1200 mg/d), gradually increasing to 50 mg/d over 2 weeks. After 4 weeks of 50 mg/d, his rituals became less frequent and intense, with improved socialization and therapy participation. Further increase of CMI to 150 mg/d to achieve therapeutic regimen, however, brought about increasing restlessness, and impulsive and agitated behavior. Reduction of CMI to 50 mg/d once again relieved the OC symptoms and improved functioning. Serial neuropsychological assessments during the study demonstrated a cognitive function change that accompanied the OC symptoms with the treatment.[8]

Patient C

Patient C is a 45-year-old white man with paranoid schizophrenia diagnosed at age 18 years, with bizarre persecutory delusions and hallucinations accompanied by impulsive and intrusive behaviors. He has had numerous hospitalizations and treatment with a variety of antipsychotic medications, with poor symptom response. During the course of illness, the patient developed bizarre, repetitive behaviors such as ritualistic touching of objects, repeated dressing and undressing, and frequent checking rituals. These rituals began several years after the onset of schizophrenic symptoms. Medical and neurological workup, including brain CT scan, revealed no abnormalities. During the current hospitalization the patient received a wide range of antipsychotic and adjunctive medication including the mood stabilizers, without significant therapeutic effects. A treatment trial with adjunctive SSRI prompted a rapid increase in anxiety, restlessness, impulsivity, and agitation. A clozapine treatment trial also promptly increased anxiety, agitation, and exacerbated impulsive and ritualistic behaviors, which caused severe distress to the patient as well as the staff. Clozapine treatment discontinuation resulted in reduction of impulsivity and ritualistic behaviors.

Patient D

A 22-year-old woman diagnosed at age 18 years with paranoid schizophrenia presented with auditory hallucinations and a thought disorder. Risperidone treatment partially improved her psychotic symptoms; however, emergence of a de novo obsessive rumination of sexual fantasy and words caused severe distress. Switching from risperidone to amisulpride significantly improved the obsessive rumination; however, the medication induced metabolic disturbances, hyperprolactinemia, and TD, which required a sequential change in antipsychotic treatment to ziprasidone and aripiprazole. However, the change in antipsychotic treatment promptly triggered an exacerbation of the obsessive symptoms, which improved on switching back to amisulpride. As the obsessive symptoms were perceived to be more distressful than the amenorrhea, TD, and even psychotic symptoms, amisulpride treatment was maintained.[45] Due to the patient's subsequent suicide attempt and worsening clinical status (TD, amenorrhea, and refractory psychotic symptoms), a clozapine treatment trial was initiated. As a precaution to minimize the potential exacerbation of the OCS, the patient was started on escitalopram, 30 mg/d and clozapine, 250 mg/d as replacements for the amisulpride, 1000 mg/d. After 4 weeks of treatment, psychotic symptoms and persistent suicidal ideations were almost fully resolved without causing an OCS exacerbation. After marked symptom reduction, escitalopram was reduced to 15 mg/d, but obsessive rumination was subsequently exacerbated. Increasing escitalopram to 20 mg/d again reduced obsession.

Case Vignette Discussion

The 4 clinical vignettes demonstrate varied clinical profiles and treatment response in patients with OC schizophrenia. These diverse clinical manifestations together with pervasive diagnostic predicament and lack of clearly defined treatment guidelines in OC schizophrenia continue to challenge the clinicians.

Patient A is a chronic, treatment-refractory OC schizophrenic who responded to adjunctive SSRI treatment, with OCS reduction and functional improvement. The specific OCS response to the anti-OCD medication and dose adjustments suggests a distinct biological pathogenesis.

Patient B demonstrated a marked OCS reduction and functional improvement with a low, subtherapeutic anti-OCD medication dose. However, the patient became markedly agitated with impulsive, ritualistic behaviors on a standard dose regimen and once again improved on returning to a low-dose SSRI regimen. The authors suspect that a pharmacokinetic interaction of the antipsychotics and antidepressants might have developed and caused the akathisia or agitation, because both fluphenazine and clomipramine are a substrate and inhibitor of CYP 2D6; thus blood levels may have increased. A standard therapeutic dose regimen of SSRI or antipsychotics can cause symptom exacerbation or adverse effects if a drug interaction develops; therefore, SSRI or antipsychotics dose adjustment should be considered when a drug interaction is expected.

Patient C illustrates a chronic treatment-refractory schizophrenia that developed de novo OCS with clozapine treatment. The OCS responded poorly to the adjunctive SSRI treatment, and improved with the dose tapering or discontinuing the offending antipsychotic medication therapy.

Patient D demonstrated sequential development of OCS following the administration of AAPs with 5-HT2a receptor antagonism, such as risperidone, aripiprazaole, and ziprasidone. In contrast, switching to amisulpride, which is a selective D2 and D3 receptor antagonist, improved the obsessive symptoms. However, clozapine was eventually used because of the refractory psychotic symptoms, TD, and suicide risk, although it had a strong potential to exacerbate the OCS. Fortunately, coadministration of escitalopram with clozapine prevented OCS exacerbation with good therapeutic efficacy. Although the use of escitalopram in schizophrenic patients with OCS has not been reported, it was selected because of its minimal drug interaction.

In summary, current evidence suggests that OC schizophrenia is a complex condition with more than one underlying pathogenesis that requires careful evaluation and individualized treatment intervention. These case vignettes illustrate some of the complexity and clinical challenges in patients with OC schizophrenia.

TREATMENT RECOMMENDATIONS

Given the current state of knowledge regarding the pathogenesis and pharmacotherapy for OCS in schizophrenia, the following recommendations may be made.

1. The OCS that develop as a part of the psychotic process might be successfully treated along with overall improvement in psychosis using antipsychotic treatment alone.

2. If the OCS is exacerbated or newly developed after using AAPs, a dosage adjustment or change in antipsychotic medications to those with a strong antidopamniergic properties and a negligible 5HT2 receptor affinity should be considered. Amisulpride seems to be promising in the management of AAP-induced OCS.
3. Use of the adjunctive anti-OCD medications such as clomipramine and SSRI seems to be effective, but clinicians must be aware of their potential pharmacokinetic and pharmacodynamic interactions with antipsychotic medications. Also, consider some reports that use of anti-OCD agents in some acutely psychotic schizophrenic patients may increase the risk of symptom exacerbation.
4. Patients receiving clozapine should be carefully assessed to determine the role of clozapine therapy on OCS. If the OCS seem to have started or worsened with clozapine treatment, clinicians should consider switching to another antipsychotic after weighing the benefits derived from clozapine against the morbidity caused by an increase in OCS. If clozapine is to be continued, its dosage may be adjusted, or SSRI considered as an antiobsessional treatment of choice, given the significant adverse effects associated with combined clozapine and CMI regimen. The novel antipsychotic drug amisulpride may offer a new treatment prospect in OC schizophrenia, however, it is not currently approved by the Food and Drug Administration (FDA) for treatment of schizophrenia in the US.
5. Finally, pharmacotherapy should be combined with the cognitive behavioral psychotherapy in treating OC schizophrenia once the patient is clinically stable or able to participate in the therapy.[82,83]

SUMMARY

Recent work in OC schizophrenia suggests far greater prevalence and continuing challenges in its clinical management. A large proportion of OC schizophrenic patients remain clinically unrecognized and often mismanaged. Unlike the earlier belief, the subgroup of OC schizophrenic patients often suffer from a worse clinical course, poor treatment response, greater neuropsychological impairments, and worse long-term outcome. In addition, the neurobiological research in schizophrenia and OCD has also established multisystem involvement in their pathogenesis, and that OC schizophrenia may involve more than one pathogenesis. Emerging evidence in recent years also suggests that the AAPs, with potent central serotonin receptor blocking properties, can cause a new onset or worsening of preexisting OCS in schizophrenia. However, amisulpride, a novel antipsychotic with potent antidopaminergic and negligible antiserotonergic effects, may offer effective pharmacotherapy without compromising the psychotic decompensation. On the other hand, adjunctive anti-OCD therapy with either typical antipsychotics or AAP seems to be effective and improves the outcome in some patients. These varying treatment response and outcomes may be related to underlying pathogenesis of the OC phenomena in schizophrenia. Further systematic studies clearly are needed to validate the earlier findings. Meanwhile, currently available evidence calls for comprehensive clinical and neuropsychological assessment aa well as individualized pharmacological treatment intervention to achieve optimal outcome in OC schizophrenic patients.

In conclusion, the emerging clinical and biological evidence in recent years has provided greater understanding and insight into OC schizophrenia. As they continue to challenge practicing clinicians, a greater understanding of pathogenesis and individualized pharmacopsychotherapeutic treatment will improve clinical course and outcome. It is clear that further work to delineate the biological and psychological pathogenesis as well as individualized treatment intervention by practicing clinicians will yield the optimum outcome.

REFERENCES

1. Hwang MY, Bermanzohn PC, Opler LA. Obsessive-compulsive symptoms in patients with schizophrenia. In: Hwang MY, Bermanzohn PC, editors. Schizophrenia and comorbid conditions. Washington (DC): American Psychiatry Press; 2001. p. 57–78.
2. Kraemer HC. DSM categories and dimensions in clinical and research contexts. In: Helzer JE, Kraemer HC, Krueger, et al, editors. Dimensional approaches in diagnostic classification: refining the research agenda for DSM-V. Arlington (VA): American Psychiatric Press; 2008. p. 5–17.
3. Westphal K. Ueber Zwangsvorstellungen. [On compulsive thoughts]. Arch Psychiatr Nervenkr 1878;8:734–50 [in German].
4. Kraepelin E. Dementia praecox, or the group of schizophrenias. NY: International University Press; 1956.
5. Stengel E. A study on some clinical aspects of the relationship between obsessional neurosis and psychotic reaction types. J Ment Sci 1945;91:166–84.
6. Bleuler E. Dementia praecox, the group of schizophrenias. NY: International University Press; 1956.
7. Kay SR, Fiszbein A, Opler LA. The positive and negative syndrome scale for schizophrenia. Schizophr Bull 1987;13:261–76.
8. Hwang MY, Opler LA. Schizophrenia with obsessive-compulsive features: assessment and treatment. Psychiatr Ann 1994;24:468–72.
9. Hollander E. Obsessive-compulsive related disorders. Washington (DC): American Psychiatric Press; 1993.
10. Eisen J, Rasmussen S. Obsessive compulsive disorder with psychotic features. J Clin Psychiatry 1993;54:373–9.
11. Thomsen PH, Jensen J. Obsessive-compulsive disorder: admission patterns and diagnostic stability. A case-register study. Acta Psychiatr Scand 1994;90:19–24.
12. Jahrreiss W. Obsessions during schizophrenia. Arch Psychiatr Nervenkr 1926;77:740–88.
13. Rosen I. The clinical significance of obsessions in schizophrenia. J Ment Sci 1957;103:778–85.
14. Insel TR, Akiskal HS. Obsessive-compulsive disorder with psychotic features: a phenomenological analysis. Am J Psychiatry 1986;143:1527–33.
15. Karno M, Golding JM, Sorenson SB, et al. The epidemiology of obsessive-compulsive disorder in five U.S. communities. Arch Gen Psychiatry 1988;45:1094–9.
16. Berman I, Kalinowski A, Berman SM, et al. Obsessive and compulsive symptoms in chronic schizophrenia. Compr Psychiatry 1995;36:6–10.
17. Hwang MY, Morgan JE, Losonczy MF. Clinical and neuropsychological profiles of OC schizophrenia. J Neuropsychiatry Clin Neurosci 2000;12:91–4.
18. Sevincok L, Akoglu A, Kokcu F. Suicidality in schizophrenic patients with and without obsessive-compulsive disorder. Schizophr Res 2007;90:198–202.
19. Buckley PF, Miller BJ, Lehrer DS, et al. Psychiatric comorbidities and schizophrenia. Schizophr Bull 2009;35:383–402.
20. Poyurovsky M, Koran LM. Obsessive-compulsive disorder [OCD] with schizotypy vs. schizophrenia with OCD: diagnostic dilemmas and therapeutic implications. J Psychiatr Res 2005;39:399–408.

21. Poyurovsky MD, Fuchs C, Weizman A. Obsessive-compulsive disorder in patients with first-episode schizophrenia. Am J Psychiatry 1999;156:1998–2000.
22. Craig T, Hwang MY, Bromet EJ. Obsessive-compulsive and panic symptoms in patients with first-admission psychosis. Am J Psychiatry 2002;159:592–8.
23. Rifkin J, Yucel M, Maruff P, et al. Psychiatric research. Neuroimaging 2005;138:99–113.
24. Kim JJ, Youn T, Lee JM, et al. Morphometric abnormality of the insula in schizophrenia: a comparison with obsessive-compulsive disorder and normal control using MRI. Schizophr Res 2003;60:191–8.
25. Kwon JS, Shin YW, Kim CW, et al. Similarity and disparity of obsessive-compulsive disorder and schizophrenia in MR volumetric abnormalities of the hippocampus-amygdala complex. J Neurol Neurosurg Psychiatr 2003;74:962–4.
26. Saxena S, Rauch SL. Functional neuroimaging and the neuroanatomy of obsessive-compulsive disorder. Psychiatr Clin North Am 2000;23:563–86.
27. Hollander E, Braun A, Simeon D. Should OCD leave the anxiety disorders in DSM-V? The case for obsessive compulsive-related disorders. Depress Anxiety 2008;25:317–29.
28. Berman I, Merson A, Viegner B, et al. Obsessions and compulsions as a distinct cluster of symptoms in schizophrenia: a neuiropsychological study. J Nerv Ment Dis 1998;186:150–6.
29. Lysaker PH, Bryson GJ, Marks KA, et al. Association of obsessions and compulsions in schizophrenia with neurocognition and negative symptoms. J Neuropsychiatry Clin Neurosci 2002;14:449–53.
30. Lysaker PH, Whitney KA, Davis LW. Associations of executive function with concurrent and prospective reports of obsessive-compulsive symptoms in schizophrenia. J Neuropsychiatry Clin Neurosci 2009;21:38–42.
31. Whitney KA, Fastenau PS, Evans JD, et al. Comparative neuropsychological function in obsessive-compulsive disorder and schizophrenia with and without obsessive-compulsive symptoms. Schizophr Res 2004;69:75–83.
32. Borkowska A, Pilaczyñska E, Rybakowski JK. The frontal lobe neuropsychological tests in patients with schizophrenia and/or obsessive-compulsive disorder. J Neuropsychiatry Clin Neurosci 2003;15:359–62.
33. Lichtenstein P, Yip BH, Björk C, et al. Common genetic determinants of schizophrenia and bipolar disorder in Swedish families: a population-based study. Lancet 2009;373:234–9.
34. Nestadt G, Samuels J, Riddle MA, et al. The relationship between obsessive-compulsive disorder and anxiety and affective disorders: results from the Johns Hopkins OCD family study. Psychol Med 2001;31:481–7.
35. Poyurovsky M, Kriss V, Weisman G, et al. Familial aggregation of schizophrenia-spectrum disorders and obsessive-compulsive associated disorders in schizophrenia probands with and without OCD. Am J Med Genet B Neuropsychiatr Genet 2005;133B:31–6.
36. Kwon JS, Joo YH, Nam HJ, et al. Association of the glutamate transporter gene SLC1A1 with atypical anitpsychotics-induced obsessive compulsive symptoms. Arch Gen Psychiatry, in press.
37. Bottas A, Cooke RG, Richter MA. Comorbidity and pathophysiology of obsessive-compulsive disorder in schizophrenia: is there evidence for a schizo-obsessive subtype of schizophrenia? J Psychiatry Neurosci 2005;30:187–93.
38. Iida J, Iwasaka H, Hirao F, et al. Clinical features of childhood-onset schizophrenia with obsessive-compulsive symptoms during the prodromal phase. Psychiatry Clin Neurosci 1995;49:201–7.

39. Fenton WS, McGlashan TH. The prognostic significance of obsessive compulsive symptoms in schizophrenia. Am J Psychiatry 1986;143:437–41.
40. Khullar A, Chue P, Tibbo P. Quetiapine and obsessive-compulsive symptoms [OCS]: case report and review of atypical antipsychoticinduced OCS. J Psychiatry Neurosci 2001;26:55–9.
41. Alevizos B, Lykouras L, Zervas IM, et al. Risperidone-induced obsessive-compulsive symptoms: a series of six cases. J Clin Psychopharmacol 2002;22:461–7.
42. Lykouras L, Alevizos B, Michalopoulou P, et al. Obsessive-compulsive symptoms induced by atypical antipsychotics: a review of reported cases. Prog Neuropsychopharmacol Biol Psychiatry 2003;27:333–46.
43. Mouaffak F, Gallarda T, Bayle FJ, et al. Worsening of obsessive-compulsive symptoms after treatment with aripiprazole. J Clin Psychopharmacol 2007;27:237–8.
44. Kim M, Park DY, Kwon JS, et al. Prevalence and clinical characteristics of obsessive-compulsive symptoms associated with atypical antipsychotics. J Clin Psychopharmacol 2007;27:712–3.
45. Kim SW, Shin IS, Kim JM, et al. The 5-HT2 receptor profiles of antipsychotics in the pathogenesis of obsessive-compulsive symptoms in schizophrenia. Clin Neuropharmacol 2009;32:224–6.
46. Alevizos B, Papageorgiou C, Christodoulou GN. Obsessive-compulsive symptoms with olanzapine. Int J Neuropsychopharmacol 2004;7:375–7.
47. Reznik I, Yavin I, Stryjer R, et al. Clozapine in the treatment of obsessive-compulsive symptoms in schizophrenia patients: a case series study. Pharmacopsychiatry 2004;37:52–6.
48. Metin O, Yazici K, Tot S, et al. Amisulpiride augmentation in treatment resistant obsessive-compulsive disorder: an open trial. Hum Psychopharmacol 2003;18:463–7.
49. Kim SW, Shin IS, Kim JM, et al. Amisulpride improves obsessive-compulsive symptoms in schizophrenia patients taking atypical antipsychotics: an open-label switch study. J Clin Psychopharmacol 2008;28:349–52.
50. Ramasubbu R, Ravindron A, Lapierre Y. Serotonin and dopamine antagonism in obsessive-compulsive disorder: effect of atypical antipsychotic drugs. Pharmacopsychiatry 2000;33:236–8.
51. Austin LS, Lydiard RB, Ballenger JC, et al. Dopamine blocking activity of clomipramine in patients with obsessive-compulsive disorder. Biol Psychiatry 1991;30:225–32.
52. van der Wee NJ, Stevens H, Hardeman JA, et al. Enhanced dopamine transporter density in psychotropic-naive patients with obsessive-compulsive disorder shown by [^{123}I]{beta}-CIT SPECT. Am J Psychiatry 2004;161:2201–6.
53. Kim CH, Cheon KA, Koo MS, et al. Dopamine transporter density in the basal ganglia in obsessive-compulsive disorder, measured with [^{123}I]IPT SPECT before and after treatment with serotonin reuptake inhibitors. Neuropsychobiology 2007;55:156–62.
54. Szechtman H, Sulis W, Eilam D. Quinpirole induces compulsive checking behavior in rats: a potential animal model of obsessivecompulsive disorder (OCD). Behav Neurosci 1998;112:1475–85.
55. Glick ID, Poyurovsky M, Ivanova O, et al. Aripiprazole in schizophrenia patients with comorbid obsessive-compulsive symptoms: an open-label study of 15 patients. J Clin Psychiatry 2008;69:1856–9.
56. Kim SW, Shin IS, Kim JM, et al. Effectiveness of switching to aripiprazole from atypical antipsychotics in patients with schizophrenia. Clin Neuropharmacol 2009;32:243–9.

57. Hwang MY, Rho J, Opler LA, et al. Treatment of obsessive-compulsive schizophrenic patient with clomipramine: clinical and neuropsychological findings. Neuropsychiatry Neuropsychol Behav Neurol 1995;8:231–3.
58. Bloch MH, Landeros-Weisenberger A, Kelmendi B, et al. A systematic review: antipsychotic augmentation with treatment refractory obsessive-compulsive disorder. Mol Psychiatry 2006;11:622–32.
59. Li X, May RS, Tolbert LC, et al. Risperidone and haloperidol augmentation of serotonin reuptake inhibitors in refractory obsessive-compulsive disorder: a crossover study. J Clin Psychiatry 2005;66:736–43.
60. Allen L, Tejera C. Treatment of clozapine induced obsessive-compulsive symptoms with sertraline. Am J Psychiatry 1994;151:1096–7.
61. Dodt JE, Byerly MJ, Guadros C, et al. Treatment of risperidone-induced obsessive-compulsive symptoms with sertraline. Am J Psychiatry 1997;154:582.
62. Haddad PM, Sharma SG. Adverse effects of atypical antipsychotics: differential risk and clinical implications. CNS Drugs 2007;21:911–36.
63. Stroebel CF, Szarek BL. Use of clomipramine in treatment of obsessive-compulsive symptomatology. J Clin Psychopharmacol 1984;4:98–100.
64. Berman I, Sapers BL, Chang HH, et al. Treatment of obsessive-compulsive symptoms in schizophrenic patients with clomipramine. J Clin Psychopharmacol 1995; 15:206–10.
65. Hwang MY, Martin AM, Lindenmayer JP, et al. Treatment of schizophrenia with obsessive-compulsive features with serotonin reuptake inhibitors. Am J Psychiatry 1993;150:1127.
66. Poyurovsky M, Isakov V, Hromnikov S, et al. Fluvoxamine treatment of obsessive-compulsive symptoms in schizophrenic patients: an add-on open study. Int Clin Psychopharmacol 1999;14:95–100.
67. Reznick I, Sirota P. Obsessive-compulsive symptoms in schizophrenia: a randomized controlled trial with fluvoxamine and neuroleptics. J Clin Psychopharmacol 2000;20:410–6.
68. Margetic B. Aggravation of schizophrenia by clomipramine in a patient with comorbid obsessive-compulsive disorder. Psychopharmacol Bull 2008; 41:9–11.
69. Bark N, Lindenmayer JP. Ineffectiveness of clomipramine for obsessive-compulsive symptoms in patients with schizophrenia. Am J Psychiatry 1992; 149:136–7.
70. Levin Z, Hwang MY. Treatment of obsessive-compulsive schizophrenic patient with clomipramine. Neuropsychiatry, Neuropsychol Behav Neurol 1996;9:2.
71. Spina E, de Leon J. Metabolic drug interactions with newer antipsychotics: a comparative review. Basic Clin Pharmacol Toxicol 2007;100:4–22.
72. Centorrino F, Baldessarini RJ, Frankenburg FR, et al. Serum levels of clozapine and norclozapine in patients treated with selective serotonin reuptake inhibitors. Am J Psychiatry 1996;153:820–2.
73. Spina E, Avenoso A, Scordo MG, et al. Inhibition of risperidone metabolism by fluoxetine in patients with schizophrenia: a clinically relevant pharmacokinetic drug interaction. J Clin Psychopharmacol 2002;22:419–23.
74. Saito M, Yasui-Furukori N, Nakagami T, et al. Dose-dependent interaction of paroxetine with risperidone in schizophrenic patients. J Clin Psychopharmacol 2005;25:527–32.
75. Crewe HK, Lennard MS, Tucker GT, et al. The effect of selective serotonin reuptake inhibitors on cytochrome P4502D6 [CYP2D6] activity in human liver microsomes. Br J Clin Pharmacol 1992;34:262–5.

76. Szegedi A, Anghelescu I, Wiesner J, et al. Addition of low-dose fluvoxamine to low-dose clozapine monotherapy in schizophrenia: drug monitoring and tolerability data from a prospective clinical trial. Pharmacopsychiatry 1999;32:148–53.
77. Hiemke C, Weigmann H, Härtter S, et al. Elevated levels of clozapine in serum after addition of fluvoxamine. J Clin Psychopharmacol 1994;14:279–81.
78. Hiemke C, Peled A, Jabarin M, et al. Fluvoxamine augmentation of olanzapine in chronic schizophrenia: pharmacokinetic interactions and clinical effects. J Clin Psychopharmacol 2002;22:502–6.
79. Weigmann H, Gerek S, Zeisig A, et al. Fluvoxamine but not sertraline inhibits the metabolism of olanzapine: evidence from a therapeutic drug monitoring service. Ther Drug Monit 2001;23:410–3.
80. Kim SW, Shin IS, Kim JM, et al. Factors potentiating the risk of mirtazapine-associated restless legs syndrome. Hum Psychopharmacol 2008;23:615–20.
81. Hwang MY, Opler LA. Management of schizophrenia with obsessive-compulsive disorder. Psychiatr Ann 2000;30:23–8.
82. Ekers D. Successful outcome of exposure and response prevention in the treatment of obsessive-compulsive disorder in patients with schizophrenia. Behavioral Cognitive Psychotherapy 2004;32:375–8.
83. Green AI, Canuso CM, Brenner MJ, et al. Detection and management of comorbidity in patients with schizophrenia. Psychiatr Clin North Am 2003;26:115–39.

The Burden of Depressive Symptoms in People with Schizophrenia

Robert R. Conley, MD

KEYWORDS

- Schizophrenia • Depressive symptoms
- Depression • Outcomes

Depressive symptoms are recognized as an important and distinct symptom domain in schizophrenia[1] and may occur at any time during the course of the illness.[2–4] Although concurrent depressive symptoms were once considered good prognostic indicators,[5] recent research has demonstrated that depressive symptoms are poor prognostic indicators of recovery and reintegration into the community.[6] Depressive symptoms worsen quality of life[7] and increase the risk of suicide,[8] psychotic relapse, and psychiatric hospitalization.[9] The prevalence of depressive symptoms among people with schizophrenia has been reported to range from 25% to 81%,[8] depending on the treatment setting, phase of the illness, and the definition of depression. It is currently unclear what proportion of people with schizophrenia treated in usual practice settings experience at least a moderate level of depressive symptoms, whether the rates of depressive symptoms change over time, or which specific functional outcomes are more adversely affected by depressive symptoms during the course of the illness.

BURDEN OF DEPRESSION IN SCHIZOPHRENIA

Prospective longitudinal data on depressive symptoms among people with schizophrenia in usual care are sparse.[2,10–13] Studies have typically monitored a few outcome measures in relatively small samples of inpatients following discharge from hospitalization. Thus, studies have usually focused on vulnerable subgroups. The objectives of this study[14] were to prospectively assess the prevalence of concurrent depressive symptoms in a large and diverse group of people with schizophrenia treated in usual practice settings across the United States, and to focus on the relationships between baseline depressive symptoms and long-term functional outcomes.

Eli Lilly and Company, US Medical Division, Lilly Corporate Center, Indianapolis, IN 46285, USA
E-mail address: conley_robert@lilly.com

Psychiatr Clin N Am 32 (2009) 853–861
doi:10.1016/j.psc.2009.09.001 psych.theclinics.com

About one third of people with schizophrenia are concurrently depressed.[14] These prevalence rates have been highly consistent over time,[2,15–22] and appear to transcend differences in study populations, phases of the illness, and measures used to define depressed status, thus bolstering the validity of the common presence of these symptoms in this disorder. Also, the more common use of so-called "second-generation" antipsychotics in the past 10 years does not seem to have affected the prevalence of these symptoms at the population level.

Depressive symptoms are associated with considerable long-term burden in the treatment of schizophrenia. Compared to those without depressive symptoms at enrollment, people with depressive symptoms have poorer long-term functional outcomes in multiple domains. The depressed were more likely to use relapse-related mental health services (emergency psychiatric services, contacts with psychiatrists); to be of greater danger to self and others (violent, arrested, victimized, suicidal); to have more substance-related problems; to evidence poorer social and family relationships; and to have a poorer quality of life, lower motivational level, poorer level of functioning, poorer mental and physical health, lower level of medication adherence, and less general life satisfaction.

The association between depressive symptoms in schizophrenia and a greater risk of psychiatric hospitalization has been frequently reported,[2,23–27] as have lower levels of activity,[2,23] greater suicidal ideations and attempts,[2,28–37] greater substance use,[38,39] poorer quality of life,[9,40–44] poorer social functioning,[2,40,43,45–47] poorer physical health,[43] poorer medication adherence,[48] and less satisfaction with life in general.[2,40]

There is a strong link between change in depression status and changes in functional outcomes in the long-term treatment of people with schizophrenia in usual care settings.[14] Persistence of depression is associated with a lack of significant changes in functional outcomes over a 1-year period, whereas subjects who changed their status have evidenced substantial improvements. Worsening or developing depressive symptoms leads to clinical worsening. Specifically, those who changed from a depressed to a nondepressed state improve on many functional outcomes, and those who changed from nondepressed to depressed have evidenced worsening in most functional outcomes. Significant functional changes include those related to medication adherence, use of alcohol and illicit drugs, suicidal thinking and attempts, family relationships, social and occupational functioning, and general life satisfaction. People with schizophrenia and depression symptoms who continued to be depressed have and maintain a 10-fold increase in suicidal thinking compared with nondepressed subjects who continued to be nondepressed (35% vs 3%).[14] The rate of suicidal thinking significantly decreases when people with depression and schizophrenia become nondepressed (from 22.8% to 9.0%), and almost double for nondepressed who become depressed (from 10.4% to 20.5%). If people with schizophrenia can avoid becoming depressed, they have improved life outcomes with chronic treatment of their schizophrenia. These improvements have personal and economic implications, such as significant decreases in rates of hospitalization and emergency psychiatric services, decreased likelihood of being arrested, increases in number of working days, increases in community activities, and increases in general life satisfaction.

The burden of depressive symptoms affects the criminal justice system in addition to the mental health system. People with schizophrenia and depressive symptoms were found to use more relapse-related mental health services and to have more frequent contacts with law enforcement agencies compared with those without concurrent depressive symptoms. This may be related to the poorer adherence to medications reported by those with concurrent depressive symptoms, thereby increasing their risk of relapse, hospitalization, and symptom exacerbation that may lead to loss of control and greater display of impulsive and hostile behaviors. Findings suggest that this relatively large subgroup of people with schizophrenia is more volatile, vulnerable, and crisis prone, and more likely to be arrested and jailed. These individuals may require, therefore, more specialized treatments and close coordination between the criminal justice and the mental health systems, as jails and prisons have become surrogate mental hospitals for large populations of severely mentally ill offenders.[49]

A recent large, 3-year, prospective, observational, study of schizophrenia assessed symptoms and functional outcomes at enrollment and at 12-month intervals.[14] Participants depressed at enrollment were compared on the trajectory of their functional outcomes during the first year of the study and across the 3-year follow-up. The depressed cohort was significantly more likely than the nondepressed to use relapse-related mental health services (emergency psychiatric services, sessions with psychiatrists); to be a safety concern (violent, arrested, victimized, and suicidal); to have greater substance-related problems; and to report poorer life satisfaction, quality of life, mental functioning, family relationships, and medication adherence. Furthermore, changes in depressed status were associated with changes in functional outcomes.

In a study[14] of over 4000 people with schizophrenia or schizoaffective disorder, 40% were depressed at baseline. Depression rates were stable over the 3 years following enrollment, with 34.1% being depressed at the end of the first year, 30.3% at the end of the second year, and 33.00% at the end of the third year. The depressed and the nondepressed had comparable attrition rates throughout the 3-year study. Compared to nondepressed subjects at enrollment, the depressed were significantly more likely to be white, previously married, less educated, with earlier age at illness onset, more common schizoaffective disorder diagnosis, more psychiatric hospitalization in the previous year, and a comorbid diagnosis of personality disorder.

During the 6 months before enrollment, the depressed were less likely to be treated with typical antipsychotics and were more likely to be treated with antidepressants, anti-anxiety agents, mood stabilizers, and hypnotics. In this 3-year study, with adjustments for age, sex, and race, the depressed cohort was more likely than the nondepressed to have poorer clinical outcomes. The depressed cohort were also more likely to use relapse-related mental health services (emergency psychiatric services, contacts with psychiatrists), to be of greater safety concern in the community (as determined by such factors as violence, arrests, victimization, suicidal thoughts, suicide attempts), to have more substance-related problems, to evidence poorer social and family relationships, and to have a poorer quality of life (overall quality-of-life measure, lower motivational level, poorer global level of functioning, poorer mental and physical health, lower level of medication adherence, and less general life satisfaction).

In this study, most subjects (77%) maintained their depressed/nondepressed status, 13% changed from depressed to nondepressed, and 10% from nondepressed to depressed. Subjects who maintained their depressed/nondepressed status tended not to evidence significant changes on functional outcomes, whereas those who changed their depressed status tended to improve if changed from depressed to nondepressed, and worsen if changed from nondepressed to depressed. The group that remained depressed maintained functional outcomes on most of their outcome measures. In contrast, those who became nondepressed improved on 62% of their functional measures, with most of the improvements occurring early in treatment. Those who became depressed worsened on 53% of their functional measures. People who maintained their nondepressed status evidenced significant improvements on several functional outcomes, such as reductions in hospitalizations, emergency psychiatric services, and arrests, in addition to significant increases in working days, in common activities, and in general life satisfaction. Depression is also associated with other serious outcomes. It has been estimated that 4.9% of all people with schizophrenia will commit suicide, usually near the time of illness onset.[50]

It is well known and widely reported that illness severity, extrapyramidal symptoms, tardive dyskinesia, and diagnosis of schizoaffective disorder influence outcomes in schizophrenia. Nevertheless, depressive symptoms were still found to be associated with the above poor outcomes even when these concurrent conditions are taken into account.[14]

TREATMENT CONSIDERATIONS

It is critical to actively attempt to treat depression associated with schizophrenia. One approach is medication. Although few practice guidelines are associated with the use of antidepressants in schizophrenia, the use of these drugs is common. It was estimated that 38% of all subjects entering the Clinical Antipsychotic Trials of Intervention Effectiveness (CATIE) for treatment of schizophrenia were being treated with a concomitant antidepressant.[24] The use of antidepressants can be effective if targeted to depressive symptoms and used at adequate dosages, typically similar to those used for major depression. The use of these drugs as general adjuncts to therapy is usually not effective, however.[51,52] Modest evidence supports the use of such drugs in this comorbid state, although most randomized trials in this area are neither large nor of the highest quality.[53] Given the current state of data in the field, the clinician must look to evidence outside of traditional clinical trials to inform good practice.[54]

A rational approach to medication treatment is critical. The following practices should maximize the likelihood of a successful outcome:

1. Identify defined target symptoms. Specific depressive symptoms, noted in language understood by the clinician, patient, and family or caregiver, are needed. Understanding the target symptoms for a specific drug trial will allow for greater clarity in defining the parameters of success and failure.
2. Systematically use drugs at sufficient dosages and for a sufficient duration to establish efficacy. This is particularly critical before adjunct drugs are used because these may complicate the therapeutic situation to the point where defining the optimal drug treatment for a patient is not possible. Consider the use of long-acting injectable antipsychotics. Partial response to antipsychotics may masquerade as depression.
3. Take into consideration the possibility that medication intolerance, noncompliance, inadequate social support, and inadequate psychosocial treatment may create the appearance of clinical depression.
4. Exhaust the utility of single agents before using adjunct agents. There is tremendous pressure for the clinician to find a drug to rapidly treat every psychological problem manifest in people. Hostility, irritability, insomnia, and anhedonia can all be secondary to psychosis and may resolve only after a patient has had a good antipsychotic drug effect.
5. Aggressively prevent extrapyramidal symptoms through the appropriate choice of primary therapy. With the arrival of antipsychotic agents clearly effective at doses

that do not produce extrapyramidal symptoms in the vast majority of patients, we should be able to almost eliminate persistent side effects as a reason for therapeutic failure.
6. Maintain a positive therapeutic attitude. Patients should be encouraged to think that there is good reason to be optimistic that some therapy will be found that will be beneficial to them, even if they have had a history of severe illness.
7. If persistent suicidality is a serious concern, consider the use of clozapine. Although this is a life-modifying medication, it is the only antipsychotic shown to be effective in the reduction of suicidal ideation.[55,56]

In addition to medication, other therapies can be very useful in the treatment of depression. Cognitive-behavioral therapy has been shown to be very beneficial in the treatment of depressive symptoms in people with chronic schizophrenia.[57] It can be easily taught to nurses and other direct-care workers.[58] This therapy works particularly well when combined with supportive employment,[57] and can enhance outcomes in supportive housing.[4] An exciting integrated approach to cognitive therapy is now under study, and will, it is hoped, provide useful methods and a greater acceptance of this therapeutic approach in the general clinic.[59,60] See **Fig.1** for a representation of depression symptoms in schizophrenia.

In conclusion, individuals with schizophrenia and concurrent depressive symptoms are common and require special treatment interventions to help increase their chances for effective recovery. Concurrent depressive symptoms are associated with significantly poorer long-term functional outcomes and substantial burden linked to greater use of emergency mental health services and the criminal justice system. Active treatment of depression in people with schizophrenia should be a standard of care.

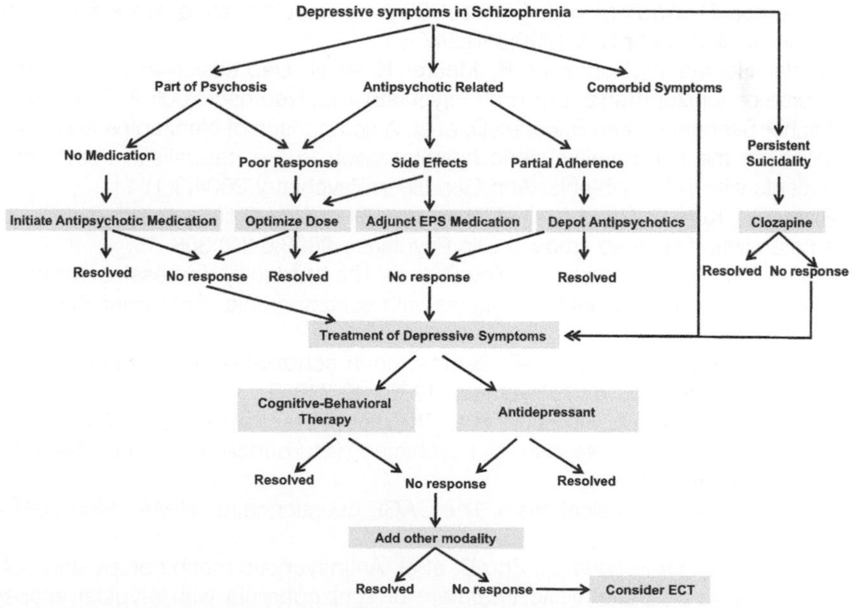

Fig. 1. Treatment algorithm for depression associated with Schizophrenia.

ACKNOWLEDGMENTS

This work represents the personal views and findings of Dr Conley. It was produced independently from his work at Eli Lilly and Company and thus does not represent the views of Eli Lilly and Company. The author would like to thank Dr S-W Kim for his assistance with the treatment algorithm. (Sung-Wan Kim, Assistant Professor, Department of Psychiatry, Chonnam National University Medical School, Korea.)

REFERENCES

1. Siris SG, Addington D, Azorin JM, et al. Depression in schizophrenia: recognition and management in the USA. Schizophr Res 2001;47(2–3):185–97.
2. Sands JR, Harrow M. Depression during the longitudinal course of schizophrenia. Schizophr Bull 1999;25(1):157–71.
3. Schooler NR, Kane JM. Research diagnosis for tardive dyskinesia [letter]. Arch Gen Psychiatry 1982;39(4):486–7.
4. Siegel CE, Samuels J, Tang DI, et al. Tenant outcomes in supported housing and community residences in New York City. Psychiatr Serv 2006;57(7):982–91.
5. Stephens JH, Astrup C, Mangrum JC. Prognostic factors in recovered and deteriorated schizophrenics. Am J Psychiatry 1966;122(10):1116–21.
6. Resnick SG, Rosenheck RA, Lehman AF. An exploratory analysis of correlates of recovery. Psychiatr Serv 2004;55(5):540–7.
7. Reine G, Lancon C, Di Tucci S, et al. Depression and subjective quality of life in chronic phase schizophrenic patients. Acta Psychiatr Scand 2003;108(4): 297–303.
8. Siris SG. Suicide and schizophrenia. J Psychopharmacol 2001;15(2):127–35.
9. Tollefson GD, Andersen SW, Tran PV. The course of depressive symptoms in predicting relapse in schizophrenia: a double-blind, randomized comparison of olanzapine and risperidone. Biol Psychiatry 1999;46(3):365–73.
10. Addington D, Addington J, Schissel B. A depression rating scale for schizophrenics. Schizophr Res 1990;3(4):247–51.
11. an der Heiden W, Konnecke R, Maurer K, et al. Depression in the long-term course of schizophrenia. Eur Arch Psychiatry Clin Neurosci 2005;255(3):174–84.
12. Ascher-Svanum H, Zhu B, Faries D, et al. A comparison of olanzapine and risperidone on the risk of psychiatric hospitalization in the naturalistic treatment of patients with schizophrenia. Ann Gen Hosp Psychiatry 2004;3(1):11.
13. Ritsner M, Kurs R, Gibel A, et al. Predictors of quality of life in major psychoses: a naturalistic follow-up study. J Clin Psychiatry 2003;64(3):308–15.
14. Conley RR, Ascher-Svanum H, Zhu B, et al. The burden of depressive symptoms in the long-term treatment of patients with schizophrenia. Schizophr Res 2007; 90(1–3):186–97.
15. Elk R, Dickman BJ, Teggin AF. Depression in schizophrenia: a study of prevalence and treatment. Br J Psychiatry 1986;149:228–9.
16. Endicott J, Spitzer RL, Fleiss JL, et al. The global assessment scale. A procedure for measuring overall severity of psychiatric disturbance. Arch Gen Psychiatry 1976;33(6):766–71.
17. Ewing JA. Detecting alcoholism. The CAGE questionnaire. JAMA 1984;252(14): 1905–7.
18. Faries D, Ascher-Svanum H, Zhu B, et al. Antipsychotic monotherapy and polypharmacy in the naturalistic treatment of schizophrenia with atypical antipsychotics. BMC Psychiatry 2005;5(1):26.

19. Harrow M, Yonan CA, Sands JR, et al. Depression in schizophrenia: are neuroleptics, akinesia, or anhedonia involved? Schizophr Bull 1994;20(2):327–38.
20. Heinrichs DW, Hanlon TE, Carpenter WT Jr. The quality of life scale: an instrument for rating the schizophrenic deficit syndrome. Schizophr Bull 1984;10(3):388–98.
21. Summers F, Harrow M, Westermeyer J. Neurotic symptoms in the postacute phase of schizophrenia. J Nerv Ment Dis 1983;171(4):216–21.
22. Swanson JW, Swartz MS, Elbogen EB. Effectiveness of atypical antipsychotic medications in reducing violent behavior among persons with schizophrenia in community-based treatment. Schizophr Bull 2004;30(1):3–20.
23. Birchwood M, Mason R, MacMillan F, et al. Depression, demoralization and control over psychotic illness: a comparison of depressed and non-depressed patients with a chronic psychosis. Psychol Med 1993;23(2):387–95.
24. Chakos MH, Glick ID, Miller AL, et al. Baseline use of concomitant psychotropic medications to treat schizophrenia in the CATIE trial. Psychiatr Serv 2006;57(8):1094–101.
25. Cuffel BJ, Fischer EP, Owen RR Jr, et al. An instrument for measurement of outcomes of care for schizophrenia. Issues in development and implementation. Eval Health Prof 1997;20(1):96–108.
26. Mandel MR, Severe JB, Schooler NR, et al. Development and prediction of post-psychotic depression in neuroleptic-treated schizophrenics. Arch Gen Psychiatry 1982;39(2):197–203.
27. Roy A, Thompson R, Kennedy S. Depression in chronic schizophrenia. Br J Psychiatry 1983;142:465–70.
28. Barnes TR, Curson DA, Liddle PF, et al. The nature and prevalence of depression in chronic schizophrenic in-patients. Br J Psychiatry 1989;154:486–91.
29. Harkavy-Friedman JM, Restifo K, Malaspina D, et al. Suicidal behavior in schizophrenia: characteristics of individuals who had and had not attempted suicide. Am J Psychiatry 1999;156(8):1276–8.
30. Kelly DL, Shim JC, Feldman SM, et al. Lifetime psychiatric symptoms in persons with schizophrenia who died by suicide compared to other means of death. J Psychiatr Res 2004;38(5):531–6.
31. Kibel DA, Laffont I, Liddle PF. The composition of the negative syndrome of chronic schizophrenia. Br J Psychiatry 1993;162:744–50.
32. Lafayette JM, Frankle WG, Pollock A, et al. Clinical characteristics, cognitive functioning, and criminal histories of outpatients with schizophrenia. Psychiatr Serv 2003;54(12):1635–40.
33. Lehman A. A quality of life interview for the chronically mentally ill. Eval Program Plann 1988;11:51–62.
34. Lehman AF, Fischer EP, Postrado L, et al. The Schizophrenia Care and Assessment Program Health Questionnaire (SCAP-HQ): an instrument to assess outcomes of schizophrenia care. Schizophr Bull 2003;29(2):247–56.
35. Liang KY, Zeger SL. Longitudinal data analyses using generalized linear models. Biometrika 1986;73:13–22.
36. Mallinckrodt CH, Sanger TM, Dube S, et al. Assessing and interpreting treatment effects in longitudinal clinical trials with missing data. Biol Psychiatry 2003;53(8):754–60.
37. Swartz RC, Cohen BN. Risk factors for suicidality among clients with schizophrenia. J Couns Dev 2001;79:314–9.
38. Baker A, Bucci S, Lewin TJ, et al. Comparisons between psychosis samples with different patterns of substance use recruited for clinical and epidemiological studies. Psychiatry Res 2005;134(3):241–50 [Epub 2005 Apr 21].

39. Patkar AA, Alexander RC, Lundy A, et al. Changing patterns of illicit substance use among schizophrenic patients: 1984–1996. Am J Addict 1999;8(1):65–71.
40. Huppert JD, Weiss KA, Lim R, et al. Quality of life in schizophrenia: contributions of anxiety and depression. Schizophr Res 2001;51(2–3):171–80.
41. Norholm V, Bech P. Quality of life in schizophrenic patients: association with depressive symptoms. Nord J Psychiatry 2006;60(1):32–7.
42. Pukrop R, Schlaak V, Moller-Leimkuhler AM, et al. Reliability and validity of quality of life assessed by the short-form 36 and the modular system for quality of life in patients with schizophrenia and patients with depression. Psychiatry Res 2003; 119(1–2):63–79.
43. Sim K, Mahendran R, Siris SG, et al. Subjective quality of life in first episode schizophrenia spectrum disorders with comorbid depression. Psychiatry Res 2004;129(2):141–7.
44. Simpson GM, Angus JW. A rating scale for extrapyramidal side effects. Acta Psychiatr Scand 1970;(Suppl 212):11–9.
45. Glazer W, Prusoff B, John K, et al. Depression and social adjustment among chronic schizophrenic outpatients. J Nerv Ment Dis 1981;169(11):712–7.
46. Jin H, Zisook S, Palmer BW, et al. Association of depressive symptoms with worse functioning in schizophrenia: a study in older outpatients. J Clin Psychiatry 2001; 62(10):797–803.
47. Kay SR, Fiszbein A, Opler LA. The positive and negative syndrome scale (PANSS) for schizophrenia. Schizophr Bull 1987;13(2):261–76.
48. Elbogen EB, Swanson JW, Swartz MS, et al. Medication nonadherence and substance abuse in psychotic disorders: impact of depressive symptoms and social stability. J Nerv Ment Dis 2005;193(10):673–9.
49. Munetz MR, Grande TP, Chambers MR. The incarceration of individuals with severe mental disorders. Community Ment Health J 2001;37(4):361–72.
50. Palmer BA, Pankratz VS, Bostwick JM. The lifetime risk of suicide in schizophrenia: a reexamination. Arch Gen Psychiatry 2005;62(3):247–53.
51. Glick ID, Pham D, Davis JM. Concomitant medications may not improve outcome of antipsychotic monotherapy for stabilized patients with nonacute schizophrenia. J Clin Psychiatry 2006;67(8):1261–5.
52. Green AI, Canuso CM, Brenner MJ, et al. Detection and management of comorbidity in patients with schizophrenia. Psychiatr Clin North Am 2003;26(1): 115–39.
53. Whitehead C, Moss S, Cardno A, et al. Antidepressants for the treatment of depression in people with schizophrenia: a systematic review. Psychol Med 2003;33(4):589–99.
54. Furtado VA, Srihari V. Atypical antipsychotics for people with both schizophrenia and depression. Cochrane Database Syst Rev 2008;(1):CD005377.
55. Meltzer HY, Alphs L, Green AI, et al. International Suicide Prevention Trial Study Group. Clozapine treatment for suicidality in schizophrenia: International Suicide Prevention Trial (InterSePT). Arch Gen Psychiatry 2003;60(1):82–91.
56. Montgomery SA, Asberg M. A new depression scale designed to be sensitive to change. Br J Psychiatry 1979;134:382–9.
57. McGurk SR, Mueser KT, Pascaris A. Cognitive training and supported employment for persons with severe mental illness: one-year results from a randomized controlled trial. Schizophr Bull 2005;31(4):898–909.
58. Turkington D, Kingdon D, Rathod S, et al. Outcomes of an effectiveness trial of cognitive-behavioural intervention by mental health nurses in schizophrenia. Br J Psychiatry 2006;189:36–40.

59. Velligan DI, Draper M, Stutes D, et al. Multimodal cognitive therapy: combining treatments that bypass cognitive deficits and deal with reasoning and appraisal biases. Schizophr Bull 2009;35(5):884–93.
60. Ware J Jr, Kosinski M, Keller SD. A 12-Item Short-Form Health Survey: construction of scales and preliminary tests of reliability and validity. Med Care 1996;34(3):220–33.

Management of Schizophrenia with Suicide Risk

Alec Roy, MD[a,*], Maurizio Pompili, MD, PhD[b,c]

KEYWORDS

• Management • Suicide • Risk • Schizophrenia • Patients

Bleuler years ago described the suicidal drive as "the most serious of schizophrenic symptoms." Even today suicidal behavior remains a major source of morbidity and mortality among schizophrenics.[1–6] For more than a decade, the literature routinely reported that 10% to 13% of schizophrenia patients die by suicide.[7] These estimates were revised by Palmer and colleagues[3] who calculated that 4.9% of schizophrenics commit suicide. However, this may represent an underestimate. Attempts at suicide are also common among schizophrenics.[8–11] For example, the National Institute of Mental Health (NIMH) Longitudinal Study of Chronic Schizophrenia found that, over a mean of 6 years, 38% of the patients made at least one suicide attempt and 57% admitted to substantial suicidal ideation.[12] Suicide is also a major issue among inpatients, with serious implication for clinical practice and patient-doctor relationships.[13]

The management of schizophrenic patients with suicide risk remains a difficult area for clinicians despite attempts to better understand it by gathering experts in the field.[14–17] Thus the aim of this article is to provide an overview with a specific focus on the management of schizophrenia with suicide risk.

MODEL OF RISK FACTORS FOR SUICIDAL BEHAVIOR IN SCHIZOPHRENIA

The stress diathesis suicide risk factor model is a helpful model for examining suicidal behavior and its management in schizophrenia.[18] In this model suicide risk factors may be either distal or proximal. Distal risk factors create a predisposing diathesis and determine a schizophrenic's response to a stressor. These factors include developmental, personality, biologic, and genetic variables. Distal risk factors affect the threshold for suicide and increase a schizophrenic's risk when he or she experiences

[a] Department of Veterans Affairs, New Jersey Healthcare System, Psychiatry Service 116A, 385 Tremont Avenue, East Orange, NJ 070818, USA
[b] Department of Psychiatry, Sant'Andrea Hospital, Sapienza University of Rome, Rome, Italy
[c] McLean Hospital, Harvard Medical School, Boston, MA, USA
* Corresponding author.
E-mail address: Alec.Roy@va.gov (A. Roy).

Psychiatr Clin N Am 32 (2009) 863–883
doi:10.1016/j.psc.2009.08.005
psych.theclinics.com

a proximal risk factor. Proximal, or trigger, factors are more closely related to the suicidal behavior and act as precipitants. These factors include life events and, relevant to schizophrenics, the stress of acute episodes of mental illness, as when relapsing into psychosis. Suicidal schizophrenics differ from nonsuicidal schizophrenics in distal risk factors (ie, more childhood trauma), and may be moved toward suicidal behavior by proximal risk factors such as exacerbation of schizophrenic illness caused by noncompliance, adverse life events, or comorbid substance abuse and depression (**Box 1**).

MANAGEMENT OF SUICIDE RISK IN SCHIZOPHRENIA THROUGH RECOGNITION OF RISK FACTORS

Analysis of risk factors for suicide in general often yields too many false positives, that is, the recognition of individuals as potential suicides when in fact they will never kill themselves. Nevertheless, suicide risk factors have a potential important impact on prevention. The schizophrenic patient at risk of suicide is young and male (except in China where schizophrenia is more prevalent among women, who are more likely to commit suicide than men[19]). Schizophrenics who commit suicide are generally white, unmarried, have good premorbid function, have postpsychotic depression, and have a history of suicide attempts and substance abuse. Hopelessness, lack of social support, and being socially isolated, along with a painful awareness of being ill and being subject to hospitalization are other important risk factors for suicide in these

Box 1
Diathesis and stress variables in schizophrenia

Diathesis/threshold variables

Aggression/impulsivity

Hopelessness

Premorbid social adjustment

Family history of suicidal behavior

Childhood abuse

Head injury

Genetics

Low serotonergic function

Chronic physical or mental illness

Chronic substance abuse

Early loss

Stress/trigger variables

Acute psychiatric episode (eg, major depressive episode, psychosis)

Acute medical illness

Stressful life event

Acute substance use

Data from Harkavy-Friedman JM. Depression and suicidal behavior in schizophrenia. In: Tatarelli R, Pompili M, Girardi P, editors. Suicide in schizophrenia. New York: Nova Science Publishers; 2007. p. 99–112.

patients. When adjustment deteriorates in schizophrenics with good premorbid functioning, suicide can result from the awareness and insight that the future may bring unacceptable changes. Also, schizophrenics who experience recent loss or rejections, along with limited support from family and community, are at high risk of suicide. These patients usually fear further mental deterioration and experience excessive treatment dependence or loss of faith in treatment.

A review by Hawton and colleagues[20] confirmed previously identified suicide risk factors for schizophrenia, and found that a reduced risk of suicide was associated with hallucinations. These investigators argued that command hallucinations were not an independent risk factor, but that they increased the risk in those already predisposed to suicide. Overall, suicide was less associated with the core symptoms of psychosis and more with affective symptoms, agitation, and awareness that the illness was affecting mental function. Reutfors and colleagues,[21] confirming already reported risk factors, recently also found that educational attainment, age 30 years or more at onset of symptoms, and a history of a suicide attempts were associated with an increased risk of suicide within 5 years after a first schizophrenia inpatient diagnosis. Alaraisanen and colleagues[22] found that suicide risk was high especially for men and in the early phase of the disease. Two-thirds of suicides occurred within 3 years after onset of illness. In a recent investigation, Pompili and colleagues[23] found several variables that in their sample constituted factors associated with suicide risk, such as agitation and motor restlessness, self-devaluation, hopelessness, insomnia, and mental disintegration.

For better management of the suicidal schizophrenia patients, clinicians should focus on state-dependent risk factors that are potentially modifiable, rather than trait-dependent risk factors that are difficult to modify (**Table 1**) as well as on protective factors (**Box 2**).

IMPORTANCE OF A PREVIOUS SUICIDE ATTEMPT

That a schizophrenic patient has previously attempted suicide is an important clinical indicator that he is at increased risk for both further attempts and completed suicide. A high percentage of schizophrenic patients who commit suicide have previously attempted suicide.[24–28] For example, a review of the literature showed that 156 of 289 schizophrenic patient suicides (54%) had made a previous suicide attempt.[9]

Table 1
State-dependent risk factors versus trait-dependent risk factors

State-Dependent Risk Factors	Trait-Dependent Risk Factors
– Clinical depression	– Younger age
– Substance abuse	– Male sex
– Hopelessness	– High socioeconomic family status
– Social isolation	– High intelligence
– Psychotic symptoms	– High premorbid level of education
– Loss of faith in treatment	– Unmarried status
– Undertreatment or noncompliance with therapy and negative attitude toward medication	– Reduced self-esteem
– Agitation and impulsivity	– Enhanced awareness of illness
	– Long duration of illness associated with multiple hospitalizations, relapses combined with treatment dependence, or loss of faith in treatment

Data from Pompili M, Lester D, Innamorati M, et al. Assessment and treatment of suicide risk in schizophrenia. Expert Rev Neurother 2008;8:51–74.

Box 2
Protective factors for suicide in schizophrenia

- Adherence to therapy
- Family support for the illness and against the stigma that arises from it
- Suitable antidepressant therapy
- Possibility of talking about the intention to commit suicide
- Family history negative for suicide
- Simple and hebephrenic subtypes of schizophrenia
- Psychological well-being—specific treatments for hopelessness and psychological pain
- Training in the development of social and cognitive skills
- Not being stigmatized

Protective factors related to interventions

- Support and programs of aftercare at discharge
- Use of atypical antipsychotics
- Regular sessions of family therapy that are able contribute to reducing the number and the duration of hospitalizations, the number of the relapses, and increased compliance to therapy
- Possibility of working and performing pleasant activities
- Limited access to the more common methods of suicide
- Programs of prevention about substance abuse
- Live in an environment adjusted to the patient's needs

From Pompili M, Lester D, Innamorati M, et al. Assessment and treatment of suicide risk in schizophrenia. Expert Rev Neurother 2008;8:51–74; with permission.

Pompili and colleagues[23] recently found that a substantial percentage of their schizophrenic suicides had previously attempted.

MANAGING SUICIDE RISK IN SCHIZOPHRENICS WITH COMORBID SUBSTANCE ABUSE

The literature suggests that nearly 50% of patients with schizophrenia have a co-occurring substance use disorder, most frequently alcohol or cannabis (at a rate about 3 times higher than that of the general population). The increased suicide risk of substance-abusing schizophrenic patients could be the result of a cumulative effect of many factors or events, such as the loss of remaining supportive social contacts through the consumption of psychotropic substances, noncompliance with antipsychotic medication, or the presence of paranoia and depression. Substance abuse worsens both the symptoms and prognosis of the schizophrenic illness, and is related to higher relapse rates.[15] Schizophrenics with dual diagnosis are best served when common etiology, risk factors, and treatments are considered. Suicide risk is therefore better managed when schizophrenic substance abusers at risk are treated in a dual diagnosis program.

MANAGING THE DEMORALIZATION SYNDROME IN THE AT-RISK SCHIZOPHRENIC

Drake and Cotton[29] described a demoralization syndrome in which schizophrenic patients become aware of their illness and its consequences. Patients then may compare their premorbid adjustment with their current state and become hopeless and depressed and, eventually, suicidal. Restifo and colleagues[30] recently provided support for aspects of the demoralization model. These investigators tested this model with 164 patients assessing depression, premorbid functioning, insight, and suicidal behavior. The study found that premorbid adjustment, insight, and past major depressive episode did not discriminate attempters from nonattempters, contrary to the model. However, consistent with the model, the interaction between good premorbid adjustment and insight predicted severity of depressive symptoms, and the psychological symptoms of depression significantly differentiated attempters from nonattempters, whereas the somatic symptoms did not. Thus, the clinician should pay particular attention to feelings of demoralization when managing suicide risk in schizophrenic patients and try foster hopeful attitudes toward the future.[31]

PSYCHOMETRIC ASSESSMENT OF SUICIDE RISK

The management of suicide risk in schizophrenia might also take advantage of information derived from psychometric instruments. For instance, Taiminen and colleagues[32] proposed the research-based 25-item schizophrenia suicide risk scale (SSRS), although the investigators noted the scale was too insensitive or too nonspecific for general use as a screening device. Turner and colleagues[33] proposed a semistructured interview for suicide in schizophrenia (ISIS) based on chart review, staff reports, and information from families. The 140-item third revision of the ISIS was tested on 270 schizophrenia patients,[34] yielding satisfactory sensitivity and specificity. More recently, (Hansen and Kingdon, personal communication) investigated 40 patients (39 with a diagnosis of schizophrenia, 1 with a diagnosis of schizoaffective disorder). Patients were tested using the health of the nation outcome scale (HoNOS), the comprehensive psychopathological rating scale (CPRS), and a validated suicidality rating scale—the InterSePT scale for suicidal thinking (ISST), a new instrument for the assessment of current suicidal ideation in patients with schizophrenia.[35] These investigators demonstrated a highly robust association between the 2 suicidality items from the CPRS and HoNOS and the InterSePT scale.

MANAGING SUICIDE RISK WITH ANTIPSYCHOTIC MEDICATION

Management of suicide risk through the use of antipsychotic medications is a key factor.[36] Typical neuroleptics do not have much evidence for suicide risk reduction.[37] The only atypical antipsychotic approved as an antisuicidal agent is clozapine. However, all atypical antipsychotics have some potential impact on suicidality in schizophrenic patients.[38,39] The distinguishing characteristic of atypical antipsychotic drugs is their fewer extrapyramidal symptoms (EPS), lower risk of tardive dyskinesia, and minimal serum prolactin increases compared with typical antipsychotic drugs.[40] Therefore, one important implication for the atypical antipsychotics and their reduction of suicide risk lies in the low incidence of EPS akathisia during treatment with these agents. The possible role of akathisia in precipitation of suicide risk for patients treated with antidepressants and antipsychotics has been reported.[41]

With regard to the atypical antipsychotics, clozapine, olanzapine, risperidone, and quetiapine have shown some power in reducing suicidality among schizophrenic patients.[38,42] According to some reports, the potential decrease in suicide mortality with clozapine treatment is estimated to be as high as 85%. In terms of benefit versus risk, whereas 1.5 of every 10,000 patients with schizophrenia who were treated with clozapine would be expected to die from agranulocytosis (evidence suggests an even lower percentage), 1000 to 1300 would have been expected to complete suicide with standard treatment.[43–45] Modestin and colleagues,[46] in a retrospective analysis, reported significant reduction of suicidal behavior and serious suicidal acts among schizophrenic patients treated with clozapine compared with other treatments, and the preventive effect disappeared after clozapine discontinuation. Hennen and Baldessarini[47] provided a meta-analysis supporting the antisuicidal effect of clozapine. A possible negative outcome associated with clozapine treatment was reported by Sernyak and colleagues[48] who, in a matched control group, found that clozapine was not associated with significantly fewer deaths due to suicide. However, one-third of the sample received clozapine for less than 6 months, even though the follow-up period was 5 to 6 years.

Meltzer and colleagues[49] organized the international suicide prevention trial (InterSePT), a prospective, randomized, masked (blinded) parallel-group study to compare the effects of treatment with clozapine versus other atypical antipsychotic drugs. Patients were seen equally frequently, with equal access to other psychotropic drugs and psychosocial treatment. During this trial, clozapine was compared with olanzapine in patients with schizophrenia or schizoaffective disorder, regardless of whether they had persistent psychotic symptoms or prior treatments, but who were at more than average risk for a subsequent suicide attempt based primarily on having made at least one suicide attempt in the 3 years before study entry or on being currently suicidal. A significant difference was demonstrated between clozapine and olanzapine in reducing suicidality, with a 24% difference in favor of clozapine. In 2003 a panel of experts in suicide prevention held a consensus conference, and provided an algorithm for effective treatment of suicidal schizophrenic and schizoaffective patients.[50] **Fig. 1** reports the full details of these guidelines. In this algorithm, there is no reference to the presence or absence of akathisia, which may lead to reduced quality of life and ultimately suicide risk.

MANAGING SUICIDE RISK IN THE SCHIZOPHRENIC WITH COMORBID DEPRESSION

Depression is an important potentially modifiable comorbid disorder often associated with suicidal behavior in schizophrenic patients. For example, one review of 270 schizophrenic suicides found that depressive symptoms were noted by their clinicians during the last period of contact before the suicide in approximately 60% of the suicides.[51] Significantly more schizophrenic suicides than schizophrenic controls have their last admission before committing suicide because of suicidal impulses or depressive symptoms. Also, significantly more schizophrenics who attempt suicide have had more depressive symptoms than schizophrenic patients who never attempt suicide.

Thus the treatment of depressive symptoms in schizophrenic patients is an important intervention for prevention of suicidal behavior. The use of antidepressants, especially tricyclics, as adjunctive agents for depressed schizophrenics has been reviewed extensively.[52–55] Antidepressants have been especially used in nonflorid psychotic patients presenting typical features of depression. Siris[56] reported that such treatments are much more successful with outpatients than with inpatients. Siris and colleagues[54,57] demonstrated that adjunctive antidepressant medication, especially in the case of imipramine, was associated with better outcome in schizophrenia patients, with fewer relapses into depression and less exacerbation of psychosis; and overall, tricyclics proved to be particularly useful in treating depressed schizophrenics. Therefore, it seems that although antidepressants may have a role as add-on therapy in amelioration of negative, depressive, and obsessive-compulsive symptoms in schizophrenia,[58–60] their specific role in preventing suicide is unclear. Combination therapy with antidepressants seems to be well tolerated, although pharmacokinetic drug-drug interactions may result in unintended elevations of antipsychotic drug concentrations, especially in the case of clozapine combined with either fluoxetine or fluvoxamine.[61]

Research suggests that monoamine oxidase (MAO) inhibitors may have a role in the treatment of depression and negative symptoms in schizophrenia. In contrast to MAO inhibitors, which strongly potentiate the catecholamine releasing effect of tyramine, (–)deprenyl (selegiline) inhibits it and is free of the "cheese effect," which makes it a safe drug. Selegiline, a selective inhibitor of MAO-B, has become a universally used research tool for selectively blocking B-type MAO and is still the only selective MAO-B inhibitor in worldwide clinical use. Data suggest that add-on therapy with selegiline is particularly helpful in schizophrenic patients presenting negative symptoms as well as depression.[62,63]

MANAGING SUICIDE RISK IN SCHIZOPHRENIA THROUGH STAFF EDUCATION

Managing the schizophrenic patient who is at risk of suicide involves the establishment of supportive relationships. Difficult relationships with the staff and difficult acclimatization to the ward environment have been reported to be risk factors for suicide.[36,64] Staff knowledge of suicidology and their readiness to deal with the anxiety and despair of suicidal schizophrenics are important in the treatment process, and uncertainties may be fatal. Increased attention to interpersonal behavior may provide a basis for more accurate recognition and more successful long-term treatment of high-risk suicidal schizophrenics. Withdrawal by a depressed schizophrenic patient and an increase in paranoid behavior should be regarded as signals of an acutely increased risk of suicide. In addition, awareness that psychological and somatic symptoms are connected may facilitate the identification of an acute risk of suicide.

Farberow and colleagues,[65] in an early study of mainly schizophrenics and manic-depressive inpatients, found that when compared with controls, the suicidal patients made more demands on hospital personnel, complained and criticized the treatment, showed marked ambivalence about leaving the security of the hospital, and had a constant need for reassurance and support. These investigators identified a pattern of behavior among the suicides, which they labeled the "dependent-dissatisfied" style. These suicidal patients showed both dependency and dissatisfaction with their lives. The "dependent-dissatisfied" person incessantly complained, demanded, insisted, and tried to control others. These patients seemed to need constantly repeated evidence of self-worth from outside sources to maintain their own self-esteem. However, their activity pushed them unrelentingly into a more difficult "bind" for, as they increased their demands, their sources of gratification became exhausted and more rejecting, forcing them to increase their demands still more. In a similar fashion, Morgan and Priest[66,67] identified what they called "terminal malignant alienation," a state derived from rejection even by the staff. Such a state is often determined by the patients' fluctuating suicidal ideation, excessive demands on staff, and complaints that lead to a distance between the patient and staff, eventually leading to final rejection.

Staff morale is crucial in identifying possible suicide risk and in determining higher risk.[68] Goh and colleagues[69] noted that a ward that counteracts suicidal tendencies is one with a calm routine, with staff who are unworried and confident. If this hypothesis is correct, inpatient suicides should occur predominantly when the calm is broken, routine disrupted, and the staff themselves disturbed. Patients should also be supervised in their initial acclimatization to the ward and when there are plans for discharge or rehabilitation. Saarinen and colleagues[70] noted that fear of the patient

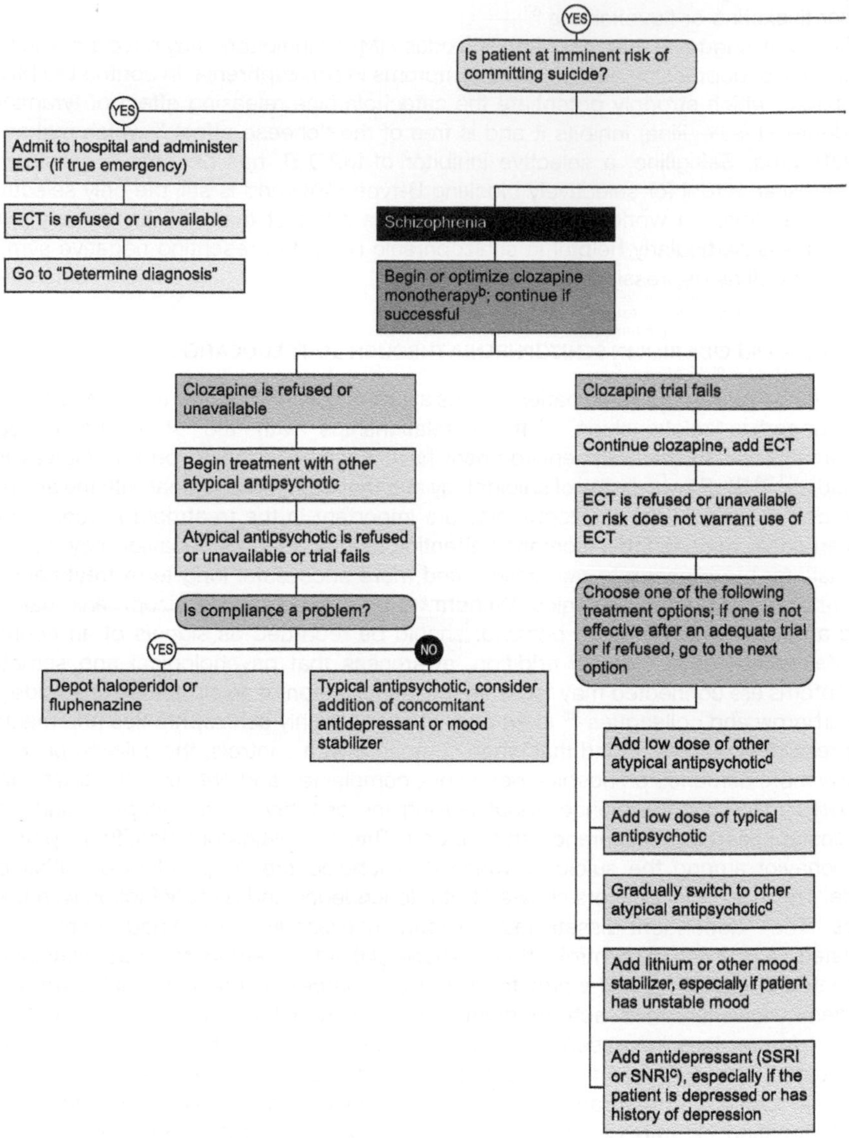

Fig. 1. Algorithm of intervention strategies for suicide. (*Reprinted from* Meltzer HY, Conley RR, De Leo D, et al. Intervention strategies for suicidality. J Clin Psychiatry Audiograph 2003;6:1–16; with permission.)

and difficulties in dealing with suicidal individuals are 2 of the most important sources of difficulty in dealing with suicidal patients in mental health environments.

MANAGING THE INCREASED SUICIDE RISK DURING AND AFTER DISCHARGE

Pompili and colleagues[13] drew attention to the importance of suitable discharge plans. A supportive, supervised living arrangement is ideal. Roy and Draper[4] also noted that

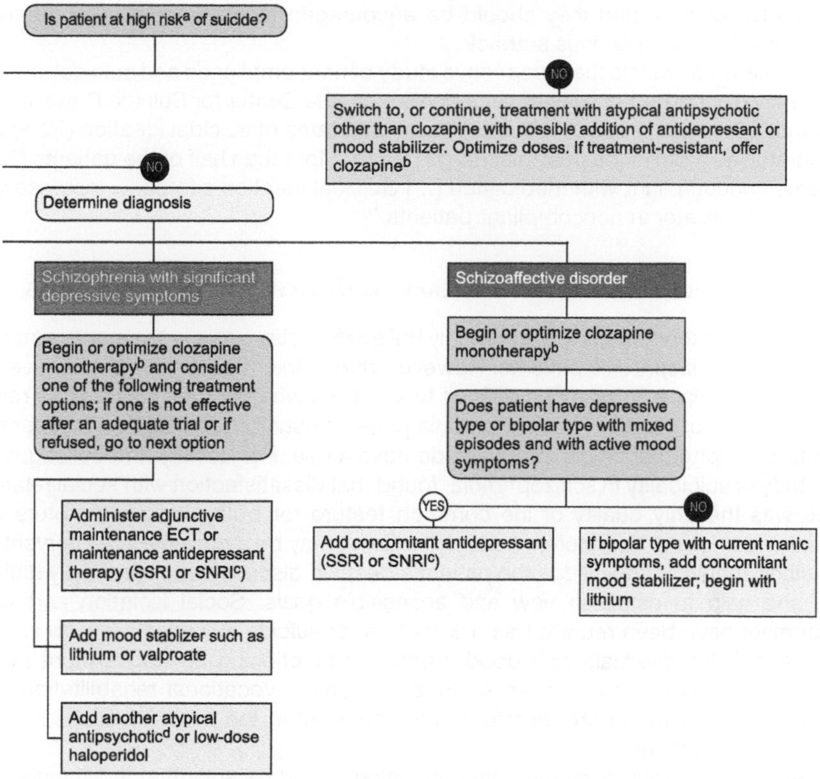

[a] A patient at high risk of suicide is one who has made a suicide attempt of at least moderate lethality within 36 months and has continued suicidal ideation or behavior.
[b] Discuss clozapine risks and benefits, including the blood monitoring schedule, with the patient and his or her caregivers. An adequate trial lasts 12–26 weeks.
[c] Be aware of possible drug interactions with clozapine, especially with fluvoxamine and fluoxetine, which can increase blood clozapine levels.
[d] If adding another atypical antipsychotic to clozapine or if switching from clozapine to another atypical antipsychotic, use one unlike clozapine, e.g., risperidone.
Abbreviations: ECT = electroconvulsive therapy, SNRI = serotonin-norepinephrine reuptake inhibitor, SSRI = selective serotonin reuptake inhibitor.

Fig. 1. (*continued*)

discharge planning was a proximal factor to suicide in several of their long-stay schizophrenics who had to deal with the painful realization that they were losing the hospital and the staff or that their family was not prepared to have them home. Rossau and Mortensen[5] found the risk for suicide greatest during the first 6 months after discharge, but suicide risk was also very high in the 5 days following discharge as well as in the first 28 days after leaving the hospital.

Staff, and especially nurses, have a crucial role in the process of suicide prevention by delivering information about preventive measures. Patients and their families should be instructed on the advisability of a return to the hospital if another disturbance occurs, and they should be encouraged to consider such a return as neither a failure nor a serious setback.

Particularly relevant is the prospective study of noncompliance and suicidal ideation in recently discharged psychiatric inpatients from the Center for Suicide Prevention in England.[71] This study found "clinically significant rates of suicidal ideation (52%) and deliberate self harm in the post-discharge period. More than half of the patients (52%) became noncompliant with medication [...] Suicidal ideation scores ... increase was significantly greater in noncompliant patients."

MANAGING SUICIDE RISK WITH PSYCHOTHERAPY AND PSYCHOSOCIAL INTERVENTIONS

Psychosocial interventions are commonly believed to play a role in the management of the suicidal schizophrenic patients. However, due to their heterogeneity and diversity from place to place, it has been difficult to establish whether they play a large role in the prevention of suicide.[72] Schizophrenia patients usually need empathic support,[73] therefore nonpharmacologic strategies do have a role. Ponizovsky and colleagues,[74] in a study of suicidality in schizophrenia, found that dissatisfaction with social relationships was the only quality of life common feature for both single attempters and multiple attempters. Therefore, social skill training may be a possible key intervention. Clinicians should acknowledge the patient's despair, discuss losses and daily difficulties, and help to establish new and accessible goals. Social isolation and work impairment have been reported as risk factors for suicide in individuals with schizophrenia.[28,75,76] Individuals with good premorbid functioning are those more at risk of suicide. Interventions such as social skill training, vocational rehabilitation, and supportive employment are therefore very important in the prevention of suicide in schizophrenic patients.

Lewine and Shriner (personal communication) found recently that individuals from higher social class who experience minimal lost potential may be at a higher risk for suicide than their counterparts with maximal lost potential; this is especially true when based on fathers' educational level. These investigators suggested that a subgroup of individuals' vocational success may depend on first addressing the cognitive conflict inherent in the phenomenon of lost potential.

It has become increasingly clear that supportive, reality-orientated therapies are generally of great value in the treatment of patients with schizophrenia. In particular, supportive psychotherapy aims at offering the patient the opportunity to meet with the therapist and discuss the difficulties encountered in daily activities. Patients are therefore encouraged to discuss concerns about medications and side effects as well as social isolation, money, stigma, and so forth. Psychosocial programs should be part of the after care programs following a hospitalization. Cognitive therapy has been reported to be helpful in one study.[77]

Overall, in the management of schizophrenic patients, involving both individual and group sessions where patients learn to cope with difficulties are key features for preventing hopeless feelings leading to suicide.[15]

Cotton and colleagues[78] outlined the importance of psychotherapy with schizophrenic patients who are at risk of suicide, and pointed to the need to appreciate hopeless awareness of chronic illness. According to Westermeyer and colleagues,[79] the surviving schizophrenic individual may be the type of patient who is able to adjust to life as a chronic schizophrenic or as a moderately and episodically impaired schizophrenic, and thus may be less likely to commit suicide. Despite major difficulties, these patients may not experience despair and an active and militant dissatisfaction with the quality of their lives.

Psychotherapies that promote insight, as in the case of psychoanalysis or psychodynamic psychotherapy, should be used carefully. These therapies may have a positive effect on symptoms, but therapists should monitor the patient's insight into illness at all times. The fear of closeness to others is often stronger than yearning for it, so the patients get locked into loneliness. Patients spend their days alone in a world where they feel isolated; they struggle to find a solution for their isolation and their inability to cope with everyday difficulties. Sometimes they try to build up patterns for self comforting through lonely activities that do not require the presence of others.[80]

INTERVENTION EARLY IN THE ILLNESS TO PREVENT SUICIDE

Nordentoft and colleagues[81] found that suicidal behavior and suicidal ideation occur frequently among patients with first-episode schizophrenic psychoses. These investigators found that suicidal ideation and reports of suicide attempts during the past year were significantly reduced after treatment, but were still at a high level compared with the general population. Melle and colleagues[82] confirmed that suicidal behavior is present in the early phases of psychotic disorders and in many cases precedes the first treatment contact. Whereas patients from communities that did not have an early psychosis detection program showed rates of suicidal behavior in the expected range, the early detection group had significantly lower rates. The study thus indicates that an early detection program, by lowering the threshold for first treatment contact and bringing patients into treatment earlier, can reduce rates of serious suicidal behavior at the point of first contact.[83] Crumlish and colleagues[84] reported that, in their sample of first-episode schizophrenia patients 6 months after presentation, the greater the recognition by individuals that they had a mental illness, the more depressed they were going to be 4 years later, and the more likely they were to attempt suicide in that period. More recently, Foley and colleagues[85] reported that suicidal ideation and suicide attempts were common features in their sample of patients with first-episode schizophrenia.

Krausz and colleagues[86] investigated suicide in patients showing symptoms of schizophrenic disorders between 14 and 18 years of age during a follow-up of between 5 and 11 years. The suicide rate of 13.1% was significantly higher than in studies of patients who developed a schizophrenic psychosis later in life. These investigators also found a significant sex difference in the rate of suicide, 21.5% in the men and 6% in the women, although the women made more attempts at suicide. Thorup and colleagues[87] investigated gender differences in age at first onset, duration of untreated psychosis, psychopathology, social functioning, and self-esteem in a group of 578 young adults with a first-episode schizophrenia spectrum disorder. This study found that the women made more suicide attempts and experienced lower self-esteem despite better social functioning.

NONADHERENCE WITH ANTIPSYCHOTICS AND SUICIDAL BEHAVIOR

A substantial percentage of schizophrenic patients who exhibit suicidal behavior are nonadherent with antipsychotic medication. The effect of poor compliance with antipsychotics on suicide rates among patients with schizophrenia was noted by an early review as well as by a recent meta-analysis, which concluded that poor compliance with antipsychotics more than triples the suicide risk in these patients.[10] Herings and Erkens[88] found that an increased suicide attempt rate was observed when comparing uninterrupted and interrupted drug use (20.0/1000 person-years vs 72.1/1000 person-years, respectively). A fourfold increased risk for attempting suicide among patients with drug holidays was found (relative risk adjusted for age and gender 4.2, 95%

confidence interval [CI]: 1.7–10.1) compared with patients without drug holidays. A review concluded that "individuals with these psychotic disorders are typically experiencing psychotic symptoms and in psychiatric treatment at the time of their attempts although frequently under-treated with respect to medication."[89]

For example, Heila and colleagues[90] found that 57% of 88 schizophrenic suicide victims were noncompliant or prescribed inadequate neuroleptic treatment. In their study, treatment noncompliance during the last 3 months of the patient's life was assessed to be present if the patient had stopped taking neuroleptic medication entirely or for most of that time. One-third of the suicide victims were assessed as neuroleptic noncompliant while others were inadequately treated. De Hert and colleagues[91] reported, in a case-control study of 63 schizophrenic suicides, that "there were several times as many patients who did not comply with treatment in the suicide group as there were in the control group (60% vs 22%, $P<.0001$)." Wolfersdorf and colleagues[92] reported that significantly fewer of 115 schizophrenic suicides were receiving depot neuroleptics than 115 living schizophrenic controls ($P<.01$), strongly suggesting that depot neuroleptics reduced the risk of suicide. This group also noted that significantly more of the other schizophrenic suicides than living schizophrenic controls were receiving low-potency neuroleptics ($P<.01$). Cohen and colleagues[93] noted that a significantly greater number of schizophrenic suicides occurred soon after discontinuation of neuroleptics, and Warnes[94] also reported that schizophrenic suicides were receiving lower doses than controls. Pompili and colleagues[23] also found that poor adherence to medications was predictive of completed suicide in their sample of schizophrenic suicides. Wilkinson and Bacon[11] reported that significantly more attempters had a history of not receiving antipsychotic medication, whereas a history of receiving antipsychotic medication was associated with a reduced risk of attempting.

MANAGING SUICIDE RISK IN SCHIZOPHRENICS WITH NEGATIVE ATTITUDES TO TREATMENT

Virkkunen[95] interviewed relatives and acquaintances of schizophrenic suicides and controls, and found that the schizophrenic suicides were significantly more noncompliant. The patients "had been more adverse to take medicines voluntarily than were the controls during the pre-suicidal months, although the relatives and acquaintances thought that the patient's condition had been relatively good while they had been taking the medicines prescribed." The patients' psychiatrists similarly reported that significantly more of the schizophrenic suicides than controls had had a negative attitude toward medication (34.5% vs 10%, $P<.01$).[96] Virkkunen concluded that "the patient ceases to use the treatment procedures made available to him. This has a general negative effect and can eventually lead to suicide."

INCREASED NUMBER OF ADMISSIONS AND SUICIDE IN SCHIZOPHRENIA

In 3 studies, schizophrenic patients who had exhibited suicidal behavior had had significantly more psychiatric admissions than schizophrenic controls who had never exhibited suicidal behavior.[8,28,97]

Hu and colleagues[24] similarly reported that schizophrenic suicides had had significantly more psychiatric admissions than controls ($P<.01$), as did Cheng and colleagues[25] when comparing 74 schizophrenic suicides with 74 schizophrenic controls. Rossau and Mortensen,[5] in a nested case-control study of 508 schizophrenic suicides, found that "increased suicide risk was also associated with multiple admissions during the previous year." Sletten and colleagues[98] and Yarden[99] also noted that the number of psychiatric admissions during the last year was associated with suicide in schizophrenic patients. Wilkinson and Bacon[11] found that both male and female schizophrenic suicides had had more admissions than schizophrenic controls.

In their review of risk factors for attempting suicide in schizophrenia, Haw and colleagues[26] concluded that "a higher mean number of psychiatric admissions was associated with an increased risk of deliberate self harm." These admission data are relevant as studies have demonstrated increased rates of relapse and readmission among schizophrenics with poor adherence as determined by pill count, self report, or blood levels of neuroleptics.[100,101]

Of relevance is that De Hert and colleagues[91] reported that their 63 schizophrenic suicides had had significantly more admissions than controls (P<.0001), and concluded that "noncompliance may lead to frequent admissions because of discontinuation of drug treatment" and that in the suicides "frequent hospitalizations are highly correlated with discontinuation of pharmacologic maintenance treatment."

Long-term compliance with atypical antipsychotics has been reported as fundamental in reducing the risk of serious adverse outcomes including suicide.[102] However, the promise of improved efficacy and tolerability of the atypical antipsychotics compared with typical or first-generation antipsychotics remains only partially fulfilled. Regardless of the shortcomings of available medications, schizophrenics who remain on antipsychotic treatment have lower rates of relapse and have milder courses of exacerbation when relapse occurs. Differential effects have been reported in the prevention of relapse between conventional and atypical antipsychotic agents. Several undesirable effects are associated with atypical antipsychotics, which seem more efficacious in the prevention of relapse (eg, worsening metabolic profile). More effective and safer treatments are needed for the prevention of recurrence of psychotic symptoms in the schizophrenic population. Moreover, adverse metabolic events, such as increased adiposity, hyperglycemia, diabetes mellitus, and dyslipidemia have been associated with treatment using atypical antipsychotic medications.

POSSIBLE FUTURE DIRECTIONS IN THE MANAGEMENT OF SUICIDE RISK IN SCHIZOPHRENIA

At the start of this article, when considering the stress diathesis model for suicidal behavior in schizophrenia, risk factors were divided up into distal and proximal. Biologic and genetic factors are distal risk factors for suicidal behavior. Some of the recent data about biology and genetics that may in the future have relevance to the management of suicide risk in schizophrenia is also discussed here.

Low Central Serotonin and Suicide in Schizophrenia

Diminished central serotonergic neurotransmission is a biologic distal risk factor for suicidal behavior.[103] In schizophrenic patients, Van Praag[104] showed that patients who attempted suicide had significantly lower cerebrospinal fluid (CSF) concentrations of the serotonin metabolite 5-hydroxyindoleacetic acid (5-HIAA) than schizophrenic patients who had never attempted suicide or normal controls.[104]

An NIMH study similarly reported that suicidal schizophrenic patients had significantly lower CSF 5-HIAAA levels.[105] An 11-year follow-up of 30 schizophrenic patients, who had CSF 5-HIAA determined at their index admission, showed that the 10 who attempted suicide during the 11-year follow-up had lower CSF 5-HIAA than the 20 who did not attempt.[106] Clozapine, which has been reported to diminish suicidal behavior in schizophrenic patients, has a marked serotonergic action.[48,49]

Heritability of Suicide in Schizophrenia

Data from clinical, twin, and adoption studies suggest that genetic factors play a role in suicidal behavior.[107] Thus it is of interest that studies from different countries show that suicidal behavior is familial in schizophrenia. For example, in one report on 5602 inpatients admitted to a Canadian psychiatric hospital, 15 of the 33 schizophrenic patients with a family history of suicide (45.4%) had attempted suicide compared with 13.5% of the schizophrenic patients without a family history of suicide.[108] De Hert and colleagues[91] reported on 870 consecutively admitted schizophrenic Belgian inpatients. The 63 who committed suicide were compared with 63 matched schizophrenic controls. Committing suicide in the schizophrenic patients was positively associated with having a family history of suicide (odds ratio = 7.39, 95% CI: 2.04–26.8). Wilkinson and Bacon[11] reported that, among 458 schizophrenics who had attempted suicide in Edinburgh, 20% had a family member who had attempted and 10% a family member who had committed suicide.

Most recently, in France Tremeau and colleagues[109] examined the influence of a family history of suicide on suicide attempt rate and attempt characteristics in schizophrenic, depressed, and opiate dependent patients. Overall, a family history of suicide was associated with a higher risk for suicide attempt, with higher lethality method, with repeated attempts, and with number of attempts, while the interaction between family history of suicide and diagnostic group was not significant. These investigators concluded that a positive family history of suicide was a risk factor for several suicide attempt characteristics, independent of psychiatric diagnosis.

The possible clinical implication of these studies in the management of suicide risk in schizophrenia is that a schizophrenic patient with a family history of suicide might be considered to be at heightened risk of suicidal behavior.

Serotonin Genes and Suicidal Behavior in Schizophrenia

Reviews conclude that the strongest current evidence for a genetic role in suicidal behavior lies with 2 serotonin genes: tryptophan hydroxylase and the serotonin transporter.[110,111]

Tryptophan hydroxylase (TPH 2) in relation to suicidal behavior

TPH is the rate-limiting enzyme in the synthesis of serotonin, a neurotransmitter implicated in suicidal behavior. TPH2 has been implicated in both completed suicide and attempted suicide.[112,113]

For example, in the authors' study Zhou and colleagues[114] examined different markers in the 5-promoter and 3-untranslated regions, and 15 SNPs spanning 106 kbp of the TPH2 gene in 1798 cases and controls. The authors reported a haplotype block of 52 kbp in size, which was associated with an increased risk of making a suicide attempt. However, there has been a negative report in schizophrenic suicides.[115]

Serotonin transporter (5-HTT) and attempting suicide

The 5-HTT proteins are responsible for the reuptake of synaptic serotonin. In a review, Lin and Tsai[111] concluded that genotypes carrying the short (s) allele of the 5-HTTLPR gene were found significantly more among patients attempting suicide than among patients who had never attempted. There was also a significant association between the SS+LS genotype and suicide attempts ($P = .003$). The frequency of the s allele was significantly higher in violent attempters, reattempters, or completers ($P = .033$). De Luca and colleagues[115] found that the intron 2-VNTR polymorphism of the 5-HTT gene was significantly associated with attempting suicide among 290 schizophrenics.

5-HTTLPR/life event interaction, and depression and suicidality

Depression is associated with suicidal behavior in schizophrenic patients, and is often precipitated by life events. Thus it is relevant that Caspi and colleagues[116] showed that the 5-HTT gene predicted an individual's sensitivity to the stressful life events precipitating depression. This group reported that an interaction between polymorphism of the 5-HTTLPR gene and stressful recent life events predicted depression and suicidal ideation and attempts in young adults with an s allele but not in l/l homozygotes. Others reported similarly in relation to depression (reviewed in Uher and McGuffin[117]). Caspi and colleagues[116] and the authors[118] also reported that 5-HTTLPR polymorphism interacted with childhood trauma to precipitate depression and suicide attempts. Particularly relevant is a recent report that in psychotic patients the ss or sl genotype of the 5-HTTLPR gene increased the risk of developing major depression during the course of their illness.[119]

Serotonin 2C receptor and suicide in schizophrenia

Dracheva and colleagues[120] recently reported a postmortem genetic study of schizophrenic and bipolar suicide victims and found 5-HT2CR mRNA editing variations that were associated with the suicides compared with controls. These investigators noted that because the VSV isoform of 5-HT2CR exhibits low functional activity, an increase in its expression frequency may significantly influence serotonin in the brain. Dracheva and colleagues concluded that overexpression of the VSV isoform in the prefrontal cortex may represent an additional risk factor for suicidal behavior in schizophrenia.

SUMMARY AND CAVEAT ABOUT MANAGING SUICIDE RISK SCHIZOPHRENICS BY ADMISSION

This article discusses the frequency of suicidal behavior in schizophrenia, offers a model for understanding it, and deals with various aspects of the management of the at-risk schizophrenic patient. However, it is noteworthy that many suicide-risk schizophrenic patients are seen in the clinic or in the emergency room, with a recent marked increase of suicide risk. These patients may present with marked suicidal ideas, or with command hallucinations telling them to harm themselves, or with a suicide plan, or even having attempted suicide. These presentations may be in the context of an exacerbation of schizophrenic-positive symptoms or in the context of comorbid depression or substance abuse. In general it is best not to hesitate but, after a complete evaluation, to admit such suicidal schizophrenics to a psychiatric ward. It may be that a short crisis admission is all that is initially required. However, it is better to be safe than sorry—and to admit.

REFERENCES

1. Miles CP. Conditions predisposing to suicide: a review. J Nerv Ment Dis 1977; 164:231–46.
2. Inskip HM, Harris EC, Barraclough B. Lifetime risk of suicide for affective disorder, alcoholism and schizophrenia. Br J Psychiatry 1998;172:35–7.
3. Palmer BA, Pankratz VS, Bostwick JM. The lifetime risk of suicide in schizophrenia: a reexamination. Arch Gen Psychiatry 2005;62:247–53.
4. Roy A, Draper R. Suicide among psychiatric hospital in-patients. Psychol Med 1995;25:199–202.

5. Rossau CD, Mortensen PB. Risk factors for suicide in patients with schizophrenia: nested case-control study. Br J Psychiatry 1997;171:355–9.
6. Harris EC, Barraclough B. Suicide as an outcome for mental disorders. A meta-analysis. Br J Psychiatry 1997;170:205–28.
7. Caldwell CB, Gottesman II. Schizophrenics kill themselves too: a review of risk factors for suicide. Schizophr Bull 1990;16:571–89.
8. Roy A, Mazonson A, Pickar D. Attempted suicide in chronic schizophrenia. Br J Psychiatry 1984;144:303–6.
9. Roy A. Suicide in schizophrenia. In: Roy A, editor. Suicide. Baltimore (MD): Williams and Wilkins; 1986. p. 97–112.
10. Drake RE, Gates C, Cotton PG, et al. Suicide among schizophrenics. Who is at risk? J Nerv Ment Dis 1984;172:613–7.
11. Wilkinson G, Bacon NA. A clinical and epidemiological survey of parasuicide and suicide in Edinburgh schizophrenics. Psychol Med 1984;14:899–912.
12. Breier A, Schreiber JL, Dyer J, et al. National Institute of Mental Health longitudinal study of chronic schizophrenia. Prognosis and predictors of outcome. Arch Gen Psychiatry 1991;48:239–46.
13. Pompili M, Mancinelli I, Ruberto A, et al. Where schizophrenic patients commit suicide: a review of suicide among inpatients and former inpatients. Int J Psychiatry Med 2005;35:171–90.
14. Tatarelli R, Pompili M, Girardi P, editors. Suicide in schizophrenia. New York: Nova Science Publishers, Inc; 2007.
15. Pompili M, Amador XF, Girardi P, et al. Suicide risk in schizophrenia: learning from the past to change the future. Ann Gen Psychiatry 2007;6:10.
16. Pompili M, Lester D, Innamorati M, et al. Assessment and treatment of suicide risk in schizophrenia. Expert Rev Neurother 2008;8:51–74.
17. Pompili M. Suicide risk in schizophrenia: an overview. In: Tatarelli R, Pompili M, Girardi P, editors. Suicide in schizophrenia. New York: Nova Science Publishers; 2007. p. 1–18.
18. Mann JJ, Waternaux C, Haas GL, et al. Toward a clinical model of suicidal behavior in psychiatric patients. Am J Psychiatry 1999;156:181–9.
19. Phillips MR, Yang G, Li S, et al. Suicide and the unique prevalence pattern of schizophrenia in mainland China: a retrospective observational study. Lancet 2004;364:1062–8.
20. Hawton K, Sutton L, Haw C, et al. Schizophrenia and suicide: systematic review of risk factors. Br J Psychiatry 2005;187:9–20.
21. Reutfors J, Brandt L, Jonsson EG, et al. Risk factors for suicide in schizophrenia: findings from a Swedish population-based case-control study. Schizophr Res 2009;108:231–7.
22. Alaräisänen A, Miettunen J, Räsänen P, et al. Suicide rate in schizophrenia in the Northern Finland 1966 Birth Cohort. Soc Psychiatry Psychiatr Epidemiol 2009, in press.
23. Pompili M, Lester D, Grispini A, et al. Completed suicide in schizophrenia: evidence from a case-control study. Psychiatry Res 2009;167:251–7.
24. Hu WH, Sun CM, Lee CT, et al. A clinical study of schizophrenic suicides. 42 Cases in Taiwan. Schizophr Res 1991;5:43–50.
25. Cheng KK, Leung CM, Lo WH, et al. Risk factors of suicide among schizophrenics. Acta Psychiatr Scand 1990;81:220–4.
26. Haw C, Hawton K, Sutton L, et al. Schizophrenia and deliberate self-harm: a systematic review of risk factors. Suicide Life Threat Behav 2005;35:50–62.

27. Drake RE, Gates C, Cotton PG. Suicide among schizophrenics: a comparison of attempters and completed suicides. Br J Psychiatry 1986;149:784–7.
28. Roy A. Suicide in chronic schizophrenia. Br J Psychiatry 1982;141:171–7.
29. Drake RE, Cotton PG. Depression, hopelessness and suicide in chronic schizophrenia. Br J Psychiatry 1986;148:554–9.
30. Restifo K, Harkavy-Friedman JM, Shrout PE. Suicidal behavior in schizophrenia: a test of the demoralization hypothesis. J Nerv Ment Dis 2009;197:147–53.
31. Haghighat R. A discourse for hope: on defenses against suicide in people with schizophrenia. In: Tatarelli R, Pompili M, Girardi P, editors. Suicide in schizophrenia. New York: Nova Science Publishers; 2007. p. 189–213.
32. Taiminen T, Huttunen J, Heila H, et al. The Schizophrenia Suicide Risk Scale (SSRS): development and initial validation. Schizophr Res 2001;47:199–213.
33. Turner RM, Korslund KE, Barnett BE, et al. Assessment of suicide in schizophrenia: development of the interview for suicide in schizophrenia. Cogn Behav Pract 1998;5:139–69.
34. Korslund KE. Psychometric evaluation of the interview for suicide in schizophrenia-third revision. Dissertation abstracts international: section B: the sciences and engineering, vol. 62; 2001.
35. Lindenmayer JP, Czobor P, Alphs L, et al. The InterSePT scale for suicidal thinking reliability and validity. Schizophr Res 2003;63:161–70.
36. Pompili M, Mancinelli I, Girardi P, et al. Making sense of nurses' role in the prevention of suicide in schizophrenia. Issues Ment Health Nurs 2004;25:5–7.
37. Carone BJ, Harrow M, Westermeyer JF. Posthospital course and outcome in schizophrenia. Arch Gen Psychiatry 1991;48:247–53.
38. Keck PE Jr, Strakowski SM, McElroy SL. The efficacy of atypical antipsychotics in the treatment of depressive symptoms, hostility, and suicidality in patients with schizophrenia. J Clin Psychiatry 2000;61(Suppl 3):4–9.
39. Montout C, Casadebaig F, Lagnaoui R, et al. Neuroleptics and mortality in schizophrenia: prospective analysis of deaths in a French cohort of schizophrenic patients. Schizophr Res 2002;57:147–56.
40. Meltzer HY. What's atypical about atypical antipsychotic drugs? Curr Opin Pharmacol 2004;4:53–7.
41. Hansen L. A critical review of akathisia, and its possible association with suicidal behaviour. Hum Psychopharmacol 2001;16:495–505.
42. Meltzer HY. Decreasing suicide in schizophrenia. Psychiatr Times 2001;18:1–5.
43. Meltzer HY, Fatemi H. Suicide in schizophrenia: the effect of clozapine. Clin Neuropharmacol 1995;18:S18–24.
44. Meltzer HY, Okayli G. Reduction of suicidality during clozapine treatment of neuroleptic-resistant schizophrenia: impact on risk-benefit assessment. Am J Psychiatry 1995;152:183–90.
45. Wagstaff A, Perry C. Clozapine: in prevention of suicide in patients with schizophrenia or schizoaffective disorder. CNS Drugs 2003;17:273–80 [discussion: 81–3].
46. Modestin J, Dal Pian D, Agarwalla P. Clozapine diminishes suicidal behavior: a retrospective evaluation of clinical records. J Clin Psychiatry 2005;66: 534–8.
47. Hennen J, Baldessarini RJ. Suicidal risk during treatment with clozapine: a meta-analysis. Schizophr Res 2005;73:139–45.
48. Sernyak MJ, Desai R, Stolar M, et al. Impact of clozapine on completed suicide. Am J Psychiatry 2001;158:931–7.

49. Meltzer HY, Alphs L, Green AI, et al. Clozapine treatment for suicidality in schizophrenia: International Suicide Prevention Trial (InterSePT). Arch Gen Psychiatry 2003;60:82–91.
50. Meltzer HY, Conley RR, De Leo D, et al. Intervention strategies for suicidality. Audiograph. J Clin Psychiatry 2003;6:1–16.
51. Roy A. Relationship between depression and suicidal behavior in schizophrenia. In: De Lisi L, editor. Depression in schizophrenia. Washington, DC: American Psychiatric Press; 1990. p. 39–58.
52. Siris SG. Depression in schizophrenia: perspective in the era of "atypical" antipsychotic agents. Am J Psychiatry 2000;157:1379–89.
53. Plasky P. Antidepressant usage in schizophrenia. Schizophr Bull 1991;17:649–57.
54. Siris SG, Bermanzohn PC, Mason SE, et al. Maintenance imipramine therapy for secondary depression in schizophrenia. A controlled trial. Arch Gen Psychiatry 1994;51:109–15.
55. Siris SG. Diagnosis of secondary depression in schizophrenia: implications for DSM-IV. Schizophr Bull 1991;17:75–98.
56. Siris SG. Suicide and schizophrenia. J Psychopharmacol 2001;15:127–35.
57. Siris SG, Morgan V, Fagerstrom R, et al. Adjunctive imipramine in the treatment of postpsychotic depression. A controlled trial. Arch Gen Psychiatry 1987;44:533–9.
58. Moller HJ. Non-neuroleptic approaches to treating negative symptoms in schizophrenia. Eur Arch Psychiatry Clin Neurosci 2004;254:108–16.
59. Rummel C, Kissling W, Leucht S. Antidepressants as add-on treatment to antipsychotics for people with schizophrenia and pronounced negative symptoms: a systematic review of randomized trials. Schizophr Res 2005;80:85–97.
60. Reznik I, Sirota P. Obsessive and compulsive symptoms in schizophrenia: a randomized controlled trial with fluvoxamine and neuroleptics. J Clin Psychopharmacol 2000;20:410–6.
61. Meltzer HY, Bobo W. Pharmacological management of suicide risk in schizophrenia. In: Tatarelli R, Pompili M, Girardi P, editors. Suicide in schizophrenia. New York: Nova Science Publishers Inc; 2007. p. 275–302.
62. Bodkin JA, Siris SG, Bermanzohn PC, et al. Double-blind, placebo-controlled, multicenter trial of selegiline augmentation of antipsychotic medication to treat negative symptoms in outpatients with schizophrenia. Am J Psychiatry 2005;162:388–90.
63. Fohey KD, Hieber R, Nelson LA. The role of selegiline in the treatment of negative symptoms associated with schizophrenia. Ann Pharmacother 2007;41:851–6.
64. Pompili M, Mancinelli I, Girardi P, et al. Nursing schizophrenic patients who are at risk of suicide. J Psychiatr Ment Health Nurs 2003;10:622–4.
65. Farberow NL, Shneidman ES, Neuringer C. Case history and hospitalization factors in suicides of neuropsychiatric hospital patients. J Nerv Ment Dis 1966;142:32–44.
66. Morgan HG, Priest P. Assessment of suicide risk in psychiatric in-patients. Br J Psychiatry 1984;145:467–9.
67. Morgan HG, Priest P. Suicide and other unexpected deaths among psychiatric in-patients. The Bristol confidential inquiry. Br J Psychiatry 1991;158:368–74.
68. Crammer JL. The special characteristics of suicide in hospital in-patients. Br J Psychiatry 1984;145:460–3.

69. Goh SE, Salmons PH, Whittington RM. Hospital suicides: are there preventable factors? Profile of the psychiatric hospital suicide. Br J Psychiatry 1989;154: 247–9.
70. Saarinen PI, Lehtonen J, Lonnqvist J. Suicide risk in schizophrenia: an analysis of 17 consecutive suicides. Schizophr Bull 1999;25:533–42.
71. Qurashi I, Kapur N, Appleby L. A prospective study of noncompliance with medication, suicidal ideation, and suicidal behavior in recently discharged psychiatric inpatients. Arch Suicide Res 2006;10:61–7.
72. De Leo D, Spathonis K. Do psychosocial and pharmacological interventions reduce suicide in schizophrenia and schizophrenia spectrum disorders? Arch Suicide Res 2003;7:353–74.
73. Drake RE, Bartels SJ, Torrey WC. Suicide in schizophrenia: clinical approaches. In: Williams R, Dalby JT, editors. Depression in schizophrenia. New York: Plenum Press; 1989. p. 153–69.
74. Ponizovsky AM, Grinshpoon A, Levav I, et al. Life satisfaction and suicidal attempts among persons with schizophrenia. Compr Psychiatry 2003;44:442–7.
75. Drake RE, Gates C, Whitaker A, et al. Suicide among schizophrenics: a review. Compr Psychiatry 1985;26:90–100.
76. Nyman AK, Jonsson H. Patterns of self-destructive behaviour in schizophrenia. Acta Psychiatr Scand 1986;73:252–62.
77. Bateman K, Hansen L, Turkington D, et al. Cognitive behavioral therapy reduces suicidal ideation in schizophrenia: results from a randomized controlled trial. Suicide Life Threat Behav 2007;37:284–90.
78. Cotton PG, Drake RE, Gates C. Critical treatment issues in suicide among schizophrenics. Hosp Community Psychiatry 1985;36:534–6.
79. Westermeyer JF, Harrow M, Marengo JT. Risk for suicide in schizophrenia and other psychotic and nonpsychotic disorders. J Nerv Ment Dis 1991;179:259–66.
80. Maltsberger JT, Pompili M, Tatarelli R. Sandro Morselli: schizophrenic solitude, suicide, and psychotherapy. Suicide Life Threat Behav 2006;36:591–600.
81. Nordentoft M, Jeppesen P, Abel M, et al. OPUS study: suicidal behaviour, suicidal ideation and hopelessness among patients with first-episode psychosis. One-year follow-up of a randomised controlled trial. Br J Psychiatry Suppl 2002; 43:s98–106.
82. Melle I, Johannesen JO, Friis S, et al. Early detection of the first episode of schizophrenia and suicidal behavior. Am J Psychiatry 2006;163:800–4.
83. Harkavy-Friedman JM. Can early detection of psychosis prevent suicidal behavior? Am J Psychiatry 2006;163:768–70.
84. Crumlish N, Whitty P, Kamali M, et al. Early insight predicts depression and attempted suicide after 4 years in first-episode schizophrenia and schizophreniform disorder. Acta Psychiatr Scand 2005;112:449–55.
85. Foley S, Jackson D, McWilliams S, et al. Suicidality prior to presentation in first-episode psychosis. Early Interv Psychiatry 2008;2:242–6.
86. Krausz M, Muller-Thomsen T, Haasen C. Suicide among schizophrenic adolescents in the long-term course of illness. Psychopathology 1995;28:95–103.
87. Thorup A, Petersen L, Jeppesen P, et al. Gender differences in young adults with first-episode schizophrenia spectrum disorders at baseline in the Danish OPUS study. J Nerv Ment Dis 2007;195:396–405.
88. Herings RM, Erkens JA. Increased suicide attempt rate among patients interrupting use of atypical antipsychotics. Pharmacoepidemiol Drug Saf 2003;12: 423–4.

89. Harkavy-Friedman JM, Nelson EA, Venarde DF, et al. Suicidal behavior in schizophrenia and schizoaffective disorder: examining the role of depression. Suicide Life Threat Behav 2004;34:66–76.
90. Heila H, Isometsa ET, Henriksson MM, et al. Suicide victims with schizophrenia in different treatment phases and adequacy of antipsychotic medication. J Clin Psychiatry 1999;60:200–8.
91. De Hert M, Mckenzie K, Peuskens J. Risk factors for suicide in young patients suffering from schizophrenia. Schizophr Res 2001;47:127–34.
92. Wolfersdorf M, Barth P, Steiner B, et al. Schizophrenia and suicide in psychiatric patients. In: Platt S, Kreitman N, editors. Current research on suicide and parasuicide. Edinburgh: Edinburgh University Press; 1989. p. 67–77.
93. Cohen S, Leonard CV, Farberow NL, et al. Tranquilizers and suicide in the schizophrenic patient. Arch Gen Psychiatry 1964;11:312–21.
94. Warnes H. Suicide in schizophrenics. Dis Nerv Syst 1968;29(Suppl):35–40.
95. Virkkunen M. Suicides in schizophrenia and paranoid psychoses. Acta Psychiatr Scand Suppl 1974;250:1–305.
96. Virkkunen M. Attitude to psychiatric treatment before suicide in schizophrenia and paranoid psychoses. Br J Psychiatry 1976;128:47–9.
97. Roy A, Schreiber J, Mazonson A, et al. Suicidal behavior in chronic schizophrenic patients: a follow-up study. Can J Psychiatry 1986;31:737–40.
98. Sletten IW, Brown ML, Evenson RC, et al. Suicide in mental hospital patients. Dis Nerv Syst 1972;33:328–34.
99. Yarden PE. Observations on suicide in chronic schizophrenics. Compr Psychiatry 1974;15:325–33.
100. Weiden PJ, Kozma C, Grogg A, et al. Partial compliance and risk of rehospitalization among California Medicaid patients with schizophrenia. Psychiatr Serv 2004;55:886–91.
101. Green AI. Treatment of schizophrenia and comorbid substance abuse: pharmacologic approaches. J Clin Psychiatry 2006;67(Suppl 7):31–5 [quiz 6–7].
102. Ward A, Ishak K, Proskorovsky I, et al. Compliance with refilling prescriptions for atypical antipsychotic agents and its association with the risks for hospitalization, suicide, and death in patients with schizophrenia in Quebec and Saskatchewan: a retrospective database study. Clin Ther 2006;28:1912–21.
103. Roy A, Linnoila M. Suicidal behavior, impulsiveness and serotonin. Acta Psychiatr Scand 1988;78:529–35.
104. van Praag HM. CSF 5-HIAA and suicide in non-depressed schizophrenics. Lancet 1983;2:977–8.
105. Ninan PT, van Kammen DP, Scheinin M, et al. CSF 5-hydroxyindoleacetic acid levels in suicidal schizophrenic patients. Am J Psychiatry 1984;141:566–9.
106. Cooper SJ, Kelly CB, King DJ. 5-Hydroxyindoleacetic acid in cerebrospinal fluid and prediction of suicidal behaviour in schizophrenia. Lancet 1992;340:940–1.
107. Roy A, Nielsen D, Rylander G, et al. The genetics of suicidal behavior. In: Hawton K, Van Heeringen K, editors. The international handbook of suicide. Chichester, Sussex (UK): John Wiley; 2000. p. 209–21.
108. Roy A. Family history of suicide. Arch Gen Psychiatry 1983;40:971–4.
109. Tremeau F, Staner L, Duval F, et al. Suicide attempts and family history of suicide in three psychiatric populations. Suicide Life Threat Behav 2005;35:702–13.
110. Rujescu D, Giegling I, Sato T, et al. Genetic variations in tryptophan hydroxylase in suicidal behavior: analysis and meta-analysis. Biol Psychiatry 2003;54: 465–73.

111. Lin PY, Tsai G. Association between serotonin transporter gene promoter polymorphism and suicide: results of a meta-analysis. Biol Psychiatry 2004; 55:1023–30.
112. Zill P, Buttner A, Eisenmenger W, et al. Single nucleotide polymorphism and haplotype analysis of a novel tryptophan hydroxylase isoform (TPH2) gene in suicide victims. Biol Psychiatry 2004;56:581–6.
113. Lopez de Lara C, Brezo J, Rouleau G, et al. Effect of tryptophan hydroxylase-2 gene variants on suicide risk in major depression. Biol Psychiatry 2007;62: 72–80.
114. Zhou Z, Roy A, Lipsky R, et al. Haplotype-based linkage of tryptophan hydroxylase 2 to suicide attempt, major depression, and cerebrospinal fluid 5-hydroxyindoleacetic acid in 4 populations. Arch Gen Psychiatry 2005;62:1109–18.
115. De Luca V, Hlousek D, Likhodi O, et al. The interaction between TPH2 promoter haplotypes and clinical-demographic risk factors in suicide victims with major psychoses. Genes Brain Behav 2006;5:107–10.
116. Caspi A, Sugden K, Moffitt TE, et al. Influence of life stress on depression: moderation by a polymorphism in the 5-HTT gene. Science 2003;301:386–9.
117. Uher R, McGuffin P. The moderation by the serotonin transporter gene of environmental adversity in the aetiology of mental illness: review and methodological analysis. Mol Psychiatry 2008;13:131–46.
118. Roy A, Hu XZ, Janal MN, et al. Interaction between childhood trauma and serotonin transporter gene variation in suicide. Neuropsychopharmacology 2007;32:2046–52.
119. Contreras J, Hare L, Camarena B, et al. The serotonin transporter 5-HTTPR polymorphism is associated with current and lifetime depression in persons with chronic psychotic disorders. Acta Psychiatr Scand 2009;119:117–27.
120. Dracheva S, Patel N, Woo DA, et al. Increased serotonin 2C receptor mRNA editing: a possible risk factor for suicide. Mol Psychiatry 2008;13:1001–10.

Schizophrenia with Impulsive and Aggressive Behaviors

J.P. Lindenmayer, MD[a,b,c,*], Isabella Kanellopoulou, MD[d]

KEYWORDS

- Schizophrenia • Impulsive behavior
- Aggressive behavior • Interventions

Impulsive and aggressive behaviors are important clinical challenges in the treatment of patients with schizophrenia. They occur both in the acute phase as well as in the chronic phase of the disorder and call for differentiated treatment interventions. It is important to always first consider behavioral and nonpharmacological interventions. High levels of structure and organization together with a nonconfrontational approach may be very successful interventions. In terms of acute pharmacological interventions, clinicians now have a broad spectrum of intramuscular antipsychotic compounds available with rapid onset of action and relatively little sedation. There is a need for new compounds with a more acceptable tolerability profile for the long-term treatment of these important syndromes.

EVALUATION AND EARLY BEHAVIORAL INTERVENTIONS

The treatment of aggressive patients with schizophrenia depends on the level of acuity and the setting where the patient is being evaluated; however, there are some general guidelines that apply to most situations. The guidelines for the management of the acutely agitated patient[1] stress the importance of collaboration between patient and clinician whenever possible in achieving the best short- and long-term outcomes. These guidelines also emphasize the importance of safety concerns in the short term (eg, control of aggressive behavior and protecting the community). The highest level of risk for acute injury during the intervention and for long-term traumatic

[a] Department of Psychiatry, New York University School of Medicine, New York University, Wards Island, New York, NY 10035, USA
[b] Psychopharmacology Research Unit, Nathan Kline Institute for Psychiatric Research, New York, NY, USA
[c] Manhattan Psychiatric Center, New York, NY, USA
[d] Mt Sinai School of Medicine, New York, NY, USA
* Corresponding author. Department of Psychiatry, Psychopharmacology Research Unit, Nathan Kline Institute for Psychiatric Research, Manhattan Psychiatric Center, New York University, Wards Island, New York, NY 10035.
E-mail address: Lindenmayer@NKI.rfush.org (J.P. Lindenmayer)

Psychiatr Clin N Am 32 (2009) 885–902
doi:10.1016/j.psc.2009.08.006 psych.theclinics.com

sequelae is associated with leaving the patient alone, followed by use of physical restraints, while voluntary medication involves the least risk.[2]

The emergency service should provide a quiet space where an agitated or violent patient can be isolated and a sense of crowding can be prevented. In most emergency rooms patients will be asked whether they have a weapon and any assessment process must halt until the patient surrenders the weapon to either an examiner or security personnel, as necessary. The most important step in the emergency room evaluation of an assaultive or agitated patient is to help the patient bring his or her agitation and violence rapidly under control. If the patient is not in restraints, it is important that he or she has enough space to move without disrupting other ongoing activities. If the patient is in restraints, the restraints can be removed only when there is evidence that the patient is in control of the aggressive impulses that result from agitation. Ventilation and talking down techniques can be used with or without parenteral medication effectively in this setting (**Box 1**).

Communication with a paranoid patient presents special problems, because usually the patient has been brought for treatment against his or her will and does not consider him or herself to be sick. The patient's position is characterized by suspiciousness, mistrust, and anger. Development of rapport with the patient requires that distrust and resentment be recognized and addressed; for example, the physician should acknowledge that the patient was brought in against his or her will. The patient then may go into a long tirade about the harmful things his or her family or the authorities are doing to the patient. The physician should permit the patient to give his or her account. Particularly, the physician should abstain from challenging the delusional state, because it would be provocative. It is more important to ask the patient reasons for him or her being the focus of perceived persecutions. If the patient directly asks the interviewer to agree with his or her delusions, the interviewer should respond that he or she can understand the interpretation of the facts by the patient, but that his or her own interpretation might be different.

EARLY INTERVENTION IN THE INPATIENT SETTING

If a patient has not yet lost control and is cooperative, "time out" in a quiet room, if available, should be offered. A quiet room will have few furnishings and none that can be moved and used as a weapon or barricade. It should be private but easily accessible and must be under close staff supervision. It offers the patient a time away from stimulation; an opportunity for reconstitution after an agitated outburst or a place to experience painful emotions. This type of isolation should not be confused with seclusion, as it is voluntary and unlocked.[2] According to the expert consensus guideline series,[1] the following have been identified as "must do" or highly desirable in the assessment of an agitated patient in the emergency setting: an assessment of

Box 1
General guidelines for the evaluation of an aggressive patient

1. Ensure safety of both patient and staff
2. Examine in open and uncrowded space
3. Bring agitation/aggression rapidly under control
4. Emphasize collaboration between patient and clinician whenever possible
5. Use ventilation and talking down techniques
6. Use pharmacological and/or restraining techniques as last resort

vital signs, a focused methodical physical examination, a cognitive examination (mini mental status examination). The following physical parameters are of paramount importance for the assessment of the physical examination: respiration and heart rhythm, possible head trauma, skin color, alcoholic odor, diameter and reactivity of pupils, lacerations, neck rigidity, breath sounds, jaundice, dyskinetic movements or tremor, level of hygiene, nystagmus, overt infectious lesions, ecchymosis, nutritional status. It is critical to remember that patients with schizophrenia can be agitated or aggressive as a result of an underlying medical condition or substance use (**Box 2**).

Laboratory tests can be very useful in assessing the general medical condition of the patient. The following tests are needed in an emergency situation: toxicology screen, blood glucose, electrolytes, complete blood count, blood or breath alcohol concentration, and urine pregnancy test.

An important goal of the emergency intervention for aggression and impulsivity is the calming of the patient without sedation. The expert consensus guidelines give third-line ratings to sleep or heavy sedation, indicating that they did not consider this an appropriate goal for emergency intervention.

Once verbal techniques and pharmacological interventions have been used, but have not succeeded in effectively treating the aggressive or violent episode, staff may have to resort to physical restraints or seclusion. These are procedures that both staff and patients usually find unpleasant; they are clearly high-risk procedures that can lead, if not done properly, to injury and psychological trauma. They should be undertaken only by well-trained staff who are accustomed to working together as a team and have trained together. The overall principle governing seclusion and restraint is to use the least restrictive alternative available to treat the episode.[2] Most treatment settings are subject to local policies, procedures, and accreditation regulations that govern the use of seclusion and restraints, which specifically dictate the duration of seclusion or a restraint episode, as well as the monitoring and documentation requirements. It is also recommended that all restraint and seclusion episodes be followed by a debriefing session for the staff involved in the episode.

SPECIFIC PROCEDURES FOR APPLYING RESTRAINTS

There are basically 3 different phases in the restraint process. After someone makes the decision to initiate restraints, a group of trained staff members physically places

Box 2
General guidelines for physical examination of an aggressive patient

1. Vital signs as level of cooperation permits
2. Focused methodical physical examination
3. Cognitive examination (mini mental status examination)
4. Check on respiration and heart rhythm
5. Rule out possible head trauma
6. Check on diameter and reactivity of pupils, nystagmus
7. Check for lacerations, dyskinetic movements, or tremor
8. Rule out signs of substance use
9. Appropriate laboratory tests

the patient in restraints. Finally, a debriefing assessment is done to evaluate the need for restraints and the staff and patient responses to it. The Centers for Medicare and Medicaid Services (CMS) interim rules state that the hospitals should have a protocol "to specify who can initiate restraints or seclusion in an emergency before obtaining a physician's or licensed independent practitioner's order."[3] Seclusion can be initiated by nursing staff, but has to be ordered within 1 hour by a physician. The physician or other licensed independent practitioner must conduct a face-to-face examination of the patient within 1 hour, which includes a review of the patient's physical and psychological state. The initial order for seclusion or restraints can have a maximum duration of only 4 hours, after which the patient has to be reevaluated by the physician and a new order has to be written. For patients younger than 18 years this duration is reduced to 2 hours. The CMS interim final rules specify continuous audio and visual monitoring while patients are in restraints. The Joint Commission on Accreditation of Healthcare Organizations (JCAHO) regulations specify continuous in-person monitoring for individuals in restraints (with continuous audiovisual monitoring allowed after the first hour for patients in seclusion). Staff is required to conduct 15-minute checks to assess vital signs, any signs of injury, and the patient's psychological state and readiness to discontinue seclusion or restraints. Full documentation in the medical record of the episode and its handling are paramount.

It is important for a successful restraint episode that the staff works as a team and that enough staff members be present both to demonstrate nonnegotiable force to the patient and to perform the procedure in a safe manner. Team members need to remove dangerous objects from themselves (eg, pens, earrings, pagers). The team needs to have a leader who assigns the task of holding a particular part: one person holds one extremity each and a fifth person is assigned to hold the patient's head to prevent any possible injury to staff and patient alike.

DIAGNOSTIC ISSUES

The importance of a full assessment of the aggressive episode cannot be overstated. In the patient with acute psychosis, medical comorbidities and substance abuse should be considered early in the differential diagnosis and treated. Violent behaviors may take different forms whether patients with schizophrenia are seen in the emergency room, an inpatient ward, or an outpatient clinic. Substance abuse is more associated with violence occurring in the community, where substances are freely available. Studies consistently find that substance abuse increases risk of violent behavior. When there is comorbidity of substance abuse with another psychiatric disorder, there is a still greater risk. Patients with paranoid schizophrenia can have prominent, systematized delusional systems, whereas disorganized, unfocused delusions are more typical of those with chronic undifferentiated schizophrenia. Organized delusional systems are often centered on a specific person who is seen as persecuting or depriving in some way. Often it is a family member or someone well known to the patient. Because patients with paranoid schizophrenia retain many cognitive functions, they can organize their behavior, and plan and carry out a serious attack with a weapon on their perceived persecutor. Among psychotic forensic patients, the more serious the violent act, the more delusions appear to have a direct role.[4] On the other hand, in disorganized psychotic patients, violence is more often unplanned, less focused, and less dangerous. Paranoid patients may respond to a bump or a shove or to physical closeness as a homosexual threat and respond immediately. Patients treated with antipsychotics may appear agitated when in reality they have akathisia as a medication side effect (**Box 3**).

Box 3
Frequent underlying causes of aggression

1. Psychosis
2. Mania
3. Dementia
4. Temporal lobe epilepsy
5. Head trauma

TREATMENT INTERVENTIONS

Both nonpharmacological and pharmacological options need to be considered in the treatment of aggression and impulsivity in patients with schizophrenia.

Nonpharmacological Interventions

Milieu therapy can start in the emergency room setting with reduction of stimulation and attempts to calm the patient by talking to the patient with a low voice. Generally the consensus is that a beneficial milieu has a low perceived level of anger and aggression and a high level of support and practical orientation, together with order and organization.

A confrontational group therapy approach in a ward setting is detrimental and individually oriented milieu therapy will be beneficial. A high mean age of patients may also contribute to a favorable trend in reducing levels of aggression. A high percentage of psychotic patients, a high number of patients, and a high staff turnover may lead to a detrimental atmosphere.[5]

A study from Norway showed that reduced group participation and increased individualized support from staff led patients to perceive the ward as having a low level of anger and aggression and a high level of order and organization. This study examined whether the level of organization was associated with improved treatment outcome. The results supported the hypothesis that the organization and milieu of brief-stay wards influence the short-term outcome of inpatient treatment of patients with schizophrenia in terms of aggression.[6]

In terms of cognitive behavioral therapy (CBT), there has been little evaluation of CBT with patients who are aggressive or violent.[7] One recent study showed some promising results in the use of CBT in patients with schizophrenia with a significant history of aggression. This was a single-blind randomized controlled trial of CBT versus social activity therapy (SAT) with a primary outcome of violence and secondary outcomes of anger, symptoms, functioning, and risk. Significant benefits were shown for CBT compared with control over the intervention and follow-up period on violence, delusions, and risk management.[8]

Psychopharmacological Treatments

In terms of pharmacologic treatments, there are several options to choose from as described in the following sections. The particular choice will be guided by patients' past response history and the side-effect profile of the drug and speed of onset. The pharmacologic treatment of acute aggression will be reviewed first followed by discussion of treatment of chronic aggression.

Acute aggression

There are several factors that need to be taken into consideration before the selection of the medication that will be administered. Three of the most important ones are the acute (immediate) effect on behavioral symptoms, the speed of onset, and the availability of an intramuscular (IM) formulation in case the patient refuses to take oral medication (**Box 4**). Other important factors include the history of past medication response, the rate of side effects, the patient preference (if the patient is currently able to express a preference or has previously completed an Advance Directive), the rate of intolerable side effects, and the availability of liquid or rapidly dissolving formulations when the patient agrees to take oral medication. In the case of oral medication, the rapidly dissolving oral formulations are the preferred choice followed by liquid formulations and tablets (**Box 5**).[1]

The medications that can be used in the case of acute aggression in a patient with schizophrenia are first-generation antipsychotics, with or without benzodiazepines, and some of the second-generation antipsychotics (SGA) that are available as IM form or rapidly dissolving tablet or liquid form. We review in the following sections the studies that are related to each of these medications (**Box 6**).

Olanzapine Olanzapine can be used for the treatment of aggression in a patient with schizophrenia both in an acute and chronic setting. It is available as a rapidly dissolving tablet, liquid, and IM form. Olanzapine IM was approved for the indication of agitation associated with schizophrenia and bipolar I mania on the basis of 1-day placebo-controlled trials in inpatients considered by the investigators to be "clinically agitated" and clinically appropriate candidates to receive treatment with IM medications.[8] In one study, recently hospitalized acutely agitated patients with schizophrenia (N = 270) were randomized to receive 1 to 3 IM injections of olanzapine (2.5, 5.0, 7.5, or 10.0 mg), haloperidol (7.5 mg), or placebo within 24 hours. A dose-response relationship for IM olanzapine in the reduction of agitation was assessed by measuring the reduction in positive and negative syndrome scale excited component (PANSS-EC) scores 2 hours after the first injection. Safety was assessed by recording adverse events and with extrapyramidal symptom scales and electrocardiograms at 24 hours after the first injection. The authors concluded that IM olanzapine at a dose of 2.5 to 10.0 mg per injection exhibits a dose-response relationship in the rapid treatment of acute agitation in patients with schizophrenia and demonstrates a favorable safety profile.[9] Wright and colleagues[10] evaluated the comparative efficacy and safety of IM olanzapine, IM haloperidol, and IM placebo for the treatment of acute agitation in schizophrenia. Hospitalized patients with schizophrenia received one to three injections of IM olanzapine, 10 mg, IM haloperidol, 7.5 mg, or IM placebo over a 24-hour period. Agitation was measured with the excited component of the PANSS-EC and two additional scales. According to scores on the PANSS-EC, both IM olanzapine and IM haloperidol reduced agitation significantly more than IM placebo 2 and 24 hours following the first injection. IM olanzapine reduced agitation significantly more than IM haloperidol 15, 30, and 45 minutes following the first injection. No patients

Box 4
First decisions

1. Choice of medication: Guided by the underlying diagnosis whenever possible
2. Route of administration: Will be determined by the level of the patient's cooperation (oral (PO) or IM)

Box 5
Flow chart of antipsychotic choice for acute treatment

First-line agents:

Ziprasidone IM or Aripiprazole IM

Or if costs are an issue: haloperidol IM with an anticholinergic.

Second-line agent:

Olanzapine IM

Third-line agents:

Risperidone M tab or haloperidol IM

treated with IM olanzapine experienced acute dystonia, compared with 7% of those who were treated with IM haloperidol. No significant QT(c) interval changes were observed in any patients. Several additional studies have documented the efficacy of olanzapine injection in the case of acutely agitated patients with schizophrenia. In a naturalistic study at San Rafael Hospital in Spain, the authors found significant improvement in the agitation in patients treated with olanzapine injection 2 hours after the medication administration.[11]

Risperidone Risperidone, like olanzapine, is available in oral rapidly dissolving form as well as a long-term IM form and can be used in the management of both acute and chronically agitated patients. Results for the oral formulation in the treatment of acute agitation support its effectiveness, whereas the use of risperidone for chronic aggression is less impressive with the exception of its possible superiority to a first-generation agent.

One of the initial studies that investigated the efficacy of the oral liquid form of risperidone compared with haloperidol injection for the treatment of acutely agitated psychotic patients was conducted by Currier and Simpson.[12] In this study, 30 patients were enrolled in each treatment group (oral risperidone liquid plus lorazepam 2 mg or haloperidol 5 mg intramuscularly plus lorazepam 2 mg). Men were significantly more likely to choose oral medication, but the other demographic characteristics did not differ significantly between the two treatment groups. Both groups showed similar improvement in agitation as measured by five agitation subitems of the PANSS, the

Box 6
Flow chart of antipsychotic choice for chronic treatment

First-line agent:

Clozapine

Second-line agent:

Olanzapine

Third-line agents:

Quetiapine; Risperidone; Valproic acid

Fourth-line agents:

First-generation antipsychotics

clinical global impressions (CGI) scale, and time to sedation. No patients receiving risperidone demonstrated any side effects or adverse events, whereas one patient receiving IM treatment with haloperidol developed acute dystonia. One subject receiving risperidone required subsequent treatment with haloperidol for ongoing agitation. A problem with this study was that the sample was one of convenience and that the patients who chose to take oral medications had to agree to take them.[12]

A European, multicenter, open-label, active-controlled trial compared oral risperidone plus oral lorazepam to standard care with IM conventional neuroleptics with or without lorazepam in the emergency treatment of acutely psychotic patients. Patients were allowed to choose either oral risperidone (a single dose of 2 mg and 2.0–2.5 mg lorazepam; 121 patients) or standard IM treatment (conventional neuroleptic with or without lorazepam; 105 patients). No additional treatment was allowed for 2 hours. Primary outcome was the percentage of patients with treatment success (asleep or at least much improved on clinical global impression–global improvement scale) 2 hours after treatment initiation. Oral risperidone plus oral lorazepam was more successful at 2 hours (66.9%) and significantly noninferior compared with standard IM care (54.3%; $P = .0003$), and the incidence of extrapyramidal symptoms (EPS) was lower (1.7%) compared with standard IM care (9.5%).[13]

Ziprasidone Ziprasidone IM formulation was approved for the indication of the treatment of acute agitation in patients with schizophrenia on the basis of two 1-day double-blind trials of hospitalized subjects considered by investigators to be acutely agitated and in need of IM antipsychotic medications.[14] In the first study, a fixed-dose clinical trial, patients were randomly assigned to receive up to four injections (every 2 hours as needed) of 2 mg (N = 54) or 10 mg (N = 63) of ziprasidone IM. The behavioral activity rating scale (BARS) measured behavioral symptoms at baseline and the response to treatment up to 4 hours after the first IM injection. Ziprasidone 10 mg IM rapidly reduced symptoms of acute agitation and was significantly more effective ($P<.01$) than the 2-mg dose up to 4 hours after the first injection. Patients were calm, but not excessively sedated, and over half were classed as responders 2 hours after the 10-mg dose. No acute dystonia or behavioral disinhibition was reported. One patient who received the 10-mg dose experienced akathisia.[15]

The second study was a prospective, randomized, double-blind, 24-hour study that assessed efficacy using the BARS and the PANSS. The mean BARS score had decreased 15 minutes after the first 20-mg IM dose and was statistically significantly lower than the 2-mg group at 30 minutes post dose. The improvement with the 20-mg dose increased until 2 hours, and was maintained until at least 4 hours post dose ($P< .001$). Two hours after the first injection, almost all of the patients receiving ziprasidone 20 mg were BARS responders compared with just one-third of those receiving 2 mg ziprasidone ($P<.001$). The calming effect of ziprasidone was also evident by the significant reduction in PANSS agitation items ($P<.05$) and CGI severity at 4 hours ($P = .008$). Both ziprasidone doses were very well tolerated. Ziprasidone IM 20 mg was not associated with EPS, dystonia, akathisia, respiratory depression, or with excessive sedation.[16]

Few studies exist that have compared ziprasidone IM to conventional antipsychotic IM formulations in the treatment of aggression in schizophrenia. In a recent study, Jangro and colleagues[17] compared the effectiveness of ziprasidone IM to haloperidol IM in an adolescent population. In this study there were only seven adolescents who were agitated because of psychosis. The authors found no difference between adolescents who received ziprasidone IM and those who received combined haloperidol and lorazepam. This was a nonrandomized, naturalistic retrospective study, in which the outcome measures were the duration of the restraints and the need for additional medications. In another study, ziprasidone was compared with haloperidol IM injection in the treatment of acute psychotic agitation. The two medications where comparable as far as their efficacy; however, haloperidol was found to have twice as many side effects as ziprasidone.[18]

Generally ziprasidone IM is well tolerated and effective in the acute management of aggression. The downside is that the IM formulation needs to be diluted and it is therefore not readily available for use.

Satterthwaite and colleagues[19] reported a meta-analysis of the risks of acute extrapyramidal symptoms in the treatment of acute agitation with IM antipsychotics. They found that the second-generation antipsychotics, which included ziprasidone, had clearly fewer side effects as far as extrapyramidal symptoms than haloperidol; however, they found only one randomized controlled trial that compared second-generation antipsychotic medication with haloperidol plus an anticholinergic agent. When they compared all studies where haloperidol and an anticholinergic agent were used, they found that IM SGAs have a significantly lower risk of acute EPS compared with haloperidol alone. The decision to use SGAs should consider other factors in addition to the reduction of EPS, which can be prevented by the use of an anticholinergic agent, such as medication availability and the patient's preference.

Aripiprazole Aripiprazole IM was approved for the indication of the treatment of acute agitation in patients with schizophrenia and bipolar I mania on the basis of three 1-day double-blind trials of hospitalized subjects considered by investigators to be acutely agitated and in need of IM antipsychotic medications.[14] In one study, 448 patients were randomized (2:2:1 ratio) to IM aripiprazole 9.75 mg, IM haloperidol 6.5 mg, or IM placebo. Patients could receive up to three injections over the first 24 hours, with second and third injections administered 2 hours or longer and 4 hours or longer, respectively, after the first, if deemed clinically necessary. The primary efficacy measure was the mean change in PANSS-EC score from baseline to 2 hours. Mean improvement in PANSS-EC at 2 hours was significantly greater for IM aripiprazole (−7.27) versus placebo (−4.78; $P<.001$); IM aripiprazole was noninferior to IM haloperidol (−7.75) on PANSS.[12] All secondary efficacy measures showed significantly greater improvements at 2 hours for IM aripiprazole and IM haloperidol over placebo.[20] In another study by Tran-Johnson and colleagues,[21] 357 patients were randomly assigned to IM aripiprazole 1.00 mg, 5.25 mg, 9.75 mg, or 15.00 mg; IM haloperidol 7.50 mg; or placebo and observed for 24 hours. The primary efficacy measure was mean change in the positive and negative syndrome scale-excited component (PEC) score from baseline to 2 hours after initial dosing. Secondary measures included the agitation-calmness evaluation scale (ACES) score. Intramuscular aripiprazole 5.25 mg, 9.75 mg, and 15.00 mg and IM haloperidol 7.50 mg demonstrated significantly greater reduction in the primary efficacy measure versus placebo. These changes were statistically significant as early as 45 minutes for the IM aripiprazole 9.75-mg group, with a trend toward significance ($P = .051$) at 30 minutes. Intramuscular haloperidol 7.5 mg first showed a significant reduction in PEC score versus placebo at 105 minutes. At 30 minutes, significantly more patients responded (defined as a greater than or equal to 40% reduction in PEC score) to IM aripiprazole 9.75 mg versus placebo (27% vs 13%, $P = .05$). IM aripiprazole 9.75 mg significantly improved agitation, without oversedation, as measured by change in ACES score from baseline to 2 hours versus placebo ($P = .003$). No patient discontinued the study because of treatment-emergent adverse events. Extrapyramidal symptoms occurred most frequently in the IM haloperidol group. The most common adverse event in IM aripiprazole recipients was headache.

First-generation antipsychotics First-generation antipsychotics continue to be useful in the treatment of acute aggression. Haloperidol is the most commonly used first-generation antipsychotic in the emergency room setting. Because of the frequent extrapyramidal side effects, it is often combined with an anticholinergic medication such as benztropine. In addition, it is usually administered with a benzodiazepine to enhance the sedative effect.

In conclusion, it appears that the intramuscular formulations of first-generation antipsychotics are gradually being replaced by second-generation compounds with fewer extrapyramidal side effects. However, the first-generation antipsychotics remain an effective and cheaper option. They are well tolerated if they are administered with an anticholinergic agent and when cost is an issue.

Chronic/persistent aggression

Both first- and second-generation antipsychotic medications have been used in the treatment of chronic aggression. There are several studies with rather contradictory results in terms of which second-generation antipsychotic is superior compared with other first- and second-generation neuroleptics with the exception of clozapine, which is considered the gold standard in the treatment of chronic and severe aggression (**Table 1**).

Clozapine The effectiveness of clozapine in the management of chronic aggression in patients with schizophrenia has been well documented. Volavka and colleagues[22] documented the superiority of clozapine in the treatment of aggression in a double-blind randomized trial. Patients with overt aggressive behavior were followed for 14 weeks and were randomly assigned treatment with clozapine, olanzapine, risperidone, or haloperidol. Clozapine was significantly superior to the other three groups in reducing the PANSS hostility score, the PANSS excitement factor, and the overt aggression scale score. In a more recent randomized study, clozapine was compared with olanzapine and haloperidol and was found to be superior to both in the treatment of aggressive behavior.[23] Chengappa and colleagues[24] also showed a decrease in seclusion/restraint in patients with schizophrenia treated with clozapine by using a mirror-image design. Another report by Spivak and colleagues[25] showed that chronic schizophrenia patients maintained on clozapine had fewer aggressive episodes and fewer suicide attempts than patients who were maintained on classical antipsychotic agents.

Olanzapine In a recent double-blind 14-week study, patients with schizophrenia and present history of physical aggression were randomized to three different groups: one treated with olanzapine (range10–30 mg), one treated with clozapine (200–800 mg), and one treated with haloperidol (up to 20 mg). The authors did a baseline cognitive and aggression assessment. At the end of 12 weeks, these assessments were repeated and the result was that the olanzapine groups showed improved cognition and impulse control compared with the clozapine and haloperidol groups.[26] One other aspect of this study was that patients' improvement of aggression on olanzapine may have been mediated by improvement in cognition, whereas patients' improvement on aggression with clozapine may have been mediated by an anti-impulsive effect of clozapine.

Interestingly, a previous study published in 2006[23] with a similar double-blind design showed that clozapine was more effective than olanzapine and haloperidol in the treatment of aggressive behavior. In this study, clozapine was superior to both olanzapine and haloperidol in the treatment of both physical and verbal aggression. Olanzapine was found to be superior to haloperidol. The PANSS improvement at the end of this 12-week study was the same for all the three groups.

Another, nonrandomized study compared olanzapine, risperidone, and clozapine in the management of chronic schizophrenia. Patients with chronic schizophrenia were assigned by the treating psychiatrist to one of these three groups. Among other measures, the authors looked at impulsivity scales. They found that all three medications were effective in decreasing the impulsivity rate without finding any significant differences between medications in the area of impulsivity. It is worth noting, however, that the clozapine group consisted of patients with more severe illness trajectory and, given that this study was not randomized, physicians' choice of medications may have been a big factor in the outcome.[27] The clinical antipsychotic trials of intervention effectiveness (CATIE) study did not show major differences in efficacy among olanzapine, quetiapine, ziprasidone, risperidone, and perphenazine in the treatment of chronic aggression in patients with schizophrenia.[28] Perphenazine showed greater effectiveness than quetiapine, but no other major differences among the different medications were detected. However, this analysis was a post hoc analysis and the study was not powered to detect differences in the occurrence of violent episodes.

Quetiapine The current data show that quetiapine may be effective in the treatment of chronic aggression; however, it is not available as an IM form for the acute treatment of aggression and needs to be titrated slowly. A post hoc analysis of three double-blind placebo-controlled trials suggests that quetiapine is beneficial in the treatment of chronic hostility/aggression and that the improvement of the hostility parameter in the PANSS coincided with the improvement of positive symptoms.[29] Another post hoc analysis published in 2003[30] showed that quetiapine was more effective than haloperidol in the treatment of aggression in schizophrenia; however, this study was designed to measure the effect of quetiapine on the psychotic symptoms in general and not in the aggressive symptoms in particular.

Quetiapine was also included in a study that was designed to assess the effectiveness of clozapine, olanzapine, risperidone, quetiapine, and haloperidol on hostile and aggressive behaviors in patients with schizophrenia. Surprisingly, this study showed that olanzapine and risperidone were superior to haloperidol and clozapine. Quetiapine was comparable to haloperidol. This study had several limitations including the fact that it was open, the administration of medications was left to the judgment of clinicians, and the patients who received clozapine were younger and more treatment refractory than the rest of the subjects.[31]

In a study done in the Mental Health Department 1 South of Turin in Italy, the authors investigated potential differences among quetiapine, olanzapine, risperidone, and haloperidol on effects on aggressive behaviors. They included patients with schizophrenia, bipolar disorder, schizoaffective disorder, delusional disorder ,and brief psychotic disorder that required management for aggressive behavior. They did not specify whether their investigation was targeting acute or chronic aggression. The authors found no differences among the medications in terms of efficacy; however, they found that the second-generation antipsychotics are better tolerated than haloperidol.[32]

Risperidone Several studies have investigated the question of whether risperidone is superior to the conventional antipsychotic medications in the treatment of chronic aggression in patients with schizophrenia. In a meta-analysis published in 2001[33] on

Table 1
Atypical antipsychotic medications that are used for the treatment of acutely aggressive schizophrenia patients

Medication	Formulation	Peak Concentration	Half-life	Common Side Effects	Warning for all Compounds
Olanzapine	2.5-, 5.0-, 7.5-, 10.0-, 15.0-, 20.0- mg tablets 5-, 10-, 15-, 20-mg rapid disintegrating tablets	6 h	21–54 h	Sedation Dizziness/Orthostatic hypotension Weight gain[a] Hyperglycemia[a]	Elderly patients with dementia-related psychosis treated with antipsychotic drugs are at an increased risk of death.
	10-mg/mL intramuscular injection	15–45 min	21–54 h	Hypercholesterolemia[a]	
Risperidone	0.25-, 0.5-, 1-, 2-, 3-, 4-mg tablets 1-mg/mL oral solution 0.5-, 1-, 2-, 3-, 4-mg orally disintegrating tablets	1–17 h	3–20 h	Sedation Dizziness/Orthostatic hypotension Weight gain[a] Hyperglycemia[a] Diabetes mellitus[a] Hyperprolactinemia[a]	
Quetiapine	25-, 50-, 100-, 200-, 300-, 400-mg tablets	1.5 h	6 h	Sedation Dizziness/Orthostatic hypotension Constipation Weight gain[a] Hyperglycemia[a] Diabetes mellitus[a]	

Ziprasidone	20-, 40-, 60-, 80-mg oral capsules	6–8 h	7 h	Somnolence Dizziness
	20-mg/mL injection	60 min	2–5 h	Akathisia Headache Weight gain[a] Hyperglycemia[a] Diabetes mellitus[a] Ziprasidone use should be avoided in combination with other drugs that are known to prolong the QTc interval
Aripiprazole	5-, 10-, 15-, 20-, 30-mg tablets 10-, 15-mg orally disintegrating tablets	3–5 h	75 h	Akathisia Hyperglycemia (rarely)[a]
	1-mg/mL oral solution 7.5-mg/mL injection	1–3 h	75 h	

[a] Appears in long-term use.

its effects on hostility and aggression, risperidone was shown to be more effective than placebo as well as the typical antipsychotics. The authors found the most statistically significant effect when they included double-blind/placebo-controlled studies. An open-label study performed by the University of Pittsburgh showed that the time spent by patients in seclusion was significantly reduced after risperidone was initiated. In this study no subjects who had been on clozapine or risperidone in the past were included. The authors concluded that risperidone appears to have had a positive impact on seclusion in this state-hospital psychiatric population.[34] Nevertheless, there are other studies that show that risperidone is not superior to conventional antipsychotics in treating aggression.[35,36]

Taken together, the published data do not suggest that risperidone is particularly more effective than other SGAs against aggression in schizophrenia patients.[37]

Ziprasidone The efficacy of ziprasidone in the management of chronic aggression in schizophrenia was studied in comparison with olanzapine, quetiapine, risperidone, and perphenazine in the CATIE study.[28] In this study there was no major difference in efficacy among these medications.

Aripiprazole To our knowledge, there are no randomized studies that have examined the role of aripiprazole in the treatment of chronic aggression in patients with schizophrenia. There are some case reports, however, that have shown that aripiprazole worsened aggressive symptoms in schizophrenia patients.[38]

Mood stabilizers Mood stabilizers have been extensively used as adjunct medication in the treatment of aggression in patients with schizophrenia; however, there is lack of good evidence for their effectiveness. In practice, however, there is a great degree of use of mood stabilizers for the treatment of aggression, which is in contrast to the paucity of available controlled efficacy data. They are also the most frequently prescribed anticonvulsants for the treatment of aggressive behaviors in patients with schizophrenia and schizoaffective disorder.[39] The rate of prescriptions of valproate formulations in patients with schizophrenia has steadily increased in the past 10 years. In New York State psychiatric hospitals alone, Citrome and his colleagues[39] report that 12.1% patients with a diagnosis of schizophrenia had valproic acid preparations co-prescribed in 1994, whereas 20.8% received it in 1996. In addition, it is used in a variety of other nonbipolar disorders for the treatment of aggressive behaviors, although it has not been tested in double-blind trials for this specific indication.[40]

Depakote A small randomized open trial compared the hostility rate of patients receiving risperidone monotherapy versus risperidone combined with depakote. The patients who completed the study in the monotherapy group were less hostile than the patients in the combination group. The authors did not find any significant differences in the hostility rating scale between the two groups.[41]

A retrospective mirror-image open-label study that was performed at a Canadian maximum security psychiatric facility showed that both topiramate and depakote can significantly lower the aggressive episodes in patients with psychosis. However, the authors did not differentiate among patients with schizophrenia or schizoaffective or bipolar disorder. Since the population was mixed, inferences about the effect of depakote on aggression in schizophrenia patients cannot be made based on these data.[42] Furthermore, a post hoc analysis of a double-blind study reported by Citrome and colleagues[43] investigated the role of depakote in hostility in patients with schizophrenia. In this study, 159 patients had been randomly assigned to four groups: treatment with olanzapine, olanzapine plus depakote, risperidone, and risperidone plus depakote. The authors show improvement in hostility rates in patients who were treated with depakote, but the results were statistically significant only on days 3 and 7 and not throughout the 25-day study.

Lithium/carbamazepine/lamotrigine Several case reports suggested that mood stabilizers could be beneficial in the management of aggression in patients by schizophrenia, but they have not been supported by controlled studies.[44]

Beta-blockers In a study done by Silver and colleagues,[45] 20 chronically aggressive hospitalized patients were administered 1 week of placebo followed by an open trial of increasing doses of propranolol. Patients who had an equivocal or definite clinical response were entered into an open add-on double-blind discontinuation study phase. Aggressive behavior was objectively documented throughout the study. After the open phase of the study, seven patients had a greater than 50% decrease in aggressive behavior. Four patients entered the double-blind discontinuation phase. The clinical course of three of those patients was consistent with the positive response to propranolol. Nevertheless, these findings need to be interpreted cautiously in the case of patients with schizophrenia, because the study population was mixed and included patients with mental retardation as well as patients with organic mental illness and severe behavioral problems. Further controlled studies are needed to investigate the effectiveness of propranolol in managing aggressive behavior in patients with schizophrenia.

SUMMARY

Impulsive and aggressive behaviors are important clinical challenges in the treatment of patients with schizophrenia. They occur both in the acute phase as well as in the chronic phase of the disorder and call for differentiated treatment interventions. It is important to always first consider behavioral and nonpharmacological interventions. High levels of structure and organization together with a nonconfrontational approach may be very successful interventions. In terms of acute pharmacological interventions, clinicians now have a broad spectrum of IM antipsychotic compounds available with rapid onset of action and relatively little sedation. Although the IM formulations of first-generation antipsychotics are gradually being replaced by second-generation ones with fewer extrapyramidal side effects, the first-generation antipsychotics remain an effective and less expensive option. The latter ones are well tolerated if they are administered with an anticholinergic agent and when cost is an issue. For pharmacological treatment of chronic aggression, clozapine is the overall gold standard; however, limited by the need for regular white blood count (WBC) monitoring and patient acceptance. Among the other SGAs that have shown efficacy in the treatment of chronic aggression is olanzapine. Its metabolic side-effect profile may also limit its usefulness and highlights the need for new compounds with a more acceptable tolerability profile for the long-term treatment of these important syndromes.

REFERENCES

1. Allen MH, Currier GW, Carpenter D, et al. The expert consensus guideline series. Treatment of behavioral emergencies. J Psychiatr Pract 2005;11(Suppl 1):5–108.
2. Lindenmayer JP, Crowner M, Cosgrove V. Emergency treatment of agitation and aggression. In: Allen MH, editor. Emergency psychiatry. Washington (DC): American Psychiatric Press; 2002. p. 115–49.

3. Restraint and seclusion: implementing the CMS hospital patients' rights conditions of participation final rule. National Association of Psychiatric Health Systems Training; February 15, 2007.
4. Taylor PJ, Leese M, Williams D, et al. Mental disorder and violence. A special (high security) hospital study. Br J Psychiatry 1998;172:218–26.
5. Vaglum P, Friis S, Karterud S. Why are the results of milieu therapy for schizophrenic patients contradictory? An analysis based on four empirical studies. Yale J Biol Med 1985;58(4):349–61.
6. Melle I, Friis S, Hauff E, et al. The importance of ward atmosphere in inpatient treatment of schizophrenia on short-term units. Psychiatr Serv 1996;47(7):721–6.
7. Haddock G, Lowens I, Brosnan N, et al. Cognitive- behaviour therapy for inpatients with psychosis and anger problems within a low secure environment. Behav Res Ther 2004;32(1):77–98.
8. Haddock G, Barrowclough C, Shaw JJ, et al. Cognitive-behavioural therapy v. social activity therapy for people with psychosis and a history of violence: randomised controlled trial. Br J Psychiatry 2009;194(2):152–7.
9. Breier A, Meehan K, Birkett M, et al. A double-blind, placebo-controlled dose-response comparison of intramuscular olanzapine and haloperidol in the treatment of acute agitation in schizophrenia. Arch Gen Psychiatry 2002;59(5): 441–8.
10. Wright P, Birkett M, David SR. Double-blind, placebo-controlled comparison of intramuscular olanzapine and intramuscular haloperidol in the treatment of acute agitation in schizophrenia. Am J Psychiatry 2001;158(7):1149–51.
11. San L, Arranz B, Querejeta I, et al. A naturalistic multicenter study of intramuscular olanzapine in the treatment of acutely agitated manic or schizophrenic patients. Eur Psychiatry 2006;21(8):539–43.
12. Currier GW, Simpson GM. Risperidone liquid concentrate and oral lorazepam versus intramuscular haloperidol and intramuscular lorazepam for treatment of psychotic agitation. J Clin Psychiatry 2001;62(3):153–7.
13. Lejeune J, Larmo I, Chrzanowski W, et al. Oral risperidone plus oral lorazepam versus standard care with intramuscular conventional neuroleptics in the initial phase of treating individuals with acute psychosis. Int Clin Psychopharmacol 2004;19(5):259–69.
14. Citrome L. Comparison of intramuscular ziprasidone, olanzapine, or aripiprazole for agitation: a quantitative review of efficacy and safety. J Clin Psychiatry 2007; 68(12):1876–85.
15. Lesem MD, Zajecka JM, Swift RH, et al. Intramuscular ziprasidone, 2 mg versus 10 mg, in the short-term management of agitated psychotic patients. J Clin Psychiatry 2001;62(1):12–8.
16. Daniel DG, Potkin SG, Reeves KR, et al. Intramuscular (IM) ziprasidone 20 mg is effective in reducing acute agitation associated with psychosis: a double-blind, randomized trial. Psychopharmacology (Berl) 2001;155(2): 128–34.
17. Jangro WC, Preval H, Southard R, et al. Conventional intramuscular sedatives versus ziprasidone for severe agitation in adolescents: case-control study. Child Adolesc Psychiatry Ment Health 2009;3(1):9.
18. Mendelowitz AJ. The utility of intramuscular ziprasidone in the management of acute psychotic agitation. Ann Clin Psychiatry 2004;16(3):145–54.
19. Satterthwaite TD, Wolf DH, Rosenheck RA, et al. A meta-analysis of the risk of acute extrapyramidal symptoms with intramuscular antipsychotics for the treatment of agitation. J Clin Psychiatry 2008;69(12):1869–79.

20. Andrezina R, Josiassen RC, Marcus RN, et al. Intramuscular aripiprazole for the treatment of acute agitation in patients with schizophrenia or schizoaffective disorder: a double-blind, placebo-controlled comparison with intramuscular haloperidol. Psychopharmacology (Berl) 2006;188(3):281–92.
21. Tran-Johnson TK, Sack DA, Marcus RN, et al. Efficacy and safety of intramuscular aripiprazole in patients with acute agitation: a randomized, double-blind, placebo-controlled trial. J Clin Psychiatry 2007;68(1):111–9.
22. Volavka J, Czobor P, Nolan K, et al. Overt aggression and psychotic symptoms in patients with schizophrenia treated with clozapine, olanzapine, risperidone, or haloperidol. J Clin Psychopharmacol 2004;24(2):225–8.
23. Krakowski MI, Czobor P, Citrome L, et al. Atypical antipsychotic agents in the treatment of violent patients with schizophrenia and schizoaffective disorder. Arch Gen Psychiatry 2006;63(6):622–9.
24. Chengappa KN, Vasile J, Levine J, et al. Clozapine: its impact on aggressive behavior among patients in a state psychiatric hospital. Schizophr Res 2002; 53(1–2):1–6.
25. Spivak B, Roitman S, Vered Y, et al. Diminished suicidal and aggressive behavior, high plasma norepinephrine levels, and serum triglyceride levels in chronic neuroleptic-resistant schizophrenic patients maintained on clozapine. Clin Neuropharmacol 1998;21(4):245–50.
26. Krakowski MI, Czobor P, Nolan KA. Atypical antipsychotics, neurocognitive deficits, and aggression in schizophrenic patients. J Clin Psychopharmacol 2008; 28(5):485–93.
27. Strous RD, Kupchik M, Roitman S, et al. Comparison between risperidone, olanzapine, and clozapine in the management of chronic schizophrenia: a naturalistic prospective 12-week observational study. Hum Psychopharmacol 2006;21(4): 235–43.
28. Lieberman JA, Stroup TS, McEvoy JP, et al. Effectiveness of antipsychotic drugs in patients with chronic schizophrenia. Clinical antipsychotic trials of intervention effectiveness (CATIE) investigators. N Engl J Med 2005;353(12): 1209–23.
29. Arango C, Bernardo M. The effect of quetiapine on aggression and hostility in patients with schizophrenia. Hum Psychopharmacol 2005;20(4):237–41.
30. Chengappa KN, Goldstein JM, Greenwood M, et al. A post hoc analysis of the impact on hostility and agitation of quetiapine and haloperidol among patients with schizophrenia. Clin Ther 2003;25(2):530–41.
31. Bitter I, Czobor P, Dossenbach M, et al. Effectiveness of clozapine, olanzapine, quetiapine, risperidone, and haloperidol monotherapy in reducing hostile and aggressive behavior in outpatients treated for schizophrenia: a prospective naturalistic study (IC-SOHO). Eur Psychiatry 2005;20(5–6):403–8.
32. Villari V, Rocca P, Fonzo V, et al. Oral risperidone, olanzapine and quetiapine versus haloperidol in psychotic agitation. Prog Neuropsychopharmacol Biol Psychiatry 2008;32(2):405–13.
33. Aleman A, Kahn RS. Effects of the atypical antipsychotic risperidone on hostility and aggression in schizophrenia: a meta-analysis of controlled trials. Eur Neuropsychopharmacol 2001;11(4):289–93.
34. Chengappa KN, Levine J, Ulrich R, et al. Impact of risperidone on seclusion and restraint at a state psychiatric hospital. Can J Psychiatry 2000;45(9):827–32.
35. Beck NC, Greenfield SR, Gotham H, et al. Risperidone in the management of violent, treatment-resistant schizophrenics hospitalized in a maximum security forensic facility. J Am Acad Psychiatry Law 1997;25(4):461–8.

36. Buckley PF, Ibrahim ZY, Singer B, et al. Aggression and schizophrenia: efficacy of risperidone. J Am Acad Psychiatry Law 1997;25(2):173–81.
37. Swanson JW, Swartz MS, Van Dorn RA, et al. Comparison of antipsychotic medication effects on reducing violence in people with schizophrenia. CATIE investigators. Br J Psychiatry 2008;193(1):37–43.
38. Lea JW, Stoner SC, Lafollette J. Agitation associated with aripiprazole initiation. Pharmacotherapy 2007;27(9):1339–42.
39. Citrome L, Levine J, Allingham B. Changes in use of valproate and other mood stabilizers for patients with schizophrenia from 1994 to 1998. Psychiatr Serv 2000;51(5):634–8.
40. Lindenmayer JP, Kotsaftis A. Use of sodium valproate in violent and aggressive behaviors: a critical review. J Clin Psychiatry 2000;61(2):123–8.
41. Citrome L, Shope CB, Nolan KA, et al. Risperidone alone versus risperidone plus valproate in the treatment of patients with schizophrenia and hostility. Int Clin Psychopharmacol 2007;22(6):356–62.
42. Gobbi G, Gaudreau PO, Leblanc N. Efficacy of topiramate, valproate, and their combination on aggression/agitation behavior in patients with psychosis. J Clin Psychopharmacol 2006;26(5):467–73.
43. Citrome L, Casey DE, Daniel DG, et al. Adjunctive divalproex and hostility among patients with schizophrenia receiving olanzapine or risperidone. Psychiatr Serv 2004;55(3):290–4.
44. Volavka J, Citrome L. Heterogeneity of violence in schizophrenia and implications for long-term treatment. Int J Clin Pract 2008;62(8):1237–45.
45. Silver JM, Yudofsky SC, Slater JA, et al. Propranolol treatment of chronically hospitalized aggressive patients. J Neuropsychiatry Clin Neurosci 1999;11(3): 328–35.

Index

NOTE: Page numbers of article titles are in **boldface** type.

Psychiatr Clin N Am 32 (2009) 903–913
doi:10.1016/S0193-953X(09)00092-6
psych.theclinics.com
0193-953X/09/$ – see front matter

F

G

H

I

L

M

N

O

Z

United States Postal Service

Statement of Ownership, Management, and Circulation
(All Periodicals Publications Except Requestor Publications)

1. Publication Title Psychiatric Clinics of North America	2. Publication Number 0 0 0 - 7 0 3	3. Filing Date 9/15/09
4. Issue Frequency Mar, Jun, Sep, Dec	5. Number of Issues Published Annually 4	6. Annual Subscription Price $230.00
7. Complete Mailing Address of Known Office of Publication (*Not printer*) (*Street, city, county, state, and ZIP+4®*) Elsevier Inc. 360 Park Avenue South New York, NY 10010-1710		Contact Person Stephen Bushing Telephone (Include area code) 215-239-3688

8. Complete Mailing Address of Headquarters or General Business Office of Publisher (*Not printer*)

Elsevier Inc., 360 Park Avenue South, New York, NY 10010-1710

9. Full Names and Complete Mailing Addresses of Publisher, Editor, and Managing Editor (*Do not leave blank*)

Publisher (*Name and complete mailing address*)

John Schrefer , Elsevier, Inc., 1600 John F. Kennedy Blvd. Suite 1800, Philadelphia, PA 19103-2899

Editor (*Name and complete mailing address*)

Sarah Barth, Elsevier, Inc., 1600 John F. Kennedy Blvd. Suite 1800, Philadelphia, PA 19103-2899

Managing Editor (*Name and complete mailing address*)

Catherine Bewick, Elsevier, Inc., 1600 John F. Kennedy Blvd. Suite 1800, Philadelphia, PA 19103-2899

10. Owner (*Do not leave blank. If the publication is owned by a corporation, give the name and address of the corporation immediately followed by the names and addresses of all stockholders owning or holding 1 percent or more of the total amount of stock. If not owned by a corporation, give the names and addresses of the individual owners. If owned by a partnership or other unincorporated firm, give its name and address as well as those of each individual owner. If the publication is published by a nonprofit organization, give its name and address.*)

Full Name	Complete Mailing Address
Wholly owned subsidiary of	4520 East-West Highway
Reed/Elsevier, US holdings	Bethesda, MD 20814

11. Known Bondholders, Mortgagees, and Other Security Holders Owning or Holding 1 Percent or More of Total Amount of Bonds, Mortgages, or Other Securities. If none, check box → ☐ None

Full Name	Complete Mailing Address
N/A	

12. Tax Status (*For completion by nonprofit organizations authorized to mail at nonprofit rates*) (*Check one*)
The purpose, function, and nonprofit status of this organization and the exempt status for federal income tax purposes:
☐ Has Not Changed During Preceding 12 Months
☐ Has Changed During Preceding 12 Months (*Publisher must submit explanation of change with this statement*)

13. Publication Title: Psychiatric Clinics of North America

14. Issue Date for Circulation Data Below: September 2009

15. Extent and Nature of Circulation			Average No. Copies Each Issue During Preceding 12 Months	No. Copies of Single Issue Published Nearest to Filing Date
a. Total Number of Copies (*Net press run*)			1860	1700
b. Paid Circulation (By Mail and Outside the Mail)	(1)	Mailed Outside-County Paid Subscriptions Stated on PS Form 3541. (*Include paid distribution above nominal rate, advertiser's proof copies, and exchange copies*)	912	831
	(2)	Mailed In-County Paid Subscriptions Stated on PS Form 3541 (*Include paid distribution above nominal rate, advertiser's proof copies, and exchange copies*)		
	(3)	Paid Distribution Outside the Mails Including Sales Through Dealers and Carriers, Street Vendors, Counter Sales, and Other Paid Distribution Outside USPS®	322	326
	(4)	Paid Distribution by Other Classes Mailed Through the USPS (e.g. First-Class Mail®)		
c. Total Paid Distribution (*Sum of 15b (1), (2), (3), and (4)*)			1234	1157
d. Free or Nominal Rate Distribution (By Mail and Outside the Mail)	(1)	Free or Nominal Rate Outside-County Copies Included on PS Form 3541	91	94
	(2)	Free or Nominal Rate In-County Copies Included on PS Form 3541		
	(3)	Free or Nominal Rate Copies Mailed at Other Classes Through the USPS (e.g. First-Class Mail)		
	(4)	Free or Nominal Rate Distribution Outside the Mail (Carriers or other means)		
e. Total Free or Nominal Rate Distribution (Sum of 15d (1), (2), (3) and (4)			91	94
f. Total Distribution (Sum of 15c and 15e)			1325	1251
g. Copies not Distributed (See instructions to publishers #4 (page #3))			535	449
h. Total (Sum of 15f and g)			1860	1700
i. Percent Paid (15c divided by 15f times 100)			93.13%	92.49%

16. Publication of Statement of Ownership

☐ If the publication is a general publication, publication of this statement is required. Will be printed in the **December 2009** issue of this publication. ☐ Publication not required

17. Signature and Title of Editor, Publisher, Business Manager, or Owner

Stephen R. Bushing – Subscription Services Coordinator — Date: September 15, 2009

I certify that all information furnished on this form is true and complete. I understand that anyone who furnishes false or misleading information on this form or who omits material or information requested on the form may be subject to criminal sanctions (including fines and imprisonment) and/or civil sanctions (including civil penalties).

Printed and bound by CPI Group (UK) Ltd, Croydon, CR0 4YY

Printed and bound by CPI Group (UK) Ltd, Croydon, CR0 4YY
03/10/2024
01040462-0020